Emergency Nursing SECRETS

Second Edition

KATHLEEN S. OMAN, RN, PhD, CNS
Research Nurse Scientist/Emergency CNS
University of Colorado Hospital
Denver, Colorado

JANE KOZIOL-MCLAIN, RN, PhD
Associate Professor
School of Nursing
Auckland University of Technology
Auckland, New Zealand

SERIES EDITOR
LINDA SCHEETZ, EdD, APRN, BC
Assistant Professor
College of Nursing
Rutgers, The State University of New Jersey
Rutgers, New Jersey

SPECIAL CONSULTANT
JEAN A. PROEHL, RN, MN, CEN, CCRN, FAEN
Emergency Clinical Nurse Specialist
Dartmouth-Hitchcock Medical Center
Lebanon, New Hampshire

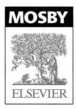

MOSBY

ELSEVIER

D0672890

MOSBY
ELSEVIER

11830 Westline Industrial Drive
St. Louis, Missouri 63146

EMERGENCY NURSING SECRETS ISBN-13: 978-0-323-04032-7
Copyright © 2007, 2001 by Mosby, Inc., an affiliate of Elsevier Inc. ISBN-10: 0-323-04032-2

Notice

Knowledge and best practice in this field are constantly changing. As new research and experience broaden our knowledge, changes in practice, treatment, and drug therapy may become necessary or appropriate. Readers are advised to check the most current information provided (i) on procedures featured or (ii) by the manufacturer of each product to be administered, to verify the recommended dose or formula, the method and duration of administration, and contraindications. It is the responsibility of practitioners, relying on their own experience and knowledge of the patient, to make diagnoses, to determine dosages and the best treatment for each individual patient, and to take all appropriate safety precautions. To the fullest extent of the law, neither the Publisher nor the Editors/Authors assumes any liability for any injury and/or damage to persons or property arising out of or related to any use of the material contained in this book.

The Publisher

ISBN-13: 978-0-323-04032-7
ISBN-10: 0-323-04032-2

Executive Publisher: Barbara Nelson Cullen
Editor: Sandra Clark Brown
Developmental Editor: Sophia Oh Gray
Publishing Services Manager: John Rogers
Senior Project Manager: Cheryl A. Abbott
Design Direction: Bill Drone

Printed in the United States of America

Last digit is the print number: 9 8 7 6 5 4 3 2 1

Working together to grow
libraries in developing countries
www.elsevier.com | www.bookaid.org | www.sabre.org

ELSEVIER   BOOK AID International   Sabre Foundation

Contributors

Pamela W. Bourg, RN, MS
Trauma Program Manager
Trauma Service
St. Anthony Central Hospital
Denver, Colorado
25. Head and Face Trauma
28. Spinal Trauma

Patricia M. Campbell, RN, MSN, CCRN, ANP, CS
Adjunct Faculty
College of Nursing—NP program
Arizona State University
Phoenix, Arizona;
Emergency Nurse Practitioner
Banner Good Samaritan Medical Center
Phoenix, Arizona
5. Self-Care for the Caregiver
6. Keeping Safe

Debra Cason, RN, MS, EMT-P
Program Director
Associate Professor
Health Care Sciences
University of Texas Southwestern Medical Center
Dallas, Texas
23. Mechanism of Injury

Sharon Saunderson Cohen, RN, MSN, CEN, CCRN
Emergency Preparedness/WMD
Clinical Nurse Specialist
Department of Emergency Preparedness
North Broward Hospital District
Fort Lauderdale, Florida
24. Shock
29. Musculoskeletal Trauma

GERALD R. CONNORS, RN, MS, CEN, LHRM
Administrative Director/Clinical Business Operations
All Children's Hospital
St. Petersburg, Florida

GRETTA J. EDWARDS, RN, CEN
Clinical Nurse
Endoscopy Laboratory
University of Colorado Hospital
Denver, Colorado

ANNE M. FELTON, RN, ND
Nurse Manager
Center for Dependency
Addiction and Rehabilitation
University of Colorado Hospital
Denver, Colorado

REGINA M. FINK, RN, PhD, FAAN, AOCN
Research Nurse Scientist
Department of Professional Resources
University of Colorado Hospital
Denver, Colorado

KATHLEEN FLARITY, ARNP, PhD, CEN, CFRN
Clinical Faculty, Physiological Nursing
University of Washington
Seattle, Washington;
Flight Nurse
Airlift Northwest
Wenatchee, Washington;
Nurse Practitioner
Wenatchee, Washington;
Flight Nurse Instructor
446th Aeromedical Evacuation Squadron
McChord Air Force Base, Washington

ANGELA HACKENSCHMIDT, RN, MS, CEN
Clinical Nurse Educator
Emergency Department
San Francisco General Hospital
San Francisco, California
   37. Underserved Patients

KRISTA M. HAUGEN, RN, MN, CEN
Flight RN
Airlift Northwest
Seattle, Washington
   21. Hematological Emergencies

KAREN HAYES, PhD, FNP, ACNP
Assistant Professor
School of Nursing
Wichita State University
Wichita, Kansas;
Emergency Department Nurse Practitioner
Via Christi Regional Medical Center
Wichita, Kansas
   35. Seniors
   38. Abused and Neglected Patients

RENEÉ SEMONIN HOLLERAN, RN, PhD, CEN, CCRN, FAEN
Nurse Manager Adult Transport Services
IHC Life Flight
Salt Lake City, Utah
   9. Resuscitation Issues

MARILYN K. JOHNSON, RN
Nursing Supervisor
Center for Safe and Healthy Families
Primary Children's Medical Center
Salt Lake City, Utah
   38. Abused and Neglected Patients

CATHERINE T. KELLY, PhD, CEN, CCRN Alumnus
Director, Consortium for Domestic Preparedness
   and Consultant, Nursing Department
SUNY Ulster
Stone Ridge, New York;
Chief Nursing Officer
Emergency Services
MedExcel USA
New Windsor, New York
   4. Death and Dying
   33. Psychosocial Aspects of Trauma

VIRGINIA M. KOZIEL, RN, BSN
Charge Nurse
Emergency Department
University of Colorado Hospital
Denver, Colorado
34. Pregnant Women

JANE KOZIOL-MCLAIN, RN, PhD
Associate Professor, School of Nursing
Auckland University of Technology
Auckland, New Zealand
38. Abused and Neglected Patients

MARY BETH FLYNN MAKIC, RN, PhDc, CNS, CCNS, CCRN
Senior Instructor
School of Nursing
University of Colorado at Denver and Health Sciences Center
Denver, Colorado;
Clinical Nurse Specialist and Educator
University of Colorado Hospital
Denver, Colorado
30. Burn Injury

RUTH E. MALONE, RN, MS, PhD, FAAN
Associate Professor of Nursing and Health Policy
Department of Social and Behavioral Sciences
School of Nursing
University of California at San Francisco
San Francisco, California
37. Underserved Patients

ELIZABETH A. MANN, RN, MS, CCRN, CCNS
Clinical Head Nurse, Major
Army Nurse Corps
United States Army Institute of Surgical Research
Burn Unit
Fort Sam Houston, Texas
30. Burn Injury

CONNIE J. MATTERA, MS, RN, EMT-P
Emergency Medical Services Administrative Director
Trauma Nurse Specialist Course Coordinator
Northwest Community Hospital
Arlington Heights, Illinois
31. Trauma During Pregnancy

REBECCA S. MCNAIR, RN, CEN
President
Triage First, Inc.
Fairview, North Carolina
1. Triage

NANCY L. MECHAM, APRN, FNP
Clinical Nurse Specialist
Emergency Department and Rapid Treatment Unit
Primary Children's Medical Center
Salt Lake City, Utah
32. Pediatric Trauma
36. Infants and Children

CHERYL MONTANIO, RN, MSN, CSPI
Clinical Nurse Educator
Rocky Mountain Poison & Drug Center
Denver Health Medical Center
Denver, Colorado
18. Ingestions and Poisonings

ROBERT MONTGOMERY, RN, ND, CNS
Assistant Professor, Anesthesiology
School of Medicine
University of Colorado Health Sciences Center
Denver, Colorado;
Acute Pain Service Clinical Nurse Specialist, Anesthesiology
School of Medicine
University of Colorado Health Sciences Center
Denver, Colorado
3. Pain Management

JANET A. NEFF, RN, MS, CEN
Trauma Program Manager
Trauma Service
Stanford University Medical Center
Stanford, California
26. Thoracic and Neck Trauma

MARGARET J. NEFF, MD, MSc
Assistant Professor of Medicine
Department of Medicine
University of Washington
Seattle, Washington;
Attending Physician
Division of Pulmonary and Critical Care Medicine
Harborview Medical Center
Seattle, Washington
26. Thoracic and Neck Trauma

KATHLEEN S. OMAN, RN, PhD, CNS
Research Nurse Scientist/Emergency CNS
University of Colorado Hospital
Denver, Colorado
2. Emergency Preparedness

BARBARA A. OVERBY, BSN, MSN, EMT-P
Adjunct Assistant Professor
School of Medicine, Emergency Medicine
University of North Carolina, Chapel Hill;
EMS Nurse Liaison
Emergency Department
University of North Carolina Hospitals
Chapel Hill, North Carolina
11. Seizures
12. Stroke

KAREN M. PICKARD, RN, LP, BSN, MS
Instructor
Quality Improvement Program Director
University of Texas Southwestern Medical School
Dallas, Texas
23. Mechanism of Injury

BARI K. PLATTER, RN, MS, CNS
Clinical Instructor
School of Nursing
University of Colorado
Denver, Colorado;
Clinical Instructor
School of Nursing
Regis University
Denver, Colorado;
Clinical Nurse Specialist/Educator
Psychiatric Services
University of Colorado Hospital
Denver, Colorado
19. Psychiatric Emergencies
39. Drug- and Alcohol-Impaired Patients

JEAN A. PROEHL, RN, MN, CEN, CCRN, FAEN
Emergency Clinical Nurse Specialist
Dartmouth-Hitchcock Medical Center
Lebanon, New Hampshire
14. Chest Pain

LORNA K. PRUTZMAN, BSN, MSN
Director
Emergency Nursing
University of Colorado Hospital
Denver, Colorado
8. Risk Management

LOIS SCHICK, MN, MBA, CPAN, CAPA
Per Diem PACU Staff Nurse
Exempla Lutheran Medical Center
Wheatridge, Colorado;
Per Diem PACU Staff Nurse
Littleton Adventist Hospital
Littleton, Colorado
10. Headache

IVY F. SHAFFER, RN
Thomas Jefferson University
Interventional Cardiology
Philadelphia, Pennsylvania
15. Respiratory Distress
20. Endocrine Emergencies

JOANN M. SORRENTINO, BSN, FNP
Denver Health and Hospital Walk-in Clinic
Denver, Colorado
22. Nonurgent Problems

DONNA OJANEN THOMAS, RN, MSN
Director Emergency Department/Rapid Treatment Unit
Primary Children's Medical Center
Salt Lake City, Utah
32. Pediatric Trauma
36. Infants and Children

CAROLEE WHITEHILL, RN, MS
Diabetes Program Administrator
University of Colorado Hospital
Denver, Colorado;
formerly Clinical Case Manager
Emergency Department
University of Colorado Hospital
Denver, Colorado
7. Case Management

JOYCE A. WRIGHT, RN, DNSc, CCRN
Assistant Professor, Director of Accelerated Nursing
Seton Hall University
South Orange, New Jersey
16. Abdominal Pain

POLLY GERBER ZIMMERMANN, RN, MS, MBA, CEN
Assistant Professor
School of Nursing
Henry S. Truman College
Chicago, Illinois
1. Triage

Reviewers

PAMELA L. ISBELL, BSN, CEN
Staff Nurse
Orlando Regional Medical Center
Orlando, Florida

MICHELLE J. KLOSTERMAN, RN, CEN
Manager, RN
Emergency Department
Adams County Hospital
West Union, Ohio

Preface

We began thinking about this second edition of *Emergency Nursing Secrets* shortly after the first edition was published. We have included additional content and topics such as resuscitation issues, endocrine and hematological emergencies, and drug- and alcohol- impaired patients that we hope will enhance the book. As we did in the first edition, we turned to leading emergency nurses and asked them to tell us their "secrets." What they have to say will impress you. They have captured the knowledge, enthusiasm, and heart of emergency nursing.

We asked the chapter authors to include concepts that inform emergency nursing practice: patient advocacy, family involvement, collaborative practice, patient teaching, ethical decision making, and evidence-based practice. They have done a wonderful job. They share with us the diversity and challenges of emergency nursing practice from caring for a child who is experiencing a febrile seizure, to balancing the competing priorities during trauma resuscitation, to making changes that better the plight of the underserved. We hope you enjoy reading the book as much as we did editing it.

Looking back over our careers as emergency nurses, the Emergency Nurses Association (ENA) has played an integral role in defining our practice. As with the first edition, we are donating a portion of our book royalties to the ENA Foundation to help support education and research in emergency nursing.

We'd like to acknowledge the authors from the first edition who were not able to contribute to this new edition: Lisa Boulais, Leslie Ste. Laurant, Sandra Rexhouse, Jill Brennan-Cook, Linda Scheetz, Maureen O'Reilly, Anne Eichhorst, Rita Kimball, Noreen Baldwin, Jean M. Montonye, Lisa Marie Bernardo, Bonnie Clemence, and Gerry B. Cancienne. Their original work was excellent and we appreciate the foundation they laid.

Finally, we'd like to thank the editors and staff at Elsevier for their support during the publishing of this second edition.

KATHLEEN S. OMAN, RN, PhD, CNS

JANE KOZIOL-MCLAIN, RN, PhD

Contents

IV   SPECIAL POPULATIONS, 409

TOP SECRETS

1. Listening to patients' stories is an important part of emergency nursing. Telling the story begins with triage and continues in various forms throughout the ED visit. ED providers may hear different aspects of the story as it unfolds, and it takes a team effort to put the pieces together to provide quality and compassionate patient care.

2. Patient advocacy, family involvement, collaborative practice, patient teaching, ethical decision making, and evidence-based practice are key concepts that inform emergency nursing practice.

3. There is a tendency to mistakenly "under triage" rather than "over triage." When unsure, always give the patient the benefit of the doubt and assign the higher of the two categories.

4. Communicate with the patient at triage in the language of symptoms, feelings, and thoughts (not "organ" talk, e.g., "How is your heart?"). Do not assume the patient is taking the medications he or she lists, and ask if the patient has anything else to say at the end of the triage encounter.

5. A clear chain of command with well-articulated roles and responsibilities is important to the success of an emergency preparedness plan.

6. Emergency nurses' accuracy in estimating patients pain intensity is less than 50%.

7. Patients with acute abdominal pain may be given opioids without fear of masking the diagnosis.

8. When patients are dying, instead of telling families "There is nothing we can do," tell families what was done, what you are doing, and what you can do.

9. Always ask the family what you can do to help them when someone has died. Every family is different and may need very different things.

10. Managing stress is key to maintaining health. Stress reducing therapies include physical exercise, meditation, humor, music, touch therapies, and guided imagery.

11. Take responsibility for your health—choose health promotion: smoking cessation, minimal alcohol intake, daily exercise, weight management, a healthy diet, healthy relationships, overcoming addictions, and practicing stress reduction activities.

12. Minimize violence in the ED through staff training and education, physical design of the ED and hospital campus, and policies and procedures for managing violent patients and visitors.

13. Prevention of infectious diseases relies on nursing education, immunizations, standard and respiratory precautions, careful hand washing, and isolation procedures and policies/procedures for safety in the workplace as outlined by the Centers for Disease Control and Prevention (CDC) and Occupational Safety and Health Administration (OSHA).

14. Latex sensitivity poses a serious problem for both staff and patients. Measures to reduce exposures include staff education, policies and procedures for caring for latex-sensitive patients and staff members, and policies regarding testing and treatment of latex-sensitive staff. Minimize exposures by reducing the use of latex products and ensuring the availability of latex-free products for sensitive patients.

15. Develop linkages to related healthcare agendas—such as public health issues, needs of the chronic care population, access to care for the medically underserved, and quality and risk issues—to incorporate established benchmarks and health-related goals.

16. When there are competing demands for nurses' time, solid teamwork and communication among all staff is necessary to reduce the risk of negligence. Remember the guiding principle of emergency nursing: "All patients are everyone's patient."

17. Electricity saves lives. Automatic External Defibrillators (AEDs) must be available in places where there are people, and the public should be educated as to their use.

18. The best way to manage a cardiac arrest is to use practice scenarios so that staff are comfortable with equipment and medications.

19. Emergency care providers need to be aware of "Do-Not-Attempt-Resuscitation" orders for the patients they care for and must respect their patients' wishes.

20. A patient who complains of the "worst headache of my life" and describes a sudden, thunderclap onset may have a potentially life-threatening subarachnoid bleed.

21. There are multiple triggers for patients developing headaches, ranging from diet, hormones, sensory stimuli, stress, and changes in their environment or habits.

22. Hypoglycemia is an easily corrected cause of seizures, so always check the glucose level in a seizing patient.

23. Status epilepticus is prolonged seizure activity for 15 to 30 minutes or two or more seizures without full recovery between seizures. This condition is life threatening, and controlling the seizures is critical.

24. Patients who experience an alcohol withdrawal seizure are also at high risk of metabolic abnormalities, subdural hematoma, and central nervous system infections.

25. Establish a stroke protocol or clinical pathway to streamline processes and avoid treatment delays.

26. TPA administration for ischemic stroke must be initiated within 3 hours from the onset of stroke symptoms.

27. TPA dose is 0.9 mg/kg IV with a maximum dose of 90 mg; 10% of the total dose should be administered as an IV bolus over 1 minute, and the remainder should be given over 60 minutes.

28. The ED environment produces anxiety for all patients, but communication with the stroke patient can be a challenge. Limit distractions, establish eye contact, speak slowly, and ask simple yes/no questions.

29. Visual acuity is the vital sign for the eye. An accurate assessment of visual acuity is essential for diagnosis and treatment.

30. Two eye emergencies require immediate initiation of treatment: chemical burns and central retinal artery occlusion (CRAO). Open eyes, acute angle closure glaucoma, and retrobulbar hemorrhage also must be treated emergently.

31. If a diagnosis of angina or acute myocardial infarction remains uncertain after nitroglycerin challenge and an ECG, treat the patient as having an acute MI. Definitive diagnosis is based on clinical presentation, presence of risk factors, ECG changes, and levels of biochemical cardiac markers.

32. Recognition and prompt treatment of exacerbations from asthma and COPD, suspected pulmonary embolism, and acute epiglottitis challenge the most seasoned clinician. The priority is always establishing and maintaining a patent airway while simultaneously ensuring adequate ventilation and perfusion.

33. As unfamiliar respiratory illnesses such as SARS, Hantavirus, and the Avian flu threaten to cause epidemic disease, it is the ED staff who will be on the front lines of recognizing, isolating, and treating these new medical enigmas. Be aware of updates from the Centers for Disease Control and Prevention, the National Institutes of Health, and the World Health Organization to be successful in this fight against emerging and potentially fatal illnesses.

34. Epiglottitis is life threatening due to sudden, unexpected airway obstruction and should always be suspected when patients present with symptoms of fever, drooling, muffled voice, and dyspnea. Though more often than not these are symptoms of a more common malady, peritonsillar abscesses, the emergency nurse must always suspect epiglottitis until ruled out.

35. Three common drugs used to relieve abdominal pain include fentanyl, morphine, and ketorolac. Research supports timely pain management that promotes patient comfort and therefore aids in establishing the diagnosis.

36. There is antivenin available for serious snakebites and stonefish and scorpion (only in Arizona) envenomation.

37. Because most tissue damage occurs during the thaw-and-refreeze cycle, rewarming of frostbite should begin when the body part can be warmed and not reexposed to cold.

38. The initial treatment for severe mountain sickness, HAPE, and HACE is immediate descent of at least 2,000 to 3,000 feet.

39. All patients, adults, and children who present with respiratory arrest or apnea should be given 2 mg of naloxone. Some patients may require larger doses, but the initial dose of 2 mg is the same for both children and adults.

40. Urine toxicology screens may fail to detect many toxins, thus the term "negative drug screen" could be misleading. Urine toxicology screens rarely change the management and are not recommended in the management of a patient who presents to the ED with a suspected overdose.

41. Routine use of syrup of ipecac as an emetic is no longer recommended for either the home setting or the ED. There is no evidence that use of ipecac syrup improves patient outcome, and it may delay administration of charcoal, antidotes, and other drugs.

42. Acetaminophen and aspirin are commonly ingested by suicidal patients. Although aspirin poisoned patients may develop acidosis, which offers a diagnostic clue, an aspirin level is recommended. Patients with acetaminophen ingestions often take more than 24 hours to show signs or symptoms that predict hepatotoxicity.

The most reliable way to exclude potential acetaminophen toxicity is to check the serum acetaminophen level.

43. Suicide contracts should not be used in the ED setting.

44. Do not assume that symptoms of psychosis are related to a psychiatric illness; instead assess for the presence of a delirium before referring the patient for psychiatric consultation.

45. Any drug can be taken as a lethal overdose. Don't assume that high-risk drugs are the only drugs used in purposeful or accidental overdoses.

46. An unexplained infection is one of the most common causes for elevated blood glucose in pediatric and adult patients with diabetes. Check patients in diabetic ketoacidosis (DKA) for sources of potential infections such as pneumonia, gastroenteritis, cellulitis, and tooth or foot infection.

47. Children less than 5 years of age in DKA with high serum osmolality are at high risk for cerebral edema. Perform neurological checks before and during hydration. Be alert for early complaints of headache and mental status changes.

48. Hematological disorders are manifestations of underlying diseases or problems.

49. Clinical presentation of hematological disorders may be subtle yet can rapidly become life threatening if not recognized and treated early.

50. The psychological and emotional toll of blood disorders, whether chronic or acute, can be extreme, and care should be taken to provide resources for education, as well as for psychosocial support.

51. Careful questioning when obtaining the history will help differentiate between a serious or emergent problem and a nonurgent problem.

52. Knowing the mechanism of injury will assist in the early identification of nonapparent injuries.

53. Mechanism of injury principles do not vary for falls in older adults, but the injuries sustained have the potential to have longer lasting, more disabling effects. They also have an associated high mortality rate.

54. Crush syndrome is a critical yet often underestimated effect of injury that will lead to renal failure and death if not recognized and treated rapidly.

55. Regardless of the precipitating cause, shock leads to decreased perfusion that is inadequate to meet the needs of the tissues.

56. Early symptoms of shock are often subtle and require extra vigilance by nursing staff so that they are not overlooked.

57. Airway obstruction continues to be a major cause of death and disability in patients with traumatic brain injuries and craniofacial injuries.

58. Discharge education following traumatic brain injury (TBI) is critical for patients. Minor TBI is a very common injury. Potential for deterioration always exists.

59. Fractures of the scapula or first rib indicate a high-energy mechanism of injury and are often associated with vascular injuries. Similarly, lower rib fractures should raise the possibility of abdominal injuries.

60. A pneumothorax (air in the pleural space) may be difficult to identify in the supine patient and seen only as a "deep sulcus sign" on a chest x-ray.

A tension pneumothorax is a life-threatening event whereby air continues to enter the pleural space but has no exit. Immediate therapy requires needle decompression followed by chest tube placement.

61. When assessing a patient with abdominal trauma, if first diagnostic exams are negative and a strong clinical suspicion of injury remains, keep looking.

62. Massive retroperitoneal hemorrhage may be present without signs of peritonitis (no rebound tenderness, guarding, or rigidity).

63. Maintenance of a patent airway should be a top priority with all immobilized patients. Suction should be readily available. If vomiting occurs, logroll the patient to facilitate airway clearance.

64. Systemic injuries can be overlooked when vital signs are altered and the assumption is made that spinal cord injury is the cause. Other injuries must be ruled out.

65. Early attention to skin care in the ED can help prevent skin breakdown in spinal cord injured patients.

66. For nurses that care for a patient with orthopedic fractures, remember to assess pulses distal to the injury before and after realignment, casting, or any repositioning or immobilization.

67. Regardless of the injury or cause of the orthopedic problem, a simple color, movement, sensation (CMS) check should be noted and trended.

68. ABCDs first, then treat the burn injuries.

69. Burn fluid administration formulas are only a guide; administer fluid to achieve physiological endpoints of adequate perfusion (i.e., urine output).

70. Children and patients with electrical or inhalation injuries require significantly more fluid resuscitation. Children need dextrose-containing maintenance fluids in addition to resuscitative fluids.

71. Prompt intubation for facial burns and suspected inhalation injury is necessary to protect the airway.

72. The challenge of major trauma to the pregnant woman is to resuscitate two lives. The best predictor of fetal survival is maternal survival.

73. Treat shock in the pregnant patient before it becomes severe. Do not wait for classic signs and symptoms. Even small amounts of supplemental oxygen to the mother can be beneficial to the fetus.

74. Due to the vasodilatory effects of hormones, the pregnant patient in shock may be warm and dry rather than cool and moist.

75. Fetal heart tones are the best indicator of fetal condition because they change before maternal vital signs. Fetal bradycardia is a grave sign and requires immediate action for fetal survival.

76. Pregnant patients in the second and third trimester should be placed in a left or right lateral recumbent position following trauma to displace the uterus from the inferior vena cava. The uterus can be displaced by tilting the patient on her side using a hip wedge or spine board or by manual manipulation.

77. Head injury is the most common type of pediatric injury, but abdominal trauma is the most commonly unrecognized cause of fatal injuries.

78. The most common psychological reaction to trauma is disorganization.

79. Following trauma, repeat information as often as possible to patients and families and "fill in" information as soon as possible.

80. Assign one team member to be the liaison for families of critically ill trauma patients.

81. Normal fetal heart tones (FHT) are 120 to 160 beats per minute and are audible with a Doppler at about 9 to 12 weeks' gestation.

82. Placenta previa causes painless, bright red vaginal bleeding with bright red discharge.

83. Placental abruption causes severe pain with no bleeding or blood that is usually dark red.

84. Forty percent of seniors leave the ED with a new prescription. Be sure patients can integrate this new medication into their already complex medication regimens.

85. Mental status change is not normal aging.

86. Atypical presentation of disease is common in older adults. Major health conditions such as myocardial infarction, pneumonia, or acute abdomen may present with simple complaints such as fatigue.

87. Infants less than 2 months of age with fever should be triaged at a more urgent acuity level even if the infant looks well. Fever can be indicative of a serious bacterial infection in this age group.

88. Always tell a child what you are going to do to avoid surprises and promote trust.

89. A child in respiratory distress who is not responding to usual interventions may be presenting with an underlying cardiac condition. Evaluate the heart rate and rhythm in all pediatric patients with respiratory distress.

90. Research has shown that families would prefer to be present during the resuscitation of their child.

91. When discharging a pediatric patient, ask the parents, "Do you feel comfortable caring for your child at home?"

92. Engaging patients and "meeting them where they are" can be an effective way to offer positive support and hope to patients who struggle with addiction and social problems. This is more likely to produce professional satisfaction than trying to control others' behavior or decisions.

93. Signs of abuse in an elderly ED patient include obvious physical signs of trauma, poor hygiene, decubitus ulcers, strained or tense relationships with caregivers, or withdrawn behavior.

94. Emergency nursing care for a patient who has been abused by a partner is based on empowerment. Focus on prior coping strategies and strengths, assess risk, offer support, plan for safety, and offer options.

95. When gathering information about mechanism of injury for children, ask only open-ended questions. Avoid leading questions.

96. Don't make assumptions in assigning responsibility for child maltreatment to a specific individual.

97. Have a high index of suspicion for reporting child maltreatment. Reporting triggers a thorough investigation, risk assessment, and intervention toward promoting child safety.

98. Suicidal ideation is a common co-morbid condition and should be assessed when taking a history from a drug- and alcohol-impaired patient.

99. Dehydration and nutritional and electrolyte imbalance are common conditions of alcoholism. Any patient with significant alcohol consumption history should be monitored carefully for withdrawal symptoms and treated appropriately.

100. This book focuses on emergency nursing secrets, but the most important secrets lie with the patient. This secret was important enough to be the first and the last: Listening to patients' stories is an important part of emergency nursing. Telling the story begins with triage and continues in various forms throughout the ED visit. ED providers may hear different aspects of the story as it unfolds, and it takes a team effort to put the pieces together to provide quality and compassionate patient care.

Section I

Practice Topics

Triage

Polly Gerber Zimmermann and Rebecca S. McNair

1. What is triage?

Triage is sorting. The original use of the French word "trier," to choose, referred to battlefield screening. The term is now commonly used to describe the concept of a rapid, focused assessment of the more than 110 million people who yearly seek emergency department (ED) care in a way that allows for the most efficient use of manpower, equipment, and facilities. ED triage systems began to evolve in the late 1950s as the number of ED visits outnumbered the available resources for immediate attention.

2. What is the purpose of triage?

The purpose of triage is to sort or classify all incoming ED patients and to set priorities for care. The goal is to get the right patient to the right place at the right time for the right reason to receive the right treatment. Beyond the historical focus of determining salvageability from war injuries, today's triage also seeks to minimize morbidity and mortality.

3. How long should the triage process take?

The commonly cited goal is about 2 to 5 minutes per patient. However, Travers (1999) found this time standard is met only 22% of the time, is extended with increasing patient age, and is significantly reduced if vital signs are not taken. Keddington (1998) found the average time spent triaging pediatric patients is 7 minutes.

4. Who should perform the ED triage function?

The Joint Commission on Accreditation of Healthcare Organizations (JCAHO) requires documentation of clinical competence for nurses but does not specifically state what that entails for triage nurses. The Emergency Nurses Association's (ENA's) 1999 Standards of Emergency Nursing Practice states that safe, effective, and efficient triage can be performed only by a registered professional nurse, educated in the principles of triage, with a minimum of 6 months' experience in emergency nursing. A registered nurse should be available to triage a patient (e.g., a visual rapid triage and formal triage interview and assessment) 24 hours per day, 7 days a week.

For departments with a large census (often around 30,000 or more patients per year), a trained technician or paramedic could assist by greeting the patient and obtaining data for quick registration (such as name, date of birth, and chief complaint), to be followed in a timely manner by emergency nurse comprehensive triage.

5. **What are the essential components of comprehensive triage?**

   - *An initial across-the-room look or visualization.* This evaluation helps to ensure stability of the ABCDs (airway, breathing, circulation, and disability). Any unstable patient is immediately sent to the treatment area for interventions. For children, the "pediatric triangle" includes a critical look at general appearance, work of breathing, and circulation.

     For stable patients, triage continues with:

   - *A rapid triage (60 seconds or less) of an appropriately elicited chief complaint, key question(s), and assessment(s), such as feeling for a pulse in the fractured extremity.* This helps rule out the worst-case scenario and determine the priority for the patient to receive a more in-depth, comprehensive triage assessment.

   - *Completion of a focused triage history and physical assessment.* This includes vital signs, pain assessment, pulse oximetry, diagnostic testing by protocol, additional department-designated information, and documentation.

   - *The triage decision, in which the patient's triage acuity or level is assigned.* This determines the urgency and order in which the patient will receive a medical screening examination (MSE) and additional assessment or treatment.

6. **What are the triage implications in systems that immediately place all patients in a treatment area?**

   In any system, an obviously critically ill individual needs to immediately go to the treatment area. In some departments, however, all individuals receive a rapid triage followed by placement in a treatment area, bypassing the waiting room. Such a system requires both an available bed and an available treating healthcare provider. It is not acceptable for a patient to sit in a room for 40 minutes before someone can obtain the initial triage nursing history and physical.

7. **What is the ENA standard for triage?**

   Comprehensive triage. However, in managing triage and patient flow, there must often be a combination of both rapid and comprehensive triage assessments.

8. **What should the triage history include?**

   The triage history typically includes the chief complaint, allergies (including food and latex), medications (prescriptions, over-the-counter medications, and complementary "natural" herbs), past medical conditions, immunizations, exposure to high-risk infection (e.g., recent travel overseas with a fever and cough), and last menstrual period or pregnancy information (if appropriate). The description of the complaint usually includes the mechanism of injury (if any), onset, and any treatment before arrival. The use of mnemonics can facilitate remembering to be thorough in information gathering.

9. **What are some examples of mnemonics to use for adult patients?**

PQRSTT

P Provokes/Palliates	What provokes the symptoms? What palliates or relieves the symptoms? Any history of trauma?
Q Quality	What does it feel like (patient's own descriptive words)?
R Radiation	Where is it located? Where does it radiate?
S Severity	Rate it on a scale of 0 to 10.
T Time	How long have you had this? Does it come and go, or is it constant? Has it ever happened before?
T Treatment	What treatment was already done (including home remedies)? What has worked before?

POSHPATE for the History of the Chief Complaint

P	Problem
O	Onset
S	Associated Symptoms
H	Previous History
P	Precipitating factors
A	Alleviating/Aggravating factors
T	Timing
E	Etiology

10. **What are some examples of mnemonics to use for pediatric patients?**

CIAMPEDS ("See, I am peds"), from the Emergency Nursing Pediatric Course

C	Chief Complaint
I	Immunizations? Need for Isolation
A	Allergies
M	Medications
P	Past medical history/Parents' impression
E	Events surrounding
D	Diet/Diapers
S	Symptoms associated with illness and injury

SAVE A CHILD

From the ENA Hawaii State Council. **SAVE** are observations to make before touching the child and **A CHILD** are key history and examination components.

S	Skin (e.g., mottled, petechiae)
A	Activity (e.g., responsive)
V	Ventilation (e.g., retractions, flaring)
E	Eye contact (e.g., glassy stare, fails to engage)
A	Abuse (e.g., unexplained bruising, inappropriate parent)
C	Cry (e.g., high-pitched)
H	Heat (e.g., fever)
I	Immunizations (e.g., up-to-date)
L	Level of consciousness (e.g., irritable, lethargic)
D	Dehydration (e.g., capillary refill, severe diarrhea/vomiting)

11. **How could the triage nurse approach the patient who is vague about the reason for coming to the ED?**

Consider asking in a sensitive, caring manner, "Why did you come to the emergency department *today*?" or "What is different about your condition *today*?" If possible, interview the patient away from family and friends because the patient may be reluctant to share the full story with others listening.

If there is still not a clear picture of why the patient came, try repeating the patient's exact words. Indicate that it is important that you understand so that you can help. This communication technique (reflection) often prompts the patient to elaborate.

If a nonmedical issue may be involved, ask, "Is there anything else going on in your life that you think could be contributing to your problem?" Sometimes patients will share, almost with relief, their current life stresses (such as the anniversary of a death).

12. **How can the nurse encourage patients to disclose healthcare practices that they may be reluctant to discuss?**

Give the patient "permission" to discuss it by bringing it into the realm of possibility. For example, if the patient is suspected of using laxatives excessively for his or her bowel problem, say, "Some people take only a tablespoon of milk of magnesia; others take two bottles a day. How much do you take?" If "natural" products are playing a role, say, "We know that up to 68% of people are using some herb or natural remedy. What remedies are you using?"

13. **Is the triage nurse liable for a Health Insurance Portability and Accountability Act (HIPAA) violation if someone inadvertently overhears a history?**

HIPAA's purpose is to limit unnecessary or inappropriate access to and disclosure of an individual's protected health information (PHI). HIPAA requires only "reasonable safeguards" to limit incidental use or disclosure. This can include lowering one's voice (or speaking close, within the patient's personal space), using curtains, turning monitor screens so they are not easily visible from a public area, and using sign-in sheets listing only the time of arrival and patient's name (not complaint). Because of the ED environment, overheard communication may be unavoidable. Examples include an emergency situation ("She's coding!"), a loud voice to overcome competing noises, a hearing-impaired patient, or a telephone conversation.

14. **What should the triage physical assessment include?**

Beyond ensuring stability of the ABCDs, include vital signs; pulse oximetry; pain assessment; weight (and height) per protocol; and a Glasgow Coma Scale score for patients who had an acute trauma or head injury, or with altered level of consciousness. Weight is essential for pediatric patients for accurate drug dosing. Many institutions omit some vital signs by policy, such as blood pressure for children younger than age 5, or temperature in a "healthy" adult with a localized extremity complaint (e.g., sprained ankle). The triage physical assessment must also include a focused assessment with regard to the chief complaint, for example, "CMS intact, + pedal pulses" for a lower extremity injury.

15. What are some discriminators that could alert the nurse that the patient's pain is from a serious etiology?

- *Comparison with past significant painful events.* For example, the patient states that it feels just like it did when he or she had kidney stones or a myocardial infarction.
- *Identification of a new distinction, particularly with ominous terms.* For instance, "the worst headache" or "excruciating, unbearable."
- *Pain begins abruptly.* The patient can recall the exact time when the ominous pain began (e.g., headache that started suddenly, "like being hit by a 2 × 4 board").
- *The pain has a maximum severity at the onset.* The greatest intensity is less than 1 minute, rather than gradually intensifying.
- *Pain is accompanied by vital sign changes or other symptoms (e.g., diaphoresis).*
- *Pain that prevents the patient from normal activities of daily living, such as work or sleep.*

16. After the nurse completes the triage focused history and physical assessment, what is involved in making a triage acuity assignment?

The ENA *Standards of Emergency Nursing Practice* (1999) indicate that triage determination is based on physical, developmental, and psychosocial needs, as well as factors influencing access to healthcare and patient flow through the emergency care system.

17. How many levels should a triage acuity scale have?

A joint American College of Emergency Physicians (ACEP) and ENA triage task force published the following statement, "ACEP and ENA believe that quality of patient care would benefit from implementing a standardized ED triage scale and acuity categorization process. Based on expert consensus of currently available evidence, ACEP and ENA support the adoption of a reliable, valid 5-level triage scale." The task force indicated that either the Canadian Triage and Acuity Scale (CTAS) or the Emergency Severity Index (ESI) is a good option. "The task force continues to encourage further research of five-level triage systems and recommends an in-depth, evidence-based review of all current five-level triage systems, as well as those under development."

18. How do CTAS and ESI differ?

The CTAS is built on the Australian method. It establishes a relationship between a group of sentinel events and the "usual" way patients with these conditions present. It includes the use of key objective data to help validate and assess the chief complaint when tiering common presentations into an appropriate triage category. The clinical descriptors for each level include high-risk historical factors, symptoms, physiological parameters, point-of-care testing, nursing assessment, and age-specific parameters.

The ESI is a triage algorithm that initially looks at high-risk indicators (mental status alteration, severe pain, or abnormal vital signs/PO_2) to arrive at the two highest levels of acuity. For patients not in those categories, the number of anticipated types of resource interventions to eventually diagnose and treat the patient is used as the discriminator to determine which of the three lower categories is most appropriate. It is unique in that it is based on acuity *and* likely resource consumption required to achieve a disposition.

19. What triage acuity level systems are U.S. EDs using most often?

In the 2001 ENA Benchmark Study, 69% of EDs were using a three-level, 12% were using a four-level, and 3% were using a five-level triage system; 12% were using no triage urgency scale at all (almost all of these were small facilities); and 4% did not respond to the item. Many EDs have since started moving toward the five-level systems; the ENA benchmark study is being repeated in 2005.

20. What if it is difficult to determine which of two acuity levels to assign to a patient?

Always give the patient the benefit of the doubt and assign the higher of the two categories. Nurses have a tendency to "under-triage" rather than "over-triage." Under-triaging presents a greater risk to the patient than over-triaging. And, if triage levels are considered in workload calculations, under-triaging may result in underestimation of ED workload.

21. Can the triage nurse ever make exceptions to the acuity system's rules in assigning a triage acuity rating?

Assign the proper rating. This is necessary for benchmarking; surveillance activities; research; legal defense; funding; case mix data; staffing levels; predictable resource consumption; budgeting; managed care decision making; and outcome measures for admission rates, ED length of stay, and complexity of care.

However, many facilities and practitioners will consider other factors and move a patient to a higher priority as a *management* decision. Some of the factors considered include:

- Presenting within 2 hours of a respiratory treatment (because the patient is experiencing a degree of "lack of response" and potential rebound)
- Experiencing severe pain (including a condition for which lying on a stretcher would help the patient's level of comfort)
- Arriving directly from a physician's office (because the patient has already been determined to be sick by a healthcare professional)
- Returning to the ED within 24 hours after ED discharge (something went wrong if the patient is back)
- Young children late at night (they do not have the coping and compensatory capacity when tired)
- Behavior that is disruptive, violent, or incompetent (the triage nurse cannot keep the patient in "control")
- Any abuse, neglect, or rape case (at risk for hidden injuries and for leaving without being seen; also because of psychological comfort and privacy needs)

22. Some EDs use a two-tier triage system. What is that?

EDs with long waiting times (either door to triage or triage to treatment) have instituted two-tier triage systems to reduce time to triage and department length of stay. In a two-tier system, the first tier involves a triage nurse rapidly assessing and categorizing all patients within 2 to 3 minutes. In the next tier, a second triage nurse conducts a more detailed assessment; implements initial treatment (such as immobilization and medication administration) and standing orders (such as laboratory and radiographic testing); and addresses family and visitor issues. Patients waiting for the second triage tier should be in a designated, observable area close to the triage station.

23. What are standing orders or protocols for diagnostic tests in triage?

Whether you have a one- or two-tier triage system, standing orders or protocols for certain diagnostic testing and medication administration have repeatedly shown to enhance timely decision making, decrease patient waiting time, and increase customer satisfaction. They are entered on the order sheet as "per protocol" or "standing order" and may qualify for reimbursement because they are appropriately applied physician orders. A collaborative process for development and implementation of these protocols should be followed with strict attention to evidence-based practice.

Numerous triage protocols have been published in the *Journal of Emergency Nursing* (e.g., Campbell, 2004; Seguin, 2004; Fry, 2001), and they are a common feature in the *Journal of Emergency Nursing's* "Managers Forum."

24. Is it essential that the triage nurse perform routine screenings?

Many screenings are required and/or desired during ED visits, including nutritional status, smoking, presence of domestic violence, alcohol or drug abuse, fall risk assessment, and/or advance directives. When it is not practical to obtain this information in the triage area it should be deferred to the treatment (primary) nurse.

25. What are some tips for better triage?

- *Look at the patient, listen, and do not write while the patient is talking to you.* Healthcare providers typically interrupt patients 23 seconds into the communication about their problem.
- *Never appear shocked by what the patient tells you.*
- *Do not discount a patient's concerns in triage.*
- *Watch people's faces.* They reflect internal emotions and will tell you when you or your questions have uncovered a painful or difficult area.
- *Ask specifically about drugs recently started.* They can cause side effects or new drug-drug interaction. Six is considered the "magic number" after which polypharmacy effects are seen. The more complex the medicine regimen, the more likely there will be confusion and errors.
- *Do not assume patients are taking their medications.* Nonadherence to some degree occurs in up to 50% of patients with chronic conditions.
- *Use the language of symptoms, feeling, and thoughts.* Avoid "organ" talk (e.g., "How are your sinuses?") and premature diagnosis (e.g., "UTI"). If the patient gives the chief complaint as a diagnosis, follow up with relevant questions, such as, "What symptoms are you having that make you think you have pneumonia?" Be a "detective" rather than a "court reporter."
- *Remember that the patient's self-diagnosis is not necessarily the correct diagnosis.* The "indigestion from something I ate" can be a cardiac symptom.

- *Exhibit concern for a higher acuity in the presence of other risk factors or co-morbidities/chronic illnesses.* The patient's physiological coping status is already stressed before this new injury or illness insult.
- *Remember that alcoholics can be sick and intoxicated.* An intoxicated person is never "just drunk" until the person is sober and assessed.
- *Ask the patient at the end of the triage encounter if there is anything else the patient wants to say.* Pay particular attention if a patient prefaces something with a statement such as, "This may not be important, but ...."

26. **What are some prioritization principles to help guide triage decisions when there are multiple patients?**

- *A (airway) is before B (breathing), which is before C (circulation), which is before D (disability), but consider the level of severity.* A severe C (e.g., rapid hemorrhage) is before a mild B (e.g., mild wheezing).
- *Systemic over local; life before limb.* Shock takes precedence over a bleeding, fractured limb.
- *Acute (recent onset) before chronic; short-term over long-term.*
- *Central pain before peripheral pain.* Pain originating within a body cavity or organ is usually more serious than pain originating in the skin, soft tissue, axial skeleton, or surface of superficial organs (e.g., eye, ear, nose).
- *Actual over potential.* The asthma condition may get worse, but treat the current hypotension. Reprioritize if and when the wheezing increases.
- *Trending.* More concern is warranted when the chief complaint is associated with other definitive changes. A worsening trend could consist of minor symptoms that tend to reoccur repeatedly, increase in severity, or indicate a steady progressive decline.
- *Potential for worsening* (e.g., an overdose or allergic response in which the final effect is not yet known). Any complaint of a throat feeling "tight" is serious.

27. **What are some common pitfalls with triage?**

- *Falling into the first come, first served mentality.* Patients should always be seen in order of need, not arrival time.
- *Using cookbook rules to make decisions.* Triage is continual critical thinking applied to *this* patient. All patients with the same complaint or demographic characteristic (e.g., all children) are not automatically assigned the same acuity level.
- *Focusing on a "red herring."* Avoid narrowing in on the most obvious symptom and missing the real problem, such as a fractured hip that was actually the result of a syncopal episode from third-degree heart block.
- *Basing the triage decision on other factors, such as the department census or "who" rather than "what."* The patient's condition should drive the acuity rating, not whether there are empty beds available or if the person is a VIP.
- *Losing objectivity.* Being unduly influenced because the patient frequently comes to the ED with similar complaints.
- *Being affected by exposure frequency.* Nurses tend to draw on their most recent, most often, or most dramatic experiences for comparison with the current patient's situation. They may forget to consider something still likely, but perhaps not as common in their department.

28. **What differences should the nurse be aware of when evaluating the physiological status of a geriatric patient?**

- *Functional or behavioral changes.* These may be related to the aging process, or the geriatric patient may exhibit behavioral symptoms with a new physical illness. For example, the primary symptom of a new urinary infection in a patient with Alzheimer's disease may be increased restlessness. New onset of confusion is sometimes the only symptom of decreased oxygenation.
- *Vague symptoms.* Older patients often do not present with classic textbook signs because of their age-related immunosuppression. For instance, in geriatric patients with pneumonia, 25% to 30% will not have fever and 20% will not have leukocytosis. The general guideline is that the atypical presentation is typical for geriatric patients.
- *High risk of polypharmacy.* The geriatric population uses 25% of all medications and 70% of all over-the-counter medications, with more than one third of this population taking eight or more different drugs each day. The risk of drug interactions rises to 100% when eight or more drugs are taken in a day.
- *Always investigate the history of a "fall."* Ask how the patient felt before the fall, because up to 40% of geriatric falls are caused by intrinsic factors such as syncope or stroke.

29. **What is most important when triaging a psychiatric patient?**

Safety needs. Determine the presence of any self-destructive thoughts, thoughts about inflicting harm on others, or disturbed thinking. It is likely that what the patient was doing outside the ED (e.g., assaulting people without provocation) is what he or she will do inside the ED. A nurse should trust his or her intuition and gut reaction. If you are feeling afraid, there is probably a good reason. Take appropriate action such as keeping the patient under observation and initiating the department's safety plan.

30. **What else will help triage psychiatric patients?**

Psychiatric expert Gail Lenehan (2006) recommends:
- *Pursue organic etiologies first if there are abnormal vital signs, pupil size, nystagmus, or a history of incontinence.*
- *Ask specific questions.* "What did you hope that we could do for you here today?" is better than a vague (therapeutic broad opening) "What's wrong?" The person may have many things wrong and a general question won't elicit the response needed.
- *Be alert to the "yes, but never this bad" syndrome.* The family or friends may initially say that the patient never did this before. Often they mean that in a quantitative sense, not qualitatively different. The patient has done it, just never to this degree.
- *Ask about awkward things* (e.g., a cooking pot upside down on the head) in a direct, but respectful, way. For example, ask the patient if he or she minds questions about the pot to better understand why it is there. The patient may be relieved to confide that it protects them from spy radiation. Avoid being patronizing.
- *Document behaviors precisely.* Include the specific cause (e.g., uttering threats to kill staff) rather than the conclusion (e.g., patient is "dangerous") that leads to controlling measures such as placing a patient in restraints.

31. What are the issues regarding language interpretation for patients with Limited English Proficiency (LEP)?

There are more than 300 languages and dialects spoken in the United States. The U.S. Civil Rights Act requires healthcare facilities to make a reasonable attempt to provide interpreter services. Similarly, the JCAHO and American Hospital Association (AHA) have made this accommodation a condition of accreditation. Federal guidelines also recommend having written materials for any group of non–English-speaking patients that constitutes 5% or more of the healthcare organization's patient volume.

Interpreters who are trained and competent must be available; telephone translation lines are an alternative. Do not automatically use family members to serve this role. The patient may not share sensitive information if a family member is serving as a translator. Also, professional translators translate exactly what the patient says without editing it in any way. Document the offer and use (or refusal) of an interpreter.

32. Should patients be told their triage acuity rating and estimated time to be seen by a physician?

Many nurses tell patients their triage rating and estimated time and provide a brochure about triage. Provide generous estimates. Patients are more satisfied when given a longer time expectation and seen sooner than when given a shorter estimated time but wait beyond it. Useful brochures include "What to Expect from Your Visit to an Emergency Care Center," which can be downloaded from the Members' Only section on the ENA website and "What you should know about the Emergency Department," available from the ACEP.

33. How can the nurse improve the patient's perception of the triage process?

Triage is often the first contact a patient or family has with the hospital. Make the triage process more positive by:
- Greeting the patient warmly.
- Using the patient's name as often as possible.
- Involving the family.
- Sharing the assessment as it is being done (e.g., "You lungs are clear right now").
- Praising what was done right (e.g., "It was good that you gave Tylenol").

34. No one likes to wait. What will help patients better tolerate a wait?

- *Advocate providing appropriate analgesics, food, and fluids.* If the patient is NPO and has a prolonged wait, consider a "rinse and spit" for comfort.
- *Give a sense of progress.* Give frequent updates and information about the wait. The individual is less likely to feel forgotten.
- *Consider scripts.* A common example is to start with an apology for the wait and let the patient know the status of the department.
- *Acknowledge feelings with empathy rather than giving factual information.* Say, "I know it is hard to wait, so we will do the best we can to make you comfortable" rather than "We are busy with sicker people."
- *Offer amenities.* Common features include multiple TVs, complimentary coffee, a fish tank, or a play area.

35. What does the phrase "waiting room etiquette" mean?

"Waiting room etiquette" is communicating and initiating appropriate infection control practices (e.g., wear a mask) to waiting patients and visitors. Tissues and hand-washing facilities (or alcohol-based waterless hand cleaner) should be available to patients in the waiting room.

36. What is the national standard for patient reassessments in the waiting room?

There is no national time standard, and defense attorneys recommend not setting a specific time limit as a rigid policy but rather as reasonable and prudent guidelines. The CTAS reflects reassessment based on acuity: Level 2 is every 15 minutes; Level 3 is every 30 minutes; Level 4 is every 60 minutes; and Level 5 is every 120 minutes. Another guideline is vital signs at least every 4 hours and a nursing note every 2 hours, with a complete reassessment every shift. A more frequent reassessment should always be initiated as warranted by a patient's condition.

37. What is the "triage out" process?

This process is also called "expedited MSE" or "referring out." Some EDs provide nonemergent patients with a next-day scheduled appointment at a clinic; others provide lists of community resources (after the MSE) but no appointment. Some protocols involve asking the patient for a downpayment (or copayment if insured) after the MSE establishes there is no emergency condition and the patient still wants to continue the visit in the ED. Those who cannot, or choose not to, pay are "triaged out" to community resources; those who pay return to the waiting room to be seen in the order indicated by their triage acuity level. There is no Emergency Medical Treatment and Active Labor Act (EMTALA) violation as long as all patients within the same category are treated the same way. "Triage out" programs claim no adverse outcomes to their process.

38. Is "triage out" a goal for every ED?

No. The process depends heavily on triage nurses being experts, operating under strict protocol, and having sufficient community resources to meet the patient's needs in a timely and appropriate manner. EMTALA expert Moy (2002) warns that the risk for violations can be high. Some also challenge the ethics of "triaging out" because the government continues to mandate that the ED is America's "safety net" for healthcare.

39. What are the EMTALA requirements related to triage?

EMTALA mandates a "decent" and "consistent" MSE for every patient who presents to the ED for care. The term MSE refers to an exam after triage, not triage itself.

40. Can patients be asked about financial information before their treatment is finished?

Yes, if the MSE is not delayed in order to obtain it.

41. What should be done if a patient leaves after triage but before the MSE?

If the triage nurse becomes aware that the patient is leaving, attempt to give risks and obtain a signature or document the impossibility of obtaining it. Documentation should illustrate that the patient is making an independent and informed decision. The percentage of patients who leave before MSE should not exceed 1% to 2% of the total patient volume.

42. When is a "fast track" option justified?

A "fast track" option can usually be justified when approximately 40% or more of the ED patient volume at an institution are classified as nonurgent. Patients appropriate for "fast track" are noninfectious; medically stable; ambulatory; do not have an anticipated need for hospital admission, IV fluids, or monitoring; and have an anticipated discharge within an hour.

43. Is it appropriate to provide telephone advice?

The ENA position (2001) is that no telephone advice is given unless a telephone triage program is in place or a life-threatening emergency is occurring. Requests that do not meet these criteria can be handled with a script that indicates an understanding of the concern, a statement that it is not in the best interest to give the caller advice over the phone, and a list of the alternatives (e.g., call 911 or private physician, go to the nearest ED).

44. What is the future of triage?

The future of ED triage is likely to be greater standardization and scientific rigor. The use of algorithms, computerized triage systems, and specialization in the triage role (with minimum requirements of education and experience) are all predicted.

Key Points

- The ENA *Standards of Emergency Nursing Practice* (1999) states that safe, effective, and efficient triage can be performed only by a registered professional nurse, educated in the principles of triage, with a minimum of 6 months' experience in emergency nursing.

- Give patients "permission" to discuss an atypical healthcare practice by bringing it into the realm of possibility. For example, "Over half of the population takes herbs every day; what do you take?"

- The ENA Comprehensive Specialty Standard (1999) indicates that triage determination is based on physical, developmental, and psychosocial needs, as well as factors influencing access to healthcare and patient flow through the emergency care system.

- The ACEP and ENA joint task force (2003) supports the adoption of a reliable, valid 5-level triage scale. Either the CTAS or ESI is a good option.

- When unsure, give the patient the benefit of the doubt and assign the higher of two acuity levels. There is a tendency to mistakenly "under-triage" rather than "over-triage."

- Communicate with the patient in the language of symptoms, feelings, and thoughts (not "organ" talk, such as, "How is your heart?"); do not assume the patient is taking the medications he or she lists; and ask if the patient has anything else to say at the end of the triage encounter.

Internet Resources

Agency for Healthcare Research and Quality, Emergency Severity Index:
www.ahrq.gov/research/esi

Canadian Association of Emergency Physicians, Canadian Triage and Acuity Scale:
www.caep.ca/002.policies/002-02.ctas.htm

Emergency Nurses Association Position Statements, *Standardized ED Triage Scale and Acuity Categorization: Joint ENA/ACEP Statement* and *Telephone Advice:*
www.ena.org/about/position

Language Line Services:
www.languageline.com

Bibliography

Brice M: Care plans for patients with frequent ED visits for such chief complaints as back pain, migraine, and abdominal pain, *J Emerg Nurs* 30(2):150-153, 2004.

Briggs JK: *Telephone triage protocols for nurses,* ed 2, Philadelphia, 2002, Lippincott.

Campbell P et al: Implementation of an ED protocol for pain management at triage at a busy level I trauma center, *J Emerg Nurs* 30(5):431-438, 2004.

Canadian Association of Emergency Physicians: Canadian Emergency Department Triage and Acuity Scale (CTAS), *J Can Assoc Emerg Phys* 1(3), 1999.

Cohen S: *101 Triage tips*, Hohenwald, Tenn, 2002, Health Resources Unlimited.

Croskerry P: The importance of cognitive errors in diagnosis and strategies to minimize them, *Acad Med* 78(8):775-780, 2003.

Diesburg-Stanwood A et al: Nonemergent ED patients referred to community resources after medical screening examination: Characteristics, medical condition after 72 hours, and use of follow-up services, *J Emerg Nurs* 30(4):312-317, 2004.

Emergency Nurses Association: *Benchmark study*. Des Plaines, IL, 2001, ENA.

Emergency Nurses Association: *ENPC provider manual*, ed 2, Des Plaines, IL, 2004, ENA.

Emergency Nurses Association: *Standards of emergency nursing practice*, ed 4, Des Plaines, IL, 1999, ENA.

Fernandes CMB et al: Five-level triage: A report from the ACEP/ENA five-level triage task force, *J Emerg Nurs* 31(1):39-50, 2005.

Fry M: Triage nurses order x-rays for patients with isolated distal limb injuries: A 12 month ED study, *J Emerg Nurs* 27(1):17-22, 2001.

Gilboy N et al: *Emergency Severity Index (ESI)*, Des Plaines, Ill, 2003, ENA.

Grossman VGA: *Quick reference to triage*, ed 2, Philadelphia, 2003, Lippincott.

Keddington RK: A triage vital sign policy for a children's hospital emergency department, *J Emerg Nurs* 24:189-192, 1998.

Lenehan GP: Triage of the psychiatric patient. In Zimmermann PG, Herr RD: *Nursing triage secrets,* St Louis, 2006, Mosby.

Macway-Jones K: *Emergency triage: Manchester Triage Group*, London, England, 1997, BMJ Publishing.

McNair R: *The nature of the beast: Comprehensive triage and patient flow workshop*, Fairview, NC, 1998-2003, Triage First.

McNair R: *A comprehensive emergency department triage course*, Fairview, NC, 2004, Triage First.

Moy MM: *The EMTALA answer book*, New York, 2002, Aspen.

Prutzman L, Oman K: Expedited medical screening exams. In Zimmermann PG: Managers forum, *J Emerg Nurs* 30(6):560, 2004.

Rutenberg CD: Telephone triage, *Am J Nurs* 100(3):77-81, 2000.

Seguin D: A nurse-initiated pain management advanced triage protocol for ED patients with an extremity injury at a level I trauma center, *J Emerg Nurs* 30(4):330-335, 2004.

Slovis CM, Wrenn KD, Meador CK: *A little book of emergency medicine rules,* Philadelphia, 2000, Hanley & Belfus.

Tipsord-Klinkhammer B, Andreoni CP: *Quick reference for emergency nursing*, Philadelphia, 1998, WB Saunders.

Travers DA: Triage: How long does it take? How long should it take? *J Emerg Nurs* 25:238-240, 1999.

Washington DL et al: Next-day care for emergency department users with nonacute conditions: A randomized controlled trial, *Ann Intern Med* 137:707-714, 2002.

Zimmermann PG: The case for a universal, valid, reliable 5-tier triage acuity scale for US emergency departments, *J Emerg Nurs* 27:246-254, 2001.

Zimmermann PG: Guiding principles at triage: Advice for new triage nurses, *J Emerg Nurs* 28(1):24-33, 2002.

Zimmermann PG: Tricks for the ED trade, *J Emerg Nurs* 29(5):453-458, 2003.

Zimmermann PG: Tips for managing pain more effectively, *J Emerg Nurs* 30(5):470-472, 2004.

Zimmermann PG and Herr RD: *Nursing triage secrets*, St Louis, Mosby (in press).

Emergency Preparedness

Gerald R. Connors and Kathleen S. Oman

1. What is a "disaster"?

A disaster is a sudden or great misfortune whereby hospital and/or community facilities are damaged and functions are impaired. Disasters may be caused by fire, weather/climate (e.g., earthquake, hurricane, tornado), explosion, terrorist activity, radiation or chemical spills, and epidemics. Disasters also can be a result of human error, which includes motor vehicle crashes, plane crashes, collapsed buildings, or similar occurrences. Disasters affect both the young and old.

2. How are disasters and their victims categorized?

Disaster situations can be classified according to the number of victims involved:
- Mass patient incident (fewer than 10 victims presenting to the emergency department—ED)
- Multiple casualty incident (between 10 and 100 victims presenting to the ED)
- Mass casualty incident (more than 100 victims presenting to the ED)

An example of a mass patient incident is a motor vehicle crash with several persons, but fewer than 10, sustaining injury. An example of a multiple casualty incident was the 1999 shooting at Columbine High School in Littleton, Colorado. Mass casualty incidents frequently occur with environmental disasters in areas of dense population. The 2001 terrorist attacks on the World Trade Center and Pentagon and 2005 Hurricane Katrina in the U.S. Gulf region are examples of mass casualty incidents. The Emergency Nurses Association (ENA) Position Statement defines a mass casualty incident as one "where sudden and high patient volume exceeds an emergency department's resources."

3. What are the phases of disaster?

- **Preimpact.** Begins before the onset of the disaster, if known in advance. It defines the time during which medical personnel anticipate and are warned. For example, the preimpact phase of a hurricane may be several days, as meteorologists track the storm and local officials order evacuations. This phase is not present in all disasters.
- **Impact.** The period during which the disaster is occurring, continuing until the initiation of the postimpact phase. This is also known as the rescue phase. At this time, several key assessments must be made, including evaluating the extent of the loss, identifying resources available, and planning the rescue of victims. This phase may be brief. It may be over in as little as 30 seconds (e.g., airplane crash) or it may be lengthy (e.g., flood).

- **Postimpact**. Also referred to as the recovery phase. During this phase, the extent of the loss has been evaluated and the rescue of victims is complete; further injuries have been minimized. This can be the lengthiest phase.

4. What are the principles of disaster management?

The eight principles of disaster management include:
- Preventing the occurrence
- Minimizing the number of casualties
- Preventing further casualties
- Rescuing the injured
- Providing first aid
- Evacuating the injured
- Providing definitive care
- Facilitating reconstruction/recovery

5. Who is responsible for disaster management?

Everyone. It is not sufficient for a few officials and planners to know their roles and responsibilities during a disaster; the roles of everyone involved must be clearly understood.

One of the lessons learned from Hurricane Katrina is that local officials and agencies have primary responsibility, especially in the early phase of the disaster. Local efforts are supplemented by state and federal aid, but if the local effort fails, the outcomes may be much worse: "Think globally, and prepare locally."

6. What are the components of disaster preparedness?

Community preparedness, field triage, hospital preparedness, and ED preparedness.

7. What is field triage?

Field triage is conceptually and operationally different than what is thought of as traditional ED triage. Field triage is a process of sorting or assessing mass casualty victims on the basis of the severity of injuries and the likelihood that they can be saved with medical intervention. The Simple Triage And Rapid Treatment (START) system is one of many that has been shown to be effective in predicting critical injury in mass casualty situations. The START system is based on a rapid (less than 30 second) assessment of respiration, perfusion, and mental status. The START algorithm is shown in the following diagram.

Triage in mass casualty incidents is not a one-time affair. Triage tags are developed so that change in status can be noted, influencing evacuation order. Immediate (red) triage category patients are always evacuated first (the so-called "Visine principle"—get the red out), followed by delayed (yellow), then minor (green, also called "walking wounded"). A modified JumpSTART triage system is available for children (www.jumpstarttriage.com).

8. What is a disaster plan and why is it important?

A disaster plan is the combination of facilities, services, equipment, personnel, procedures, and communication operations needed to ensure quality patient care during an incident. The goal of this plan is to maintain safe operations of

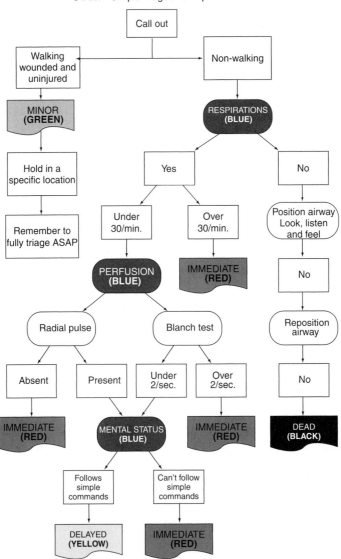

START - Simple Triage and Rapid Treatment

START—Simple Triage And Rapid Treatment. Evacuation/transport priority: *RED*, Immediate; *YELLOW*, delayed; *GREEN*, minor. *(Modified from Community Emergency Response Team [CERT] Los Angeles [www.cert-la.com/triage/start.htm].)*

the healthcare facility and meet the healthcare needs of the community during a disaster incident.

A disaster plan is developed to promote the consistency of emergency plans in times of crisis. The disaster plan can create an orderly response to an emergency situation (e.g., fire, bombing, hurricane), providing the flexibility to expand or contract, depending on the type of event and the severity and duration of the emergency. In any disaster plan, refinement and improvements are ongoing.

9. How should a hospital evaluate the effectiveness of its disaster plan?

Barring a real disaster, the best way for a hospital to evaluate the effectiveness of its disaster plan is through periodic disaster drills or disaster preparedness exercises. The benefits of conducting disaster drills are numerous. Not only do these exercises allow a hospital to evaluate the effectiveness of its plan, they also provide personnel the opportunity to practice the plan and help hospital staff prepare themselves for a real disaster.

Hospitals should evaluate their disaster preparedness plan as often as necessary but at least annually. Some hospitals conduct disaster preparedness exercises as often as four times a year. Because disasters can be unpredictable and untimely, disaster drills should be conducted not only on day shift but on evening and night shifts as well. Having these exercises on all shifts will provide for greater staff exposure, allowing more hospital personnel the opportunity to participate in the drill. A critique of the drill is an important way to continually improve on areas needing attention. The critique allows evaluation of key components: communication, supplies and staffing.

10. What are the roles of emergency nurses in disaster management?

ED nurses have multiple roles, including how to care for multiple victims in an ED that may be overwhelmed, effective communication, effective utilization of available resources, safety and security, coordination of resources and care to victims, and documentation. To address these needs, the creation of a hospital-wide disaster/safety committee is paramount. This group should be multidisciplinary and address issues such as supplies, equipment, evacuation, and staffing needs. The committee should have emergency personnel as members and include them in decision making. Clearly defined roles for members of the ED team should be understood by all those involved.

11. What are the emergency nurse's responsibilities in the event of a disaster?

It is important to understand your role *before* a disaster occurs. A hospital's disaster plan should clearly delineate responsibilities for personnel working in the ED as well as other departments throughout the facility. The plan should identify specific duties for all ED staff, including the charge nurse, triage nurses, resuscitation nurses, treatment nurses, physicians, unit secretaries, and admitting or registration personnel. Documentation of these duties should be clearly outlined and easily accessible.

For optimal success, it is best to continue normal patient processing through the ED. ED staff are well versed in the routine daily functioning of the department. Maintaining routine patient processes will allow the staff to perform at their most effective levels during a time that can be stressful and chaotic. The hospital disaster preparedness plan should strive to maintain the integrity of routine patient flow to the extent possible.

12. What should be included in a disaster critique?

Begin the critique with identifying information, such as date and time of the event, type of disaster, location of disaster, number of anticipated victims, and number of patients in the ED at the time the disaster was announced. Also include the information provided in the following table.

Criteria for disaster management critique

Activity	Specific questions
Triage	Was triage accurate?
Patient flow	Where were ED patients sent?
	How many patients were sent to each area of the hospital?
	How many patients were discharged home?
Communication	Was the initial communication from the county EMS appropriate?
	Was administration properly notified?
	Was paging audible?
	Was interdepartmental communication adequate?
Staff response	Was ED nursing staff prepared?
	Was ED physician staff prepared?
	Was the OR prepared?
	Were the inpatient nursing units prepared?
	Were ancillary services (respiratory, lab, radiology) prepared?
	Were other key areas (pastoral care, social work, security) prepared?
Family members	Were family members informed and handled appropriately?
Media	Were the media handled appropriately?
Documentation	Was the registration process effective?
	Was the medical record accessible?
Command	Was the command center initiated?
	Were space and phone lines adequate?
Medical supplies	Were medical supplies accessible?
	Were medical supplies adequate?

13. **What additional supplies should be available to care for patients involved in a disaster?**

The majority of supplies that will be needed in a disaster are probably already stocked in the ED. The quantity of supplies available may need to be augmented, including materials required to maintain airway, breathing, and circulation, as well as items to treat soft tissue injuries. In the four major hurricanes that hit the southern United States in 2004, the most predominant injuries of survivors were soft tissue injuries, such as lacerations and abrasions. To prepare for large-scale disasters, large quantities of bandage materials, suture sets, tetanus toxoid, and irrigation fluid should be available. Additional materials that may prove beneficial in a disaster include patient care packets with a preassigned medical record number, name band, and ED chart. Because the hospital's water supply may be interrupted, potable water and waterless hand cleaner should be available.

Supplies that will be needed immediately should be housed in an area where they can be quickly and easily obtained. Larger quantities of backup materials can be housed at another location, such as a warehouse. Depending on the type of disaster, available transportation, and condition of the supply warehouse, it may be difficult to access backup materials. Because of the potential inaccessibility of additional supplies, lists of alternative supply vendors should be included in the hospital's disaster plan.

14. **Should the ED have specialized medical equipment to provide care to disaster patients?**

Because a disaster can interrupt central power, oxygen, and vacuum, the ED may need medical equipment that is portable and battery-operated. Many departments already have battery-operated portable cardiac monitors and defibrillators, suction devices, infusion pumps, and vital sign monitoring systems. EDs should examine critical equipment, such as ventilators, to determine whether they are battery-powered. To maintain the ability to function without electricity, all battery-operated medical equipment should be fully charged. Additional portable equipment that may prove beneficial in a disaster includes hand-operated sphygmomanometers, flashlights for all patient care areas, portable beds or cots to allow for an increased patient load, and portable oxygen tanks.

For disasters involving chemical contamination or hazardous material exposure, decontamination equipment will be needed: personal protective equipment, including protective respirators for healthcare providers; a field shower; and a means for handling hazardous waste.

Another reason for having equipment and supplies portable is that a disaster might affect the integrity of the ED (and hospital). A fire, explosion, or flood could necessitate relocation of emergency services.

15. **How should communication be maintained during a disaster?**

The hospital's disaster preparedness plan should include a well-defined, clearly outlined method for transmitting information. The plan should address internal communication, external communication, and the appropriate flow of information. An established communication hub will help to minimize information difficulties that can occur in a disaster. The hospital's emergency operations center is typically the center of the communication network. The hospital's disaster plan should strive to eliminate or minimize unnecessary communication traffic, which can obstruct telephone lines.

Because routine telephone service may be interrupted, provisions must be made to institute alternative methods of communication. Information can be transmitted through the use of mobile or cellular phones, radio communication systems, bullhorns, runners, signs, and flyers. Local television and radio stations can be of great assistance in maintaining communication between the disaster site, the hospital, and the general public. In the event that this form of communication is used, the hospital's public relations officer should be involved.

16. If not at work when a disaster strikes, where should an emergency nurse report?

Report to the ED or other designated area identified in the hospital's disaster plan. Most departments will activate their telephone alert roster, telling personnel where to report. Realizing that they will probably be needed, many staff members will not wait for the alert notification.

Reporting to the disaster site is generally *not* recommended. Scene response should be left to prehospital experts. Prehospital personnel have been trained in scene assessment and field care. ED-based nurses will be most comfortable and most effective working in the hospital, an environment with which they are familiar.

17. How can local community agencies assist the hospital in the event of a disaster?

Local private and community agencies can assist in a variety of ways. As previously discussed, television and radio stations can be an integral part of maintaining communication. The local American Red Cross chapter may assist in providing shelter for disaster victims not requiring hospitalization. Hospitals may have contracted with area businesses to ensure sufficient quantities of food and potable (drinkable) water. Additional medical care can be provided by disaster medical assistance teams located throughout the country.

The National Guard, police departments, and fire agencies will likely be involved at the disaster site. However, EMTs, paramedics, community nurses, and physicians may approach the hospital, volunteering their professional skills. Provisions should be made to verify practitioner licenses and credentials. The Health Resources and Services Administration (HRSA) is developing a national system for registration of healthcare professionals (the Emergency System for Advance Registration of Volunteer Health Professions—ESAR-VHP). Health professionals who wish to assist during a disaster may apply through the county health department; credentials are verified and methods of contact are established (see www.hrsa.gov/bioterrorism/esarvhp).

18. What additional resources are available to assist with disaster response?

- Federal Emergency Management Agency (FEMA)
- National Disaster Medical System (NDMS)
- Joint Commission on Accreditation of Healthcare Organizations (JCAHO)

As in the state of Florida, some states have developed agencies to assist in disaster relief, for example, Disaster Aid Services to Hospitals (DASH).

19. **What is FEMA's role in disasters?**

FEMA's mission is "to reduce loss of life and property and protect our nation's critical infrastructure from all types of hazards through a comprehensive, risk-based, emergency management program of mitigation, preparedness, response and recovery" (www.fema.gov/about). In carrying out its mission, FEMA works with federal and state government officials and with community groups to:
- Protect lives and prevent the loss of property from disaster
- Reduce the economic impact from disaster
- Reduce human suffering and enhance the recovery of communities after disaster strikes

20. **Where is quick information about disaster preparedness and management available?**

FEMA maintains an online, searchable database, the Global Emergency Management System (GEMS), with links to worldwide disaster resources. The database can be accessed at www.fema.gov/gems.

21. **What considerations are important with respect to weapons of mass destruction and bioterrorism?**

The threat of intentional release of chemical and biological agents is real. The ED must have a system to manage this type of incident. The following considerations should be evaluated:
- Appropriate personal protective equipment for staff, including respiratory protection
- Availability of proper decontamination services and procedures
- Established biochemical triage process
- Staff competency in the identification of bacterial agents, viruses, and biological toxins, including symptoms and care
- Regular drills to measure the facility's and staff's responsiveness to this threat

22. **What are Class A biological agents and how are they recognized and managed in the ED?**

These agents are easily transmitted from person to person, cause high mortality, might cause public panic and social disruption, and require a coordinated action response for public health preparedness. Examples of these agents and their typical presentation are listed in the following table.

23. **What chemical agents are of concern?**

Chemical agents have been used as weapons and are highly likely to cause major morbidity and mortality. Categories of chemical agents include:
- Nerve agents (tabun, sarin, soman)
- Blood agents (cyanide)

Class A biological agents

Agent	Clinical presentation	Medical management
Anthrax (*Bacillus anthracis*), inhaled	The initial symptoms most often reported are fever, nonproductive cough, myalgia, and malaise, resembling those of a viral upper respiratory tract infection. Early in the course of the disease, chest radiographs show a widened mediastinum, which is evidence of hemorrhagic mediastinitis, and marked pleural effusions. After 1 to 3 days, the disease takes a fulminant course with dyspnea, strident cough, and chills, culminating in death.	Intravenous penicillin and doxycycline are recommended.
Botulism toxin (*Clostridium botulinum*)	Symptoms range from subtle motor weakness or cranial nerve palsies to rapid respiratory arrest. The initial symptoms of foodborne botulism may be gastrointestinal and can include nausea, vomiting, abdominal cramps, or diarrhea; after the onset of neurological symptoms, constipation is more typical. Dry mouth, blurred vision, and diplopia are usually the earliest neurological symptoms. These initial symptoms may be followed by dysphonia, dysarthria, dysphagia, and peripheral muscle weakness. Paralysis begins with the cranial nerves, then affects the upper extremities, the respiratory muscles, and finally the lower extremities. Onset usually occurs 18 to 36 hours after exposure (range, 6 hours to 8 days). In severe cases, extensive respiratory muscle paralysis leads to ventilatory failure and death unless supportive care is provided.	Supportive therapy with mechanical ventilation. Ventilatory support is most commonly needed for 2 to 8 weeks. The administration of antitoxin is the only specific pharmacological treatment available for botulism. One vial (7500 International Unit of type A, 5500 International Unit of type B, and 8500 International Unit of type E antitoxins) per patient is administered, and it is believed that no additional doses are necessary.
Plague (*Yersinia pestis*)	Aerosolized plague may cause fever, cough, chest pain, and hemoptysis with signs consistent with severe pneumonia 1 to 6 days after exposure. Rapid evolution of disease occurs in the 2 to 4 days after symptom onset and leads to septic shock with high mortality without early treatment.	Early treatment and prophylaxis with streptomycin or gentamicin or the tetracycline or fluoroquinolone classes of antimicrobials are advised.

Continued

Class A biological agents—cont'd

Agent	Clinical presentation	Medical management
Smallpox (*Variola major*)	The incubation period for smallpox is 7 to 17 days (mean, 10 to 12 days). The prodromal phase, which lasts for 2 or 3 days, is characterized by severe headache, backache, and fever, all beginning abruptly. The rash begins as small, red macules, which become papules with a diameter of 2 to 3 mm over a period of 1 or 2 days; the papules become vesicles with a diameter of 2 to 5 mm. The lesions occur first on the face and extremities and eventually cover the body. Pustules that are 4 to 6 mm in diameter develop about 4 to 7 days after the onset of the rash and remain for 5 to 8 days. The pustules then crust over into scablike lesions. Smallpox lesions are generally all at the same stage of development.	A suspect case of smallpox should be managed in a negative-pressure room and the patient should be vaccinated if the illness is in an early stage. Strict respiratory and contact isolation are imperative. There is no treatment approved by the Food and Drug Administration (FDA) for orthopoxviruses. Penicillinase-resistant antimicrobial agents should be used if smallpox lesions are infected. Patients need adequate hydration and nutrition, because substantial amounts of fluid and protein can be lost by febrile persons with dense, often weeping lesions.
Tularemia (*Francisella tularenis*)	Onset is usually abrupt, with fever, headache, chills and rigors, body aches, and sore throat. A dry cough and chest pain frequently occur. Sweats, fever and chills, progressive weakness, malaise, anorexia, and weight loss characterize the continuing illness. Disease may be complicated by pneumonia, sepsis, and meningitis.	Streptomycin and IV gentamicin are drugs of choice. In a mass casualty setting, oral doxycycline and ciprofloxacin are preferred.
Viruses (Ebola hemorrhagic fever, Marburg hemorrhagic fever, Lassa fever, Argentine hemorrhagic fever)	Common presenting complaints are fever, myalgia, and prostration; clinical examination may reveal only conjunctival injection, mild hypotension, flushing, and petechial hemorrhages. Full-blown viral hemorrhagic fever (VHF) typically evolves to shock and generalized bleeding from the mucous membranes and often is accompanied by evidence of neurological, hematopoietic, or pulmonary involvement.	Supportive treatment of shock and bleeding. Ribavirin is a nonimmunosuppressive nucleoside with broad antiviral properties and is of proven value for some VHF agents.

- Blister agents (lewisite, nitrogen, and sulfur mustards)
- Heavy metals (arsenic, lead, mercury)
- Volatile toxins (benzene, chloroform)
- Pulmonary agents (phosgene, chlorine)
- Pesticides, dioxins, and acids

For more information about chemical agents, symptoms, and treatment, see the Centers for Disease Control and Prevention (CDC) website (www.cdc.gov) and the Center for the Study of Bioterrorism (CSB) website (www.bioterrorism. slu.edu). The local Poison Control Center can also provide information about the management of specific agents.

24. What is the best way for an ED to prepare for a bioterrorism or chemical attack?

Training, training, and more training. Gone are the days when the department had one nurse designated as the "disaster" nurse. ED staff need to be prepared and competent to deal with a variety of bioterrorism events to keep themselves safe and provide effective patient care. Links with public health agencies and authorities responsible for environmental sampling and decontamination are also key aspects of a coordinated plan.

25. Is bioterrorism the most common method used by terrorists?

During the period from 1980 to 2001, bombings accounted for nearly 70% of all terrorist attacks in the United States. Blast injuries among bombing survivors are most common to the lungs, eyes, abdomen, and brain.

Key Points

- Preparation is the key to emergency management.
- A sound emergency preparedness plan addressing both internal and external situations is valuable.
- A clear chain of command with clearly articulated roles and responsibilities is important to the success of the plan.
- Supplies and equipment for the ED are the hallmark of a prepared department able to render care to those needing it the most.
- A defined triage process is paramount; the process should include decontamination (if needed), documentation of care, and prioritization of patients.
- A continued refinement of emergency preparedness skills is required to maintain touch with current threats.
- Regular drills and practice sessions ensure that emergency nurses are prepared when the need arises.

Internet Resources

American Nurses Association and U.S. Department of Health & Human Services National Nurses Response Team:
www.nursingworld.org/news/disaster/response.htm

Centers for Disease Control and Prevention, Emergency Preparedness & Response:
www.bt.cdc.gov

Emergency Nurses Association Position Statement, *Mass Casualty Incidents* (pdf document):
www.ena.org/about/position/PDFs/MassCasualtyIncidents.pdf

Federal Emergency Management Agency:
www.fema.gov

National Disaster Medical System:
www.oep-ndms.dhhs.gov

Bibliography

Bernardo LM and Veenema TG: Pediatric emergency preparedness for mass gatherings and special events, *Disaster Manag Response* 2(4):118-122, 2004.

Connors G and Boulais L: Disaster management. In Oman K, Koziol-McLain J, and Scheetz L: *Emergency nursing secrets*, Philadelphia, 2001, Hanley & Belfus.

Goodwin Veenema T: *Disaster nursing and emergency preparedness for chemical, biological, and radiological terrorism*, New York, 2003, Springer Publishing.

Hohenhaus SM: Practical considerations for providing pediatric care in a mass casualty incident, *Nurs Clin North Am* 40(3):523-533, 2005.

Hsu EB et al: *Training of hospital staff to respond to a mass casualty incident*, AHRQ Pub No 04-E015-2, Rockville, Md, 2004, Agency for Healthcare Research and Quality.

Laskowski-Jones L: Emergency and mass casualty nursing. In Ignatavicius DD and Workman ML: *Medical surgical nursing*, ed 5, St Louis, 2006, Elsevier.

Pain Management

Robert Montgomery and Regina M. Fink

1. What is pain and what is its impact on the emergency department (ED)?

According to the International Association for the Study of Pain (IASP) (1986), pain is "an unpleasant sensory and emotional experience associated with actual or potential tissue damage or described in terms of such damage." McCaffery (1999) defines pain more globally as "whatever the experiencing person says it is, existing whenever he or she says it does." Pain is one of the leading causes of ED visits; studies have shown that up to 80% of patients present with pain. Unfortunately, 35% to 60% of patients leave the ED with their pain unrelieved. Pain must be assessed and treated within a developmental and multidimensional framework that encompasses physiological, sensory, affective, cognitive, behavioral, sociocultural, and environmental dimensions. The Emergency Nurses Association (ENA) has identified pain management as a chief clinical issue and a high priority, requiring research.

2. What is the difference between acute and chronic pain?

Acute pain is generally classified as pain that is of short or predictable duration, has an identifiable cause, and subsides as healing takes place. Chronic pain worsens and intensifies with the passage of time and is further subclassified into malignant and nonmalignant pain.

Acute vs. Chronic pain

Pain type	Characteristics	Causes
Acute	Serves as a warning Follows injury to body Disappears over time May be associated with objective signs of autonomic nervous system activity Usually a single, easily discernible cause Degree and intensity "make sense" based on recent injury or disease process Anxiety common	Trauma Surgery Infection Fracture Pancreatitis Bowel obstruction

Continued

Acute vs. Chronic pain—cont'd

Pain type	Characteristics	Causes
Chronic	Serves no purpose Worsens/intensifies with passage of time Rarely accompanied by sympathetic nervous system arousal Degree and intensity don't "make sense" Usually has multiple causes Frustration and depression common	Malignant Cancer HIV/AIDS Nonmalignant Low back pain Sickle cell anemia Rheumatoid arthritis Osteoarthritis Pelvic pain Diabetes Migraine

3. How can a nurse differentiate among the various pain types?

Pain can be classified as neuropathic or nociceptive. Neuropathic pain is usually caused by peripheral or central nervous system damage, whereas nociceptive pain refers to pain traveling along normal nerve conduction pathways and may be further subclassified into visceral or somatic pain. Acute pain is usually of nociceptive origin. Chronic pain may be both nociceptive and neuropathic. Some of the common types of pain seen in the ED are back pain, migraine, chest pain, and abdominal pain. The following table describes various pain types a clinician may see in the ED.

Types of pain seen in the ED

Pain type	Words used to describe pain	Etiology	Examples	Treatment
Neuropathic	Burning, shooting, numbness, radiating, lancinating, "like a fire," electrical jolts	Peripheral or central nervous system damage	Postherpetic neuralgia, peripheral neuropathy secondary to diabetes, HIV, cancer and its treatment (radiation, chemotherapy), chronic pelvic pain, fibromyalgia, reflex sympathetic dystrophy (RSD)	Antidepressants, anticonvulsants, benzodiazepines, +/− opioids

Types of pain seen in the ED—cont'd

Pain type	Words used to describe pain	Etiology	Examples	Treatment
Visceral (poorly localized)	Squeezing, cramping, pressure, distention, bloated feeling, stretching	Pain occurs in deep organs and is often referred along dermatomes	Bowel obstruction, venous occlusion, ischemia, post abdominal or thoracic surgery, ascites, chest pain, ovarian cyst, appendicitis	Opioids (use caution in patients with bowel obstruction)
Somatic (well localized)	Achy, throbbing	Cutaneous or deep tissue inflammation or bone injury	Degenerative joint disease, bone metastasis from cancer	NSAIDs, muscle relaxants, +/− opioids

4. **What are barriers to optimal pain management for patients in the ED?**

Barriers are similar to those found in other healthcare settings, but with the added factor of diagnosing and quickly treating patients whose conditions include trauma, life-threatening injuries, abdominal pain, and chest pain. Widely recognized healthcare provider barriers include:
- Limited knowledge of analgesics
- Inadequate pain assessment, especially in those patients who are unable to self-report pain
- Lack of understanding of the differences among the terms "addiction," "tolerance," and "dependence"
- Fear of causing or contributing to addiction
- Concerns about causing side effects and inducing tolerance
- Fear of masking symptoms that could be diagnostic
- Ethnic and/or cultural differences and language barriers between healthcare providers and patients

Populations requiring special consideration are patients who are elderly, children, minorities, cognitively impaired, or have a history of active substance abuse. These patients are routinely undermedicated because of fears of addiction, adverse effects, and possible bias. There is evidence to suggest that healthcare professionals often make treatment decisions based on preconceived ideas regarding diagnosis, age, ethnicity, and socioeconomic status. A unique barrier in the ED is the concern that administration of pain medications may adversely affect the ability to accurately evaluate the patient's physical condition, coupled with the belief that analgesics should be withheld until diagnoses have been made. These concerns are not substantiated with research or clinical data and need to be abandoned.

5. What are common patient and family concerns about pain medications?

It is important to solicit patients' and families' worries about pain control and medications to legitimize and clarify their concerns. A patient may fail to report pain in an attempt to be a "good" patient or because of the following myths about opioids:

- If I take pain medicine (opioids) regularly, I will get hooked or addicted.
- Pain is expected. I just need to bear it or hang in there.
- I should wait to take pain medicine until I really need it, or it won't work later.
- I'd rather have a bowel movement than take pain medicine and become constipated.
- I have nausea or itching with pain medicine, so I must have an allergy.
- My family thinks that I take too much pain medicine, so I should hold back.

6. How should pain be assessed in the ED?

The quality and utility of any assessment tool are only as good as the assessor's ability to listen, believe, and understand the patient's pain. Pain assessment must be continuous, individualized, and documented so that all healthcare providers involved will have an understanding of the patient's pain. Emergency nurses' accuracy in estimating patients' pain intensity has been shown to be less than 50% across all pain complaints, and patients with musculoskeletal pain had their pain intensity underestimated 95% of the time. The Joint Commission on Accreditation of Healthcare Organizations' (JCAHO's) standards call on hospitals and other healthcare agencies to recognize the patient's right to appropriate pain assessment and management, to assess pain in all patients, and to record assessment results in a manner that facilitates regular reassessment and follow-up. In many institutions, pain has been equated to the "fifth vital sign" to emphasize its importance in patient care. Remember, the patient's self-report of pain is most accurate. Nurses should not attempt to "estimate" a patient's pain. Pain assessment should include asking the patient about the following five key components of pain:

- Words used to describe the pain
- Intensity of the pain
- Location of the pain
- Duration of the pain
- Aggravating and alleviating factors

No pain assessment is complete unless patients are asked about the presence of symptoms or side effects associated with pain or its treatment. These include nausea and vomiting, decreased appetite, constipation, pruritus, confusion, sedation, and urinary retention. Additionally, inquiring about how pain affects a patient's activities of daily living, previous pharmacological and nonpharmacological approaches used (what has worked and what hasn't), and the patient's knowledge of the etiology of pain will be helpful in determining treatment modalities.

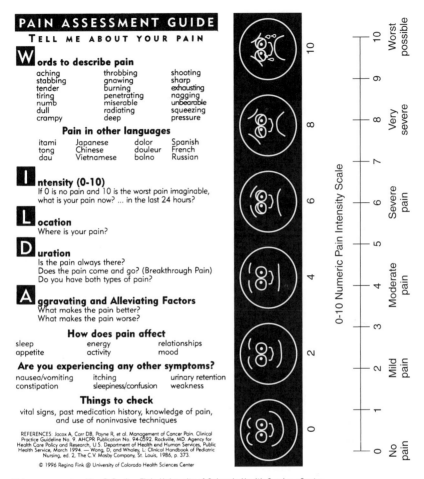

Pain assessment guide. © Regina Fink, University of Colorado Health Services Center.

7. What is the best pain intensity scale to use in the ED?

Assessing pain intensity captures only one aspect of the pain experience. However, it is the most frequently used parameter in clinical practice. Pain intensity should be evaluated not only at the present level, but also at its least, worst, and with movement. Patients should also be asked how their pain compares with yesterday or with their worst day they can remember. Comfort goals (where they want their pain to be) are also important to assess.

Pain intensity can be measured quantitatively with a numeric rating scale, verbal descriptor scale, faces scale, or pain thermometer. No single scale is appropriate for all patients. Having the availability of more than one scale in the ED will allow patients to choose which scale will work best for them. Staff should carefully document which scale the patient used so that all members of the healthcare team will be aware of the appropriate scale to use.

8. If a patient is sedated, nonverbal, or cognitively impaired, can he or she still have pain?

The gold standard or primary source of pain assessment is the patient's self-report. However, pain instruments relying on verbal self-report may not be practical for use with patients who cannot verbalize pain or in patients with advanced disease when delirium or cognitive failure is prevalent. The potential for unrelieved and unrecognized pain is greater in patients who cannot verbally express their discomfort. The inability to communicate effectively because of impaired cognition and sensory losses is a serious problem for many patients with trauma and life-threatening illness. Clearly, pain assessment techniques and tools are needed for patients, whether mentally incompetent or nonverbal, who communicate only through their unique behavioral responses. It is important for nurses to remember that pain is communicated through both verbal and nonverbal behaviors.

It may be more complicated to assess nonverbal cues in the ED setting because in contrast to patients with acute postoperative pain, patients with chronic pain or pain caused by trauma may not demonstrate any specific behaviors indicative of pain. It is also erroneous to assess pain by reliance on involuntary physiological reactions, such as increases in blood pressure, pulse, or respiratory depth. Elevated vital signs may occur with sudden, severe pain but not with persistent pain when the body reaches physiological equilibrium. The absence of behavioral or involuntary cues does not negate the presence of pain. Nonverbal patients should be empirically treated for pain if there is preexisting pain or evidence that an individual in a similar condition would experience pain. Family members and significant others who know the patient may be helpful in the pain assessment process.

Trauma patients who are paralyzed with neuromuscular blocking agents and placed on a ventilator may still experience pain but will be unable to communicate with their healthcare providers. While they may be receiving sedation with the use of a benzodiazepine, these patients still require analgesics for pain management purposes. It is imperative that these patients be adequately medicated for pain with the use of short-acting intravenous (IV) pain medications without active metabolites such as fentanyl and hydromorphone. These medications may be easily reversed with IV naloxone if excessive sedation occurs, although this is highly unlikely.

9. Is there a tool that can be used to assess pain in the ED patient who is nonverbal or cognitively impaired?

There have been a variety of instruments that have been used to observe and measure the frequency of pain behaviors in the elderly, demented, children, and infants but their use has been limited in the ED population. The Pain Assessment Behavioral Scale (PABS), developed and validated by Campbell, Renaud, and Vanni (2005), has been used to assess pain in adult patients unable to self-report (nonverbal, cognitively impaired [encephalopathic, hypercalcemic, neurologically impaired], intubated/sedated, demented, end of life). The following behavior parameters are assessed and scored on a scale of 0 to 2 and totaled (possible score 0 to 10): facial expression, restlessness, muscle tone, vocalization, and consolability. Patients should be observed at rest and with movement; reposition the patient during assessment and score the higher score. The PABS may not be valid in patients who are neuromuscularly blocked or are exhibiting decorticate and/or decerebrate posturing. Additionally, intubated patients may have limited vocalizations; thus, nurses need to use their clinical judgment when scoring patients' behaviors.

Pain assessment behavioral scale

	0	1	2	
Face	Facial muscles relaxed	Facial muscle frown, tension, grimace	Frequent to constant frown, clenched jaw	**Face Score:**
Restlessness	Quiet, relaxed appearance; normal movement	Occasional restless movement, shifting position	Frequent restless movement; may include extremities or head	**Restlessness Score:**
Muscle Tone	Normal muscle tone, relaxed	Increased tone, flexion of fingers and toes	Rigid tone	**Muscle Tone Score:**
Vocalization*	No abnormal sounds Endotracheal tube (ETT): comfortable on awakening	Occasional moans, cries, whimpers, or grunts Attempting to talk around ETT	Frequent or continuous moans, cries, whimpers, or grunts Anxiously attempting to talk around ETT	**Vocalization Score:**
Consolability	Content, relaxed	Reassured by touch or talk Distractible	Difficult to comfort by touch or talk	**Consolability Score:**

PAIN ASSESSMENT BEHAVIORAL SCALE TOTAL (0-10):   /10

How to use the pain assessment behavioral scale:

Observe behaviors at least 2-5 minutes, with patient uncovered. Mark the appropriate number for each category. Total the numbers in the Pain Assessment Behavioral Score Total column.
No evidence of pain = 0. Mild pain = 1-3. Moderate pain = 4-6. Severe pain = ≥7.

*Vocalization is difficult to measure in patients with artificial airways. Nurse should use clinical judgment in scoring to assess whether patient appears comfortable on awakening.
Adapted for use at the University of Colorado Hospital from Margaret Campbell, RN, MS, Detroit, October 2000, Detroit Medical Center.

Continued

Pain assessment behavioral scale—cont'd

Considerations:

Use the WILDA (words, intensity, location, duration, aggravating/alleviating factors) pain scale when ever possible to obtain the patient's self-report of pain. Self-report is the best indicator of the presence and intensity of pain.

Use the PABS for patients who are unable to provide a self-report of pain (e.g., cognitively impaired, intubated).

Observe patient at rest and with movement, repositioning patient during assessment if possible, and then score the higher score. (For example, if while resting, patient's muscle tone is 0, but with reposi tioning, the muscle tone becomes rigid, score 2 on muscle tone.) Assess muscle tone in patients with a spinal cord lesion or injury at a level above the lesion or injury. Assess patients with hemiplegia on the unaffected side.

The PABS may not be valid in patients receiving neuromuscular blockade or exhibiting posturing.

A "proxy pain evaluation" from family, friends, or clinicians close to the patient may be helpful to evaluate pain based on previous knowledge of patient response.

When in doubt, provide an analgesic.

10. Should placebos be used to assess pain in the ED?

No. The American Society for Pain Management Nursing (ASPMN) states that "placebos should not be used by any route of administration in the assessment and/or management of pain in any individual regardless of age or diagnosis." Placebos should never be used to determine if the pain is "real" or to diagnose psychological symptoms such as anxiety associated with pain or drug-seeking behavior. The American Nurses Association's (ANA's) Code for Nurses includes basic ethical values such as truth telling, trust, and respect for patients. Administering a placebo not only deceives a patient but also raises ethical concerns and compromises the therapeutic healthcare professional/patient relationship. The only time a placebo is warranted is when a patient has given informed consent to its use as part of an Institutional Review Board (IRB)–approved clinical trial.

11. Are patients addicted when they keep asking for more pain medication or increasing the dose they are taking?

No. They are probably exhibiting signs of "tolerance," a normal pharmacological effect in which the patient requires higher doses of a drug to maintain adequate pain relief. Physiologically, the body requires more opioid to continue to provide the same analgesic effect. This state of adaptation to opioids is variable in occurrence and is not easily predicted. Signs of tolerance should be treated by increasing the drug dose, decreasing the interval between doses, or switching to another drug. It is important, however, to carefully evaluate the need for dose escalation. In the patient with chronic pain, recurrence of disease or development of a new pathology is the most likely cause for dose escalation. Patients treated with prolonged opioid therapy do not usually develop addictive disorders.

12. When patients experience withdrawal signs and symptoms, does it mean they are addicted to pain medication?

No. The patient is probably showing signs of physical dependence, which develops when opioids are taken for an extended period (usually 1 week or more). Like tolerance, physical dependence is a normal body response. If an opioid is abruptly stopped, the patient may experience withdrawal symptoms: nervousness or jittery feelings, anxiety, chills alternating with hot flashes, excessive salivation, lacrimation, rhinorrhea, diaphoresis, piloerection, nausea, vomiting, abdominal cramps, or insomnia. Reassure patients that physical dependence is not unique to opioids. The abrupt discontinuation of beta blockers, corticosteroids, and antidepressants can also produce withdrawal symptoms. The fastest method to treat withdrawal symptoms is to restart the patient's opioid drug. To prevent withdrawal symptoms, discontinuing opioids should be done gradually.

In contrast, addiction or psychological dependence is an abnormal behavior involving an overwhelming desire to obtain the medication for its psychological effects. More specifically, opioid addiction is a pattern of impaired control over drug use, compulsive use, continued use despite harm, craving, and the need to use the opioid for effects other than pain relief. Patients who take opioids for pain relief are using them therapeutically. Confusion regarding the differences between physical dependence and addiction is a significant barrier to effective pain management for the person with chronic pain.

13. How should opioids be tapered to prevent withdrawal from occurring?

Postoperative or trauma patients sometimes present to the ED with withdrawal symptoms because their pain has decreased and they have abruptly stopped taking their pain medications. It is common for these patients to have been taking opioids regularly for longer than 2 weeks. To prevent withdrawal, a gradual tapering schedule should be discussed with the patient. The tapering rate of opioids varies by patient. The following guidelines are usually used.
- Decrease the total 24-hour opioid dose by 50% and administer in divided doses according to duration of action for 2 to 3 days.
- Decrease the dose by 25% every 2 to 3 days thereafter until the total daily dose is roughly equal to 20 to 30 mg of oral morphine per day.
- After 2 days on the final dose, stop the medication. If a patient experiences anxiety or withdrawal symptoms, a clonidine patch may be helpful to lessen or alleviate the side effects. The usual dose of the patch is 0.1 to 0.2 mg/day; it is changed every 7 days.

14. How can a healthcare professional differentiate between a person who is "drug seeking" and a person who has chronic pain?

"Drug seeking" is a set of behaviors in which an individual makes a directed and concerted effort to obtain medication. These behaviors may include obtaining medication from multiple providers; repeated episodes of prescription loss; multiple requests for early refills; requesting analgesics by name, dose, interval, or route; "clock watching"; asking for an analgesic in advance of when it is due; preferring the "needle to the pill"; "hitting the PCA button too much"; and a patient claiming allergy to everything except a particular opioid. These behaviors do not in themselves constitute addiction and may occur when pain is under treated. Patients with chronic pain may take extraordinary steps to ensure adequate medication supply; rather than indicating addictive disease, this may represent an appropriate approach to obtaining pain relief. This is called "pseudoaddiction." It can be distinguished from true addiction in that the behaviors resolve when pain is effectively treated. The patient with chronic pain who repeatedly accesses the ED for pain management can be particularly stressful for staff and may be labeled a "repeater" or "frequent flyer" or be suspected of abusing medications. Short-term interventions aimed at quick discharge can feed into the patient looking for a "cure" and do not address the need for appropriate referral and long-term management. The case for determining true addictive disease is a difficult one because the severity of pain suffered cannot be objectively quantified but only subjectively reported. Referral to providers trained in addiction diagnosis and treatment should be made when needed.

15. How is pain treated in a patient with a history of substance abuse?

Just because a patient has a history of alcohol or drug abuse does not mean that he or she should not be given opioids for pain relief. Pain should still be treated with opioids as indicated. In fact, it is not uncommon to administer higher than usual starting doses to provide adequate analgesia in active substance abusers or in persons on a methadone maintenance program because these patients have developed significant drug tolerance. Additionally, a shorter dosing interval may be appropriate for patients who have addiction and pharmacological tolerance. For example, morphine, which has a usual duration of action of 3 to 4 hours, may need to be dosed every 1 to 2 hours in a person with opioid addiction.

The use of opioids should be openly discussed with the patient who may fear addiction relapse. These patients should be encouraged to express concerns and fears. A patient's wish to decline opioids should be honored. In addition, patients and healthcare providers should contact the recovery or methadone maintenance program for advice and collaboration. Explicit guidelines should be established for the following situations: prescription renewals, procedure to be followed with lost or stolen prescriptions or medications, procedure to ensure that only one clinician is prescribing analgesics, and urine drug testing. Failure to comply with guidelines should be delineated. For example, if medications are "lost" or the patient has "run out," the patient may be required to come to the treatment facility to obtain daily doses or may need to be admitted to the hospital for pain medication adjustment. Patients should be reassessed frequently and prescribed a set amount of opioids. Nonopioids or adjuvant drugs may be helpful in decreasing opioid requirements.

16. **How is the appropriate analgesic chosen for a patient?**

Analgesic choice is usually based on the patient's pain type (acute or chronic, neuropathic, visceral or somatic), the pain intensity, the duration of the pain (whether it is always there or comes and goes), the patient's ability to take medication by mouth, history of previous exposure to analgesics (avoiding those with side effects), and overall patient status. Patient status includes the patient's age, diagnosis, functional or performance state, hepatic or renal insufficiency, and any possible interactions of the analgesic with other medications that may be taken. With greater emphasis on providing appropriate pain assessment and management, pain management triage protocols are beginning to be developed and utilized. These protocols allow nurses to administer analgesics before physician evaluation.

17. **What is the best route for administration of opioids?**

Regardless of the type of pain being treated, opioids should be administered by the least invasive and safest route capable of producing satisfactory analgesia; generally only one route of administration at a time should be used. The oral route is the preferred route of opioid administration and should always be considered before other routes because it is relatively safe, convenient, and inexpensive. However, when rapid onset of analgesia is desired, as is often the case in the ED setting, the IV route is used. The patient is transitioned to the oral route when pain is under control and the patient is able to retain oral medications. Other effective routes of administration for certain opioids include subcutaneous, rectal, transdermal (fentanyl [typically used in patients with chronic pain] or lidocaine patch), transmucosal (fentanyl unit), epidural, and intrathecal (using an implantable drug-infusion pump).

Although commonly used, the intramuscular (IM) route of administration is not recommended for pain management. The IM route has many disadvantages and essentially no advantages. Disadvantages include painful administration, unreliable absorption with a 30- to 60-minute lag time to peak effect, and a rapid drop in action compared with oral administration.

18. **What is the adjuvant analgesic of choice for use in patients with musculoskeletal pain?**

Adjuvant drugs are nonopioid medications that enhance analgesia. Nonsteroidal antiinflammatory drugs (NSAIDs) are effective for the relief of musculoskeletal pain when used alone or as an adjuvant to opioids. Management of mild to moderate pain should begin, unless there is a contraindication, with an NSAID. Moderate to severe pain is routinely treated initially with an opioid analgesic. NSAIDs can have a significant opioid dose-sparing effect on musculoskeletal pain and can be useful in reducing opioid side effects. NSAIDs decrease levels of inflammatory mediators generated at the site of tissue injury. The concurrent use of opioids and NSAIDs often provides more effective analgesia than either drug class alone. Ketorolac (Toradol) is a parenteral NSAID that is indicated for short-term use (less than 5 days) in the management of moderate to severe pain. The risks associated with ketorolac are similar to those of oral NSAIDs: renal impairment, gastrointestinal (GI) bleeding, and platelet dysfunction (but with

C O M M O N L Y   U S E D   A N A L G E S I C S

The following equianalgesic doses are drug and route conversions approximately equal to a single morphine 10 mg IM dose. Keep in mind that the equianalgesic dose is not the usual starting dose; it is just an estimate. Individualize and titrate dose according to the patient's age, condition, response, and clinical situation. **USE CHART AS GUIDELINE ONLY.** Unless otherwise stated, t 1/2 of opioids ranges from 2-3 hours. Rescue dose for breakthrough pain is usually calculated at 10-20% of the 24 hour dose. Use 1/4 to 1/2 the IM dose for single IV bolus.

Equianalgesic Conversion Equation

$$\frac{\text{Current Opioid (single conversion dose \& route)}}{\text{New Opioid (single conversion dose \& route)}} = \frac{\text{Total 24° dose of current opioid}}{\text{Total 24° dose of new opioid}}$$

Example
Patient's receiving a total 24° dose of morphine 180 mg PO.
What is the equivalent 24° dose of PO hydromorphone?

$$\frac{\text{Equianalgesic Dose}}{} = \frac{\text{Total 24° Dose}}{}$$

$$\frac{\text{morphine 30 mg PO}}{\text{hydromorphone 7.5 PO}} = \frac{\text{morphine 180 mg PO}}{x}$$

x = hydromorphone 45 mg PO. The patient will receive hydromorphone 6-8 mg PO q 4°

ANALGESIC OPIOID AGONIST	EQUIANALGESIC DOSES Parenteral (IV,IM,SQ) (mg)	Oral (mg)	Dose Interval (hours)	COMMENTS
				COMMENTS UCH formulary items are in **BOLD**. Comparative costs ($$$$ most - $ least).
Morphine	10	30	3-6	Active metabolite, Morphine-6-glucuronide, (M6G), more potent and longer half-life than morphine. Sublingual: 20-30% bioavailability. Systemic vasodilation due to histamine release. Injection: **0.5, I, 1, 2, 3, 4, 5, 8, 10, 15** mg/ml. Oral solution **10** and **20 mg/5 ml; 20 mg/1 ml.** Suppository: 5, 10, 20, 30 mg. **($$)**
Morphine Sustained Release Capsules	—	30	24	Kadian® 20, 30, 50, 60, 100 mg capsules should be administered every 24 hr; not PRN. Capsules and its contents should not be chewed, crushed or dissolved but may be opened and given by G-tube or sprinkled over food (e.g. applesauce) immediately prior to ingestion. **($$$)**
Morphine Controlled/ Sustained Release Tablets	—	30	8-12	Do not crush. Give every 8-12 hr around the clock, not PRN. **MS Contin® 15, 30, 60, 100, 200 mg; Oramorph SR® 15, 30, 60, 100 mg;** Morphine sulfate XR (generic MS Contin) 15, 30, 60, 100, 200. **($$$)**
Hydromorphone (Dilaudid®)	1.5	7.5	3-4	No clinically active metabolites. Injection: 1, 2, 3, 4, **10** mg/ml. Tablet: 1, **2, 3, 4, 8** mg. Suppository: 3 mg. Oral solution: 1 mg/ml. **($$)**
Fentanyl (Sublimaze®, Innovar®)	100 μg (0.1 mg)	1000 μg OT	0.5-I	Drug of choice in patients with renal and liver disease. Injection: **50** μg/ml. Actiq, oral transmucosal (OT) fentanyl, approved for breakthrough pain; 200, 400, 600, 800, 1200, 1600 μg units. Use only up to 4 Actiq doses for breakthrough pain episodes/day. Consume one unit; may repeat at 30 minutes. **($$$$)**
Transdermal Fentanyl (Duragesic®)	—	—	72	**Transdermal (Duragesic®)** patch, **25, 50, 75, and 100** μg/hr. Change patch every 48-72 hr. Approximate equianalgesic conversion: divide total 24-hour oral morphine dose (mg) by 2 to get fentanyl dose in μg/hr. Reaches therapeutic serum level 12-16 hr after initial application; lasts 17 hr after removal. Rate of drug release can be increased by fever. May cause less constipation than oral controlled/sustained release opioids. **($$$)**
Levorphanol (Levo-Dromoran®)	2	4	3-6	Careful titration due to long t 1/2 of 12-16 hr; accumulates with repetitive doses. Maintenance dose may be one-twentieth the equianalgesic dose of oral morphine dose. Injection: **2** mg/ml. Tablet: **2** mg. **($$)**
Meperidine (Demerol®)	75	300 NR	3-4	Normeperidine (toxic metabolite) accumulates with repetitive doses, causing CNS excitation. Normeperidine t 1/2 = 15-40 hr. Avoid use for chronic pain longer than 48 hr; doses > 600 mg/24 hr. Contraindicated in patients with impaired renal function. Injection: 10, **25, 50, 75, 100** mg/ml. Tablet: 50 or 100 mg. Oral solution: 10, 50 mg/5 ml. **($$)**
Methadone acute pain chronic pain	10 2-4	20 2-4	4-6 12-24	Careful titration and monitoring due to long t 1/2 of 24-36 hr; accumulates on days 2-5. Consider dose reduction after 12-24 hr. Maintenance dose of oral methadone may be one-tenth the equianalgesic dose of oral morphine. Injection: 10 mg/ml. Tablet: **5 or 10** mg. Oral solution 1, 2, 10 mg/ml. **($)**
Oxycodone	—	30	3-6	Tablet: 5, 15, 30 mg **(Roxicodone®)** with **acetaminophen 500 mg (Roxicet®, Tylox®)**, acetaminophen 325 mg **(Percocet®)**, or aspirin 325mg **(Percodan®)**. Oxy IR® capsules 5 mg. Oral solution **(Roxicodone®):** 1 and 20 mg/ml, 5 mg/ml. **($$)**
Oxycodone Controlled Release Tablets	—	20	12	Do not crush. Give every 12 hr around the clock, not PRN. **Oxycontin® 10, 20, 40, 80, 160 mg. ($$$)**
Codeine	130	200 NR	3-6	Use for mild to moderate pain, constipating. Injection: **15, 30, 60 mg/ml. Tablet: 15, 30, 60** mg; 30 mg with 300 mg acetaminophen **(Tylenol #3®)**; 60 mg with 300 mg acetaminophen (Tylenol #4®). Oral solution: **2.4** mg/ml with acetaminophen 24 mg/ml. **($$)**
Hydrocodone	—	30 NR	3-4	Use for mild to moderate pain. Available only in compounded formulation. Tablet: **5 mg with 500 mg acetaminophen (Vicodin®)**; 7.5 mg with 750 mg acetaminophen (Vicodin ES®); 7.5 mg with 200 mg ibuprofen (Vicoprofen®); 5 or 10 mg with aspirin 325 or 650 mg (Lortab®); 5, 7.5, 10 mg hydrocodone with 400 mg acetaminophen (Zydone®). **($$)**
Tramadol (Ultram®)	—	—	4-6	Weak mu opioid agonist for mild to moderate acute and chronic pain, 25-100 mg PO q 4-6 hr (not to exceed 400 mg/day or 300 mg/day in patients > 75 years). Decrease dose by 50% in patients with renal impairment. **($$$)**
AGONIST-ANTAGONIST Nalbuphine (Nubain®)	10	—	3-6	May produce withdrawal in opioid dependent patients. Decreases respiratory depression and pruritus due to opioids while maintaining analgesia. Opioid receptor binding: agonist at sigma, partial agonist at mu and kappa; antagonist at mu. Injection: **10** and **20** mg/ml.

NR = not recommended at that dose.

Commonly used analgesics. *(Copyright 2001. Developed by: Regina Fink, RN, PhD, AOCN; Rose A. Gates, RN, MSN, CNS/NP; Robert Montgomery, RN, ND, OCN; Clark Lyda, RPH. Reviewed by: Andrea Iannucci, PharmD; Jerry Hall, MD; Jennifer Biekert, RN, ND. Approved by: Pharmacy and Therapeutics Committee, University of Colorado Hospital.) DISCLAIMER: The intent of this guide is to provide a brief summary of commonly used analgesics. It is not a complete pharmaceutical review. All medications should be administered only with physician or authorized allied health provider orders. Absolutely no liability will be assumed for use of this guide.*

an additional risk for patients who are hypovolemic, because these patients may develop acute renal failure very quickly). Patients at increased risk for GI bleeding, in particular the elderly, should avoid NSAIDs or use as needed with caution.

Another risk recently recognized with use of all NSAIDs is for cardiovascular events. The Food and Drug Administration (FDA) has recently issued warnings and new requirements for labeling on both prescription and over-the-counter NSAIDs, and two of the selective cyclooxygenase-2 (COX-2) inhibitors drugs have been take off the market. The largest cardiovascular risk has been identified with long-term use. There has been no quantification of risk with short-term use of NSAIDs for acute or traumatic pain, although recommendations are to use the smallest effective dose for the shortest time possible. One undisputed difference with the COX-2 drugs (e.g., Celebrex) is they have no platelet inhibition effect.

19. What is the best way to switch from one opioid to another?

Becoming familiar with an equianalgesic chart is helpful to convert medication doses from one route to another or from one drug to another. Equianalgesic doses are approximate conversions of one drug to another with doses decreased to allow for incomplete cross-tolerance. Medication doses should be adjusted according to the patient's pain intensity and overall health status (including age and organ failure). The following case exemplifies how an equianalgesic chart can be used.

M.K. presents to the ED with pain associated with a fractured femur after a motor vehicle crash. After 5 to 10 mg IV morphine is given, M.K. complains of nausea and vomiting and relates that he has had problems with nausea associated with morphine administration in the past. How would an equianalgesic dose of hydromorphone (Dilaudid) be established? Per the equianalgesic chart in the following table, 10 mg IV morphine is roughly equivalent to 1.5 mg IV hydromorphone. Administering 1 to 2 mg IV hydromorphone as a starting dose in place of morphine would be an appropriate action.

20. What is breakthrough pain and how is it managed?

Breakthrough pain is a transitory exacerbation or flare of pain occurring in patients already on a stable or regularly scheduled dosage of long-acting opioid. Breakthrough pain occurs in approximately 65% of patients. It is treated with short-acting opioids. The dose of a short-acting opioid is usually 10% to 20% of the total 24-hour long-acting opioid dose. For example, a patient with breast cancer has bone pain associated with metastatic disease. She has been taking 60 mg of long-acting morphine PO bid (every 12 hours around the clock). Short-acting morphine elixir should be available for breakthrough pain at a dose of 10 to 20 mg PO every 2 hours PRN.

21. Can a patient-controlled analgesia (PCA) pump be used in an ED?

A PCA pump is a useful tool in the management of many painful conditions in the ED. Usually, when a patient reports to the ED, pain is at a moderate to severe level, especially for someone with a history of chronic pain and/or trauma. One of the best ways to treat severe pain is to titrate IV push opioids while carefully monitoring patient response. After the pain is reduced to a tolerable level, a PCA

Initial PCA dosage recommendations for adults

Opioid (Concentration)	Loading range	Basal range	Incremental range	Lockout
Morphine (1 mg/ml)	1-4 mg	0-3 mg	0.5-3 mg	6-10 min
Hydromorphone (0.2 mg/ml)	0.2-0.4 mg	0-0.3 mg	0.1-0.6 mg	6-10 min
Fentanyl (10-25 mcg/ml)	25-50 mcg	0-50 mcg	10-100 mcg	6-8 min

pump can be initiated. This might be especially useful for a patient who may be a surgical candidate and must remain NPO, or the patient with chronic malignant or nonmalignant pain who is having an acute pain exacerbation and whose ultimate dosage needs cannot yet be predicted, such as a person with sickle cell anemia. The dosing of the PCA should take into account the amount of medication that it took to achieve an adequate level of analgesia via IV push, commonly referred to as the "loading dose." A basal or continuous infusion rate may be used in patients who are not opioid naive or who require increased doses of pain medication. The table above can be used to guide selection of a PCA dosing schedule. The use of a PCA pump not only provides a sense of control for patients but also decreases their waiting time for analgesic doses. When initiating a PCA pump or changing an existing PCA order, two nurses or licensed healthcare providers should always check the pump programming to ensure the proper analgesic dose is being administered because incorrect programming has been associated with medication overdosage and possible adverse patient events.

22. Can analgesics be given to alleviate abdominal pain before a surgery evaluation?

Yes. It has been a widely held belief that an acute abdomen should be evaluated by a surgeon before any pain medication is given for fear of masking symptoms that could be diagnostic or because of concern about the patient's ability to provide an informed consent after taking pain medication. However, studies have shown that patients with acute abdominal pain may be given opioids without fear of masking the diagnosis. In fact, in one study the trend was toward more accurate diagnoses in the patients who received morphine compared with the control group who received normal saline; a better abdominal examination is performed in the group receiving IV opioids. The choice of analgesic to administer should be based on the clinical presentation and the amount of pain reported. A short-acting opioid (e.g., fentanyl) may be an option until the surgeon can evaluate the patient. The American Pain Society (APS), American College of Emergency Physicians (ACEP), and Canadian Association of Emergency

Physicians (CAEP) have policy statements that encourage early pain relief in nontraumatic acute abdominal pain patients.

23. Why is meperidine a poor choice for pain relief?

Meperidine (Demerol) has been a popular opioid analgesic for decades. Meperidine has a rapid onset, short half-life, and duration of action of approximately 2 to 3 hours. Many clinicians are not aware that meperidine has active metabolites such as normeperidine that can accumulate and cause restlessness, tremors, seizures, and convulsions in patients who take more than 400 mg/day or in persons with renal insufficiency. Although the half-life of meperidine is 3 to 4 hours, the half-life of normeperidine is 15 to 40 hours.

24. What analgesics should be avoided in persons with kidney or liver failure?

Opioid analgesics with long half-lives (12 to 35 hours), such as methadone (Dolophine), levorphanol (Levodromoran), and propoxyphene (Darvon), and opioids with active metabolites such as meperidine (Demerol) and morphine should be avoided in patients with renal or liver impairment. Additionally, NSAIDs are contraindicated in patients with renal failure. They must be used with extreme caution, if at all, in patients with compromised renal function.

25. What adjuvant analgesic medications should be considered in patients with neuropathic pain?

Tricyclic antidepressants (e.g., nortriptyline, desipramine, amitriptyline [avoid in the elderly]) and anticonvulsants (e.g., gabapentin, clonazepam, oxcarbazepine, topiramate) are the most effective medications for the management of neuropathic pain. They may be used alone or in combination with opioids for moderate to severe pain. Antidepressant doses to control pain are usually much less than needed to treat depression. Pain can be reduced within days after taking a few doses. Gabapentin has relatively mild side effects. Dosing starts at 100 to 300 mg/day and is titrated according to patient tolerance with doses as high as 2400 to 3600 mg/day in tid divided doses. Clonazepam not only helps neuropathic pain but also has the added benefit of reducing anxiety. Common starting doses are 0.5 mg at bedtime, increasing to 0.5 to 1.0 mg PO tid.

26. Is an epidural catheter indicated in the ED for the management of pain in flail chest?

Initial management of the severe pain that can occur with rib fractures in flail chest should be done with IV opioids. This is the fastest method to provide analgesia and allows the most flexibility to evaluate the patient's condition. The goals of pain control in this population are to ensure adequate vital capacity and inspiratory force and to encourage coughing to clear secretions. After the patient has been stabilized and a satisfactory level of analgesia attained, placement of an epidural catheter may be considered if there are no contraindications. Although adequate analgesia could be provided through the use of PCA, the majority of patients cannot tolerate the pain induced by deep breathing and coughing, even when provided with optimal IV opioid therapy. They would rather avoid the pain by lying still than treat the pain associated with deep breathing and coughing with the IV opioids. An anesthesiologist should be consulted to evaluate the patient for catheter placement in the ED or to see the patient upon arrival to the inpatient nursing unit.

27. What should be considered in the evaluation and treatment of a patient with an implanted neurostimulator system or intrathecal drug pump?

Neurostimulation systems, also called spinal cord stimulators, are implantable devices used by pain specialists to treat chronic pain. The system typically consists of an implanted battery power source, usually located in the lower back or abdomen, that is connected to a stimulating electrode in the epidural space that delivers electrical impulses along the spinal cord to block pain signals. If a patient with a stimulator is involved in a trauma, the electrode may migrate, disconnect, or fracture, resulting in a change in stimulation pattern or cessation of stimulation altogether. Each patient has a handheld programmer to turn the system on and off. When a system stops working, pain should be controlled with supplemental medication and the patient should follow up with the managing physician for system troubleshooting and repair. Magnetic resonance imaging (MRI) is contraindicated for patients who have a neurostimulator; computed tomography (CT) scan is used instead.

Intrathecal drug pumps are also implantable devices used in treating chronic pain. The combined pump/reservoir is usually located in the lower abdomen and is connected to a tunneled catheter that terminates in the intrathecal space. Medications such as an opioid (e.g., morphine, fentanyl, hydromorphone), baclofen, bupivacaine, and clonidine are either used alone or in combination and are delivered in a small continuous daily amount. Problems with the system because of trauma, malfunction, or mismanagement can result in withdrawal or overdose. The pump is programmed through a special computer and the reservoir is accessed with a specific manufacturer's needle kit. Resources for the evaluation, troubleshooting, and management of these implantable devices include the managing pain physician, the device manufacturer, and possibly pain specialists. Patients are given a device identification card to carry at all times and are also usually given a printout of their pump medications and rate, or stimulator settings by their managing physician. MRI is usually allowable with an implanted pump, but the pump should be checked afterward to ensure it is infusing properly because the test may temporarily slow the pump down and set off the alarm.

28. Are there any particular analgesics that should be avoided in an elderly population?

Avoid opioids with long half-lives, such as methadone and propoxyphene. Use caution with morphine because the active metabolite, morphine-6-glucuronide, may accumulate and lead to confusion and disorientation. Long-term use of NSAIDs may cause renal impairment, GI bleeding, and cardiovascular events.

Always be aware of other drugs the patient may be taking, because combinations may lead to delirium or disorientation. When administering opioids and adjuvant medications, the recommendation is to "start low and titrate slow." Be careful not to start more than one analgesic medication at the same time, because of possible drug interactions. Provide easy-to-read instructions to the patient and family member.

29. How common is opioid-induced respiratory depression?

Fear of respiratory depression ranks high among factors that limit nurses' and other healthcare professionals' administration of opioids. Patients on chronic opioid therapy, such as persons with chronic malignant or nonmalignant pain, rarely experience respiratory depression. Opiate-naive patients, particularly those in the postoperative setting, are most vulnerable. Being knowledgeable about risk factors that may predispose an individual to opioid-induced respiratory depression allows clinicians to plan pain management strategies and increase nurse monitoring in accordance with the degree of risk. The following are risk factors associated with respiratory depression.

METABOLIC ALTERATION
- Liver impairment or failure
- Renal impairment or failure
- Sepsis
- Hypovolemia

RESPIRATORY COMPROMISE—CONDITIONS LIMITING AIR EXCHANGE
- Pulmonary disease (asthma, chronic obstructive pulmonary disease—COPD)
- Sleep apnea
- Intrathecal analgesia

CONCURRENT ADMINISTRATION OF MEDICATIONS WITH SEDATIVE EFFECTS
- Other opioids
- Sedatives/hypnotics
- Antidepressants (e.g., amitriptyline)
- Benzodiazepines (e.g., diazepam, lorazepam)
- Antihistamines (e.g., diphenhydramine, hydroxyzine)
- Antiemetics (e.g., promethazine [Phenergan], prochlorperazine)

OTHER FACTORS
- Obesity
- First opioid dose

30. If respiratory depression does occur, how should naloxone be administered?

Naloxone (Narcan) is an opioid antagonist that is administered to patients with apnea or significant respiratory depression (fewer than 6 or 7 respirations per minute) suspected from opioids. When administered for respiratory depression, one ampule of naloxone (0.4 mg/ml) is diluted with 9 ml of normal saline with 40 mcg or 1 ml administered every 2 to 3 minutes until the desired effect is achieved. The goal is to reverse respiratory depression without reversing analgesia. The duration of action of naloxone is shorter than that of opioids, so repeated doses or continuous infusion may be needed in certain cases. The naloxone doses used for apnea, respiratory arrest, or in the comatose patient are generally higher (i.e., 2 mg).

31. A.K. is a 25-year-old African-American woman with sickle cell crisis who presents to the ED with excruciating pain. What should be done to alleviate her pain?

First, an accurate pain assessment must be done to determine the source and characteristics of A.K.'s pain. It is important to know what doses of analgesics A.K. has used to alleviate her pain in the past and what has occurred recently to exacerbate her pain. Typically, patients with chronic pain may be followed by a case manager who will be able to inform the ED staff of the patient's plan of care. It may be advantageous to have written or computerized pain care plans for patients with chronic pain who frequently visit the ED. Some of the following questions may be useful to include in the pain assessment:

- Tell me about your pain.
- What words would you use to describe it?
- On a scale of 0 to 10, with 0 being no pain and 10 being the worst pain imaginable, what is your pain now? What has your pain been in the past 24 hours? In the past week?
- Where is your pain?
- Is it always there or does it come and go?
- What makes your pain better and what makes it worse?
- What have you been using to decrease your pain?
- What medications have you been taking?
- How often do you take the pain medication?
- When you take it, does it work? How long does it take to work?
- Are you having any side effects such as constipation, nausea, or sleepiness?
- Have you tried anything else such as heat or cold, relaxation therapy, or massage to help alleviate your pain?

A.K. is experiencing deep muscular, bone, and joint pain particularly in her legs and back. She describes her pain as achy and throbbing and rates it as a 9 on scale of 0 to 10 at the present time. It usually subsides to a 2 or 3 on a scale of 0 to 10. A.K. consistently takes long-acting oxycodone 80 mg tid (every 8 hours) with oxycodone 20 mg every 3 hours PRN for severe pain. Additionally, she uses heat to help the painful episodes. The pain has worsened with the change in the weather and because A.K. has decreased her medication because of constipation. A.K. is given 10 to 30 mg IV morphine in the ED over 2 hours for acute pain and is restarted on her oral pain medication regimen. Her pain has decreased in intensity to a 5 on a scale of 0 to 10. A rectal examination is done to determine if A.K. is impacted, and stool softeners and laxatives are instituted for the constipation. A.K. is instructed to make an appointment with her hematologist the next day for a follow-up appointment.

32. What is the role of nonpharmacological approaches to relieve pain in the ED?

Nonpharmacological modalities include physical and psychosocial interventions that can be used to augment, not replace, drug therapy. Physical modalities used to reduce pain include cutaneous stimulation (heat, cold, massage, vibration), transcutaneous electrical nerve stimulation (TENS), reflexology, therapeutic touch, and acupressure or acupuncture. Psychosocial interventions help patients gain a sense of control by using cognitive techniques that affect how pain is interpreted and behavioral techniques that provide the patient with skills to cope with and modify responses to pain. Examples of psychosocial interventions include relaxation, imagery, meditation, deep breathing, hypnosis, distraction and reframing (replacing negative thoughts with more positive ones), music therapy, psychotherapy, biofeedback, and pastoral counseling.

33. What special considerations are necessary in the assessment and management of pain in children?

Children are recognized as one of the groups of patients who have been traditionally under treated for pain. Specific misconceptions about pain management include:
- Children do not experience as much pain as adults do.
- Assessing pain in children is unreliable and inconsistent.
- The use of opioids causes respiratory depression and addiction.

Because of the complexity of the pain experience and the problems of measurement in children, pain assessment and analysis require a multifaceted approach. The healthcare provider must use every available means of assessment and consider all findings in the analysis of a child's pain.

Assessment procedures include:
- Pain history from the child and parents
- Child's self-report
- Direct observation
- Proxy report
- Physiological indicators
- Response to analgesics

Assessment tools should be appropriate for the child's age and cognitive development. As with adults, a child's self-report is the most accurate indicator of pain. Self-reports can be used for developmentally normal children over the age of 4. Self-report tools for children over age 4 include the Oucher (Beyer, 1988), the Poker Chip Tool (Hester, 1979), and Faces (Wong, 2001) scales. Generally children over the age of 7 can use a numerical rating scale, a visual analog scale, or a horizontal word-graphic rating scale.

The Face, Legs, Activity, Cry, Consolability (FLACC) scale is a behavioral scale that was originally used to measure pain severity in young children experiencing postoperative pain. It may be useful with preverbal children. Each of the five categories is scored from 0 to 2, resulting in a total score between 0 and 10.

FLACC behavior scale

	0	1	2
Face	No particular expression or smile	Occasional grimace or frown	Frequent to constant frown, clenched jaw, quivering chin
Legs	Normal position or relaxed	Uneasy, restless	Kicking, legs drawn up, tense
Activity (Body Position)	Lying quietly, normal position	Squirming, shifting back and forth	Tense, arched, rigid, or jerking
Cry	No cry (awake or asleep)	Moans or whimpers; occasional complaint	Crying steadily, screams or sobs, frequent complaints
Consolability	Content, relaxed	Reassured by occasional touching, hugging or "talking to"	Difficult to console or comfort

Interventions to control and relieve pain involve measures to reduce fear and anxiety, strategies to enhance the child's sense of control, and pharmacological and nonpharmacological measures. The use of pharmacological measures in children is similar to the approach used in adults. A stepwise approach is used with nonopioids such as acetaminophen and ibuprofen for mild to moderate pain, progressing to opioids for severe pain. As with adults, but especially with children, IM injections should be avoided because of the associated pain and anxiety they can produce. The dose of analgesic should be based on the clinical situation and the maximum recommended therapeutic dose. Dosage determination in children is more difficult than in adults because of the use of body weight and requires professional decision making.

Nonpharmacological approaches may be helpful in alleviating pain in children. Distraction is most commonly used and may come in the form of music, movies, kaleidoscopes, bubbles, and talking stuffed animals that tell stories.

Key Points

- Pain is one of the leading causes of ED visits.
- Emergency nurses' accuracy in estimating patients' pain intensity is less than 50%.
- One of the top barriers to optimal pain management is healthcare professionals' fear of causing or contributing to addiction.
- Pain assessment should include five key parameters: words, intensity, location, duration, and aggravating and alleviating factors.
- Analgesic choice is based on the patients' pain type, pain intensity, duration of pain, patient's ability to take medications, patient's previous analgesic use, and patient status.
- Patients with acute abdominal pain may be given opioids without fear of masking the diagnosis.
- Assessment of five pain behaviors (facial grimace, restlessness, muscle tone, vocalization, consolability) should be observed in the nonverbal or cognitively impaired patient.

 Internet Resources

American Pain Foundation:
www.painfoundation.org

American Pain Society:
www.ampainsoc.org

American Society for Pain Management Nursing:
www.aspmn.org

International Association for the Study of Pain:
www.iasp-pain.org

Joint Commission on Accreditation of Healthcare Organizations, *Pain Assessment and Management Standards—Hospitals*, 2001:
www.jcrinc.com/subscribers/perspectives.asp?durki=3243&site=10&return=2897

University of Wisconsin Comprehensive Cancer Center, Pain & Policy Studies Group:
www.medsch.wisc.edu/painpolicy

Bibliography

American Academy of Pain Medicine, American Pain Society, American Society of Addiction Medicine: *Definitions related to the use of opioids for the treatment of pain*, Consensus Document, Glenview, Ill, 2001, Author.

American College of Emergency Physicians: Clinical policy for the initial evaluation and management of patients presenting with a chief complaint of nontraumatic acute abdominal pain, *Ann Emerg Med* 36:406–415, 2000.

American Pain Society: *Principles of analgesic use in the treatment of acute pain and cancer pain*, ed 5, Glenview, Ill, 2004, Author.

American Society for Pain Management Nursing: *Pain management in patients with addictive disease*, Position Statement, Pensacola, Fla, 2002, Author.

American Society for Pain Management Nursing: *Use of placebos in pain management*, Position Statement, Pensacola, Fla, 2005, Author.

Bayley EW et al: ENA's Delphi study on national research priorities for emergency nurses in the United States, *J Emerg Nurs* 30(1):12–21, 2004.

Beyer J, Aradine, C: Convergent and discriminate validity of a self-report measure of pain intensity for children, *Child Health Care*, 16(4), 274–282, 1988.

Blank F et al: Adequacy of pain assessment and pain relief and correlation of patient satisfaction in 68 ED fast-track patients, *J Emerg Nurs* 27:327–334, 2001.

Campbell ML, Renaud E, Vanni L: *Psychometric testing of a pain assessment behavior scale.* Paper presented at the Midwest Nursing Research Society annual meeting, Cincinnati, April 2005.

Campbell P et al: Implementation of an ED protocol for pain management at triage at a busy level I trauma center, *J Emerg Nurs* 30(5):431–438, 2004.

Gates RA, Fink RM: Pain management. In Gates RA and Fink RM, editors: *Oncology nursing secrets*, Philadelphia, 2001, Hanley & Belfus.

Hester NKO: The Preoperational Child's Reaction to Immunization, *Nurs Res* 28, 250–254, 1979.

Loveridge N: Ethical implications of achieving pain management, *Emerg Nurs* 8(3):16–21, 2000.

McCaffery M, Pasero C: *Pain: Clinical manual*, ed 2, St Louis, 1999, Mosby.

Merkel S: The FLACC: A behavioral scale for scoring postoperative pain in young children, *Pediatr Nurs* 23(3):293–297, 1997.

Miaskowski C et al: *Guideline for the management of cancer pain in adults and children*, APS Clinical Practice Guideline Series, No 3, Glenview, Ill, 2005, American Pain Society.

Puntillo K et al: Accuracy of emergency nurses in assessment of patients' pain, *Pain Manag Nurs* 4(4):171–175, 2003.

Seguin D: A nurse-initiated pain management advanced triage protocol for ED patients with an extremity injury at a level I trauma center, *J Emerg Nurs* 30(4):330–335, 2004.

Tanabe P, Buschmann M: A prospective study of ED pain management practices and the patient's perspective, *J Emerg Nurs* 25:171–177, 1999.

Taxonomy Subcommittee for the IASP; Merskey H et al. *Pain*. 1986(suppl 3):S1–226.

Wong DL et al: *Wong's essentials of pediatric nursing*, ed 6, St Louis, 2001, Mosby.

Death and Dying

Catherine T. Kelly

1. In some instances, patients die in the emergency department (ED) without resuscitation measures being attempted. How can the families be helped during this time?

Instead of telling families, "There is nothing we can do," use the aggressive comfort treatment (ACT) approach, which stresses what *can* be done for patients and families. First, ask if there is anything special the family would like done, including cultural and religious practices. Then, describe what can be done to decrease pain, hunger, and discomfort. Focus on caring activities and try to eliminate useless procedures such as arterial blood gases (ABGs) when the decision has been made to limit interventions. Allowing the family to assist with comfort care, such as placing a cool cloth on the patient's forehead, holding hands, or singing a favorite song, may decrease the family's feelings of helplessness. The ability to help in some way may contribute to a "good" death and help the family move through the grief process.

2. Who should notify the family that someone has died?

Many families have stated that they want a physician to inform them about the death. However, family members prefer that a nurse stay with them to answer questions and provide comfort. Nurses are perceived as compassionate, acknowledging the significance of the death for the family.

3. Can anyone else help with death notification?

Yes. Explore developing a collaborative group that can be called on to assist families in the ED when death occurs. Team members may include social workers, clergy, psychiatric staff, and trained volunteers.

4. What is the first thing a nurse should say when he or she has to tell a family someone has died?

Do *not* start with "I'm sorry" or "I have bad news for you." Statements like these do not give families enough time to assimilate and process information. Sit close to the family and speak directly to them. Use the sequential notification process to tell families about death or any other critical situation. This notification process provides guidelines to help inform family members of deaths and critical situations in a short period of time. The staff member should:

- Find out what the family already knows. Talk briefly with other staff members and first responders to determine what the family has seen or been told.
- Give them a brief description of what has happened during the time the patient was receiving care, bridging their knowledge of events. Begin with simple information and then provide more complex details.
- Explain what resuscitation efforts were made.
- Conclude the description with a statement that describes the patient's response to treatment, and explain the cause of death. It is important to use the word "died" when describing the patient's response to treatment, such as he died because he lost so much blood or he died because his heart stopped. Do not explain death to a child as if the deceased person is sleeping. This statement may cause a child to fear sleep because they or a loved one may not wake up.

5. **What is the best way to tell someone about a death over the telephone?**

Try any way possible to have the person come to the ED. If notification of a death must be made over the telephone, the sequential notification process works well. Each case is different, so rely on institution policy. In some situations it may be good to first call with basic information, such as, "There has been an accident and the staff is working with Mrs. X. I'll call you back in 5 to 10 minutes to tell you how things are going; can you call someone to stay with you?" When this two-step process is used to handle notification, the person who was called may then have someone with him or her when he or she is told about the death. If there is a list of resources, such as counselors, support groups, or clergy, who are available to go to the survivor's home, contacting them will provide an additional source of support for the bereaved.

6. **Should the call be made during the middle of the night or wait until a reasonable hour?**

Family members prefer to be called as soon as possible, no matter what the time. Waiting to notify a family of a critical injury or death may make it harder for the family to trust the caregivers. Moreover, the family may feel that they were cheated out of precious last moments to spend with the deceased.

7. **How should the body be prepared if the family wants to see it?**

The body should be cleaned of all blood, secretions, and dirt *if forensic evidence is not needed.* Gelfoam or wound glue can be applied to oozing wounds to decrease the amount of drainage, and clean dressings applied. Intravenous (IV) lines, catheters, and endotracheal tubes (ETTs) should be removed *if approved by the medical examiner.* Medical equipment should be cleaned but left by the bedside. This helps families know that appropriate interventions were performed.

8. **What should the family be told before they go in to see the body?**

Clearly describe everything they will see, including ETTs, obvious wounds, and medical equipment. This information may need to be repeated several times because people need time to understand new material, especially during an extremely stressful situation such as this. Ask the family and friends if they are ready to see the body after describing what the family will see. Give them time to process all of the information and have them indicate when they are ready to see the body. Selecting the time to view the body gives them some control and "permission" to take the time they need to be adequately prepared.

9. **Is there a "best way" to position the body?**

Yes. The body should be positioned with the head elevated. Placing a small towel under the head will bring the chin closer to the chest; this helps keep the mouth closed. Place the body near the door, feet first. This prevents the family from having to walk across a large open area to approach the body. Give the family "permission" to touch the body if they want to. Before they touch their loved one, prepare them for how the skin may feel different. If possible, place one of the patient's hands outside the sheet or blanket. If the body is totally deformed, or can't be touched because of the need for forensic evidence, the family may be able to touch the patient's hair. Always check with law enforcement before having anyone else come in contact with the body.

10. **How should the room be prepared and the lighting adjusted when a family wants to spend some time with the body, especially if it is a child who has died?**

Although a child's death is tragic, every death may be thought of as a significant loss and all people, regardless of age, can experience death in a supportive way with the help of healthcare personnel. If time and space in the ED permit, the family should be allowed to stay as long as possible. The room should be lighted normally; dim lights can create a surrealistic experience. Also, make sure the room smells "normal." The use of air fresheners may cause the family to always associate that specific smell, such as vanilla, with the person's death. Place several chairs next to the stretcher so that the family can sit if they choose, or need, to do so. A rocking chair will be welcomed by parents of infants or small children who want to hold and rock the baby one last time.

11. **Should the nurse stay with the family when they see the body?**

Every case is different. Assess the situation by asking the family what they prefer. Most often, staff will stay the first few minutes to answer questions, and then ask the family if they want to be alone for a while.

12. **What if the ED is busy and there is no time or space to provide family support?**

Be proactive. Talk with supervisory personnel to identify other areas, preferably near the ED, where families can stay with loved ones who have died. This is also a good opportunity to identify personnel who can become part of a collaborative team that will respond when needed to stay with a grieving family.

13. **What should children be told when someone they care about dies?**

Children should be told the truth. It is important that the adults who are with the child hear what is said so they can repeat the explanation later to the child.

Use simple terms and speak directly to the child. Be careful to avoid common phrases, such as "gone to sleep," because the child may become afraid to sleep, or "You're the man or woman of the house now," which places tremendous stress on a grieving child.

14. Is there anything special that can be done to help parents when a child dies?

Yes. The most important thing to do is provide the family with as much time as they need to say good-bye, even if this means the child must be moved out of the ED to a quiet place. It can be very hard for families to leave a loved one's side because they don't want to leave the deceased person alone in a morgue. Parents sometimes find comfort in leaving a child's favorite toy or blanket with him or her. Offer the parents the opportunity to comb their child's hair or wash their child's face while they spend time with their child. Parents may also appreciate a lock of hair, a footprint or handprint, or a Polaroid photo to take with them. If the parents decline these mementos, see if you can have them stored with the medical record in case the parents change their minds later.

15. Should the family be present during resuscitation?

Controversy still exists regarding this topic. Robinson (1998) studied 25 patient resuscitations, 13 with families present and 12 without, and concluded that there were no adverse psychological effects on family members who witnessed the resuscitation. The family members all claimed to be satisfied with their decision to stay. Since then many studies have been done in this area with diverse populations. Moreland (2005) did an extensive literature review of this topic and noted significant differences in how institutions addressed this issue. Most family members wanted to be present. Hospital staff and physicians appear to be more uncomfortable with family presence. However, if families are present, one staff member must be assigned to stay with the family to provide explanation and support. The presence of family members during resuscitation is supported by the Emergency Nurses Association (ENA).

16. When someone dies suddenly, is the death more difficult for the survivors to accept?

Friends and family often have difficulty believing that someone who was healthy is now dead. This period of disbelief can last several days. Sudden deaths are commonly related to trauma, but other deaths from myocardial infarction, asthma, or overwhelming infection result in the same type of disruption for the survivors. Survivors often experience anger and confusion. Their normal world has been shattered and they need immediate help organizing activities during the initial postdeath period. Help them identify immediate needs and focus on short-term goals. Information may need to be repeated several times before it is understood.

17. How can people call a death sudden if the patient was chronically or terminally ill?

Chronically or terminally ill patients may die sooner than expected, resulting in a sudden death scenario. The survivors may not have had enough time to integrate the person's impending death into their lives, and therefore the death is unexpected. Survivors may have believed they were prepared for the death and are surprised at the intensity of their reactions. The amount of confusion the survivors experience may be similar to that experienced by survivors who have been through the sudden traumatic death of a loved one.

18. What can a healthcare provider do to help people who are faced with sudden death?

In addition to providing support, information, and guidance, a written instruction sheet for the family and friends can be helpful. This written information can include how to contact a funeral director, relevant support programs, community agencies, emergency telephone numbers, and the name and phone number of someone at the hospital whom they may contact if they need further information.

19. What is the best way to talk with families about organ donation?

This is often a difficult situation with uniquely individual reactions. However, these guidelines help ED staff work with potential organ donors and families:
- First, follow the hospital's protocol for organ procurement. The hospital's protocol will identify who serves as a liaison between the family and the transplant program staff.
- Health Care Financing Administration (HCFA) guidelines (effective August 1998 and enforced August 1999) require that hospitals inform their organ procurement office of all deaths that occur and that trained staff discuss organ donation and obtain consent.
- Arrange for regional transplant program (RTP) personnel to provide annual updates on organ donation. Doing so will ensure that staff members have current information about caring for the potential donor and updated information regarding state legislation.
- Respect each staff member's individual beliefs. Identify which staff believes in organ donation and work with them to enhance the skills needed to speak with families and provide care to the donor. Some staff members are "good" in certain situations, such as starting IVs; find out who is "good" with organ donation.
- Be knowledgeable about state and federal regulations; post guidelines in a conspicuous place where staff can easily access them.

Keeping up to date with information provided by RTP personnel will help the nurse talk with families so they can make an informed decision about donation.

20. Will donating organs make the family's grief more difficult to resolve?

Each family will respond in unique ways. Some families may need time to acknowledge the patient's death before dealing with organ donation. It is important to separate the events of death notification and request for organs into two separate conversations. Early consultation by the emergency care provider with the local organ procurement team can help the family transition from a death to donation focus. Early referral and collaborative family care has a positive effect on donations and subsequent family well-being. Many donor families state that they receive some comfort from knowing that someone else may benefit from the death of their loved one. What appears to be important for the family's grieving process is that they have all the information they need to make a decision with which they will be comfortable.

It is important to refer to the potential donor by name as the death notification and organ procurement process continues. Families should be informed of everything that is being done for their loved one. Families should be asked about what would best help them at this time. They may desire a quiet space, time alone with the patient, or time to talk with other loved ones. It is difficult to balance the need for family support and time because time is so critical for organ viability. One major benefit of calling in the transplant team is that they are well trained in helping families move through the decision process as quickly as possible. The transplant team is the best resource to utilize.

Patients may present to the ED with donor cards, motor vehicle licenses, or other documents stating that they wish to donate their organs. Each state and U.S. territory has different regulations regarding the legal status of these documents; these legal regulations should be included in the official ED policy. The ENA Position Statement, *Role of the Emergency Nurse in Tissue and Organ Donation*, also provides excellent guidelines.

21. What is the most important thing to remember when caring for dying patients and their families?

Take a quiet moment to think about what you would want to happen for yourself or your loved ones in a death situation. It is acceptable to ask people what is important to them; follow their wishes as much as possible. Survivors describe remembering the first 2 hours after being informed of a death as a videotape that keeps replaying. The survivors often are able to describe every detail of the notification event or witnessing of the death, so it is important to be as supportive as possible during this time.

22. Should ED staff send cards or contact families of deceased patients?

Many hospitals have developed organized programs, such as the Death Notification and Survivor Care Program at the University of California at San Francisco, to assist staff and families through the year following a patient's death. An integral part of such a program is to send a sympathy card or letter to the bereaved family. Other programs incorporate a follow-up telephone call to the family to validate their loss and offer support.

Initiating family contact after a patient death adds another dimension to the healthcare provider's practice. The patient death is no longer seen as the final point of patient care. Instead, there is a continuing connection with the family that may help the healthcare provider deal more effectively with cumulative grief. Individuals who are designated to contact families must receive special training from professionals who are skilled in working with bereaved families. Follow-up cards and telephone calls must be made by staff members who genuinely like working with bereaved families. Specific bereavement intervention training is available through organizations such as the Association for Death Education and Counseling (ADEC), the National Association of Social Workers (NASW), and local ministries.

23. Should staff attend the funeral of a patient who has died in the ED?

Many times staff will choose to go to a funeral of a patient they have known for a long time or one in which they were involved in a prolonged resuscitation. This is an individual decision. Staff should be given the opportunity to attend funerals, if they choose to do so. For some staff, attending the funeral may help them to process the death and enhance their own grief regarding the death. Other staff will have no desire to attend a patient's funeral, and this choice must also be respected.

When deciding to grant a staff member time off to attend a funeral, the most important question a manager can ask is, "Will attending the funeral help this staff member?" The ultimate goal is to make whatever time investment is necessary to enhance the long-term mental health and productivity of each staff member.

24. After supporting a family through death in the ED, is it normal for the nurse to feel emotionally drained?

Yes. It takes a tremendous amount of emotional energy to care for a dying patient and the family. Many healthcare providers experience cumulative grief reactions because of the number of patient deaths they encounter. Each provider may handle this type of stress in many ways. There is no "correct" way to deal with patient death. The challenge is to find a healthy way to deal with the stress. These mechanisms may include exercise, meditation, reading, and talking with a colleague. Unhealthy responses may include excessive alcohol intake, drug use, overeating, and altered sleep patterns.

Larson (1993) wrote about the effects of facing grief, loss, and life-threatening illness on a routine basis. Nurses must understand their own stress responses and determine what reduces their stress. The foundation of Critical Incident Stress Debriefing (CISD) also addresses the emergency care provider's possible reactions to crisis situations such as patient death.

Each facility that provides emergency services should have access to teams trained in CISD (also called Critical Incident Stress Debriefing). For many years, CISD was used only for prehospital care personnel, such as paramedics and firemen. Now, we know that ED personnel may benefit from the debriefing process. It is important for the staff to hear about all aspects of a critical event; there is a need to know what happened. Providing the staff with time to discuss their perceptions and feelings leads to greater understanding of the event. This type of understanding is believed to enhance the long-term mental health of the healthcare provider who routinely encounters critical situations.

The CISD process begins with a confidential review of the critical event by those people who were involved with the situation. Everyone has the opportunity to describe what they experienced and felt as the event unfolded. Clarification and information related to the event are shared by all participants. Additional opportunities to meet as a group or individually with a CISD counselor are provided.

Some literature supports that persons may need to use their usual support systems first. This initial support may be enough for some people; others may need additional resources as time goes by.

25. How should the nurse deal with unresolved concerns about other staff practicing certain procedures on newly deceased patients or prolonging resuscitation for those patients whose prognosis is futile?

Work with the ED management team, legal counsel, and perhaps the ethics committee at the facility to address this issue. After discussing the ramifications of this practice, written guidelines should be developed and followed by all staff who may be involved in these situations.

The major issues related to practicing procedures on the newly dead, which create emotional discomfort for staff, include choosing whether to tell the family, obtaining consent, disfigurement, and religious implications. Recommendations regarding these topics are conflicting. Iserson (1993) argues that consent to practice on a dead body is not necessary, whereas Goldblatt (1995) states that family consent must be obtained. Oman (1996) interviewed interns, residents, attending physicians, nurses, and clergy at a large teaching hospital to determine their experience with practicing procedures on the newly dead and found evidence of moral conflict, concerns about maintaining secrecy, lying in the medical record, and fear of disfiguring the body. In a later study, Oman surveyed the public and found that adults viewed this as an acceptable practice and felt that consent should be obtained (Oman, Armstrong, and Stoner, 2002).

26. What does it mean when the deceased's body is released by the medical examiner?

This means that the medical examiner or his or her representative has been informed of the patient's death and he or she has determined that a postmortem exam is not needed. The funeral home can come to pick up the body. Of significance in the ED, all tubes and devices can be removed in preparation for the family to view the body.

It may be helpful to create a form that can be used by staff to record what information was relayed to the medical examiner's office, including the staff member who notified the medical examiner, date, time, and action desired by the medical examiner.

27. When is it appropriate to transport the deceased patient to the morgue?

First, the body must be released by the medical examiner. Second, find out if the family is coming in and their approximate arrival time. If there is time and space in the ED, consider keeping the deceased there until the family has visited. If time and space are not available, the body may need to be moved to another location for family viewing if the morgue is not designed for family visits.

Ensure that the body and belongings are labeled appropriately. The body should be wrapped according to protocol and identifying tags must be securely attached. After the body is taken to the morgue, document the date, time, and personnel who took the body to the morgue. Document the disposition of valuables and personal belongings.

28. Who arranges for the body to be picked up from the morgue?

This arrangement is made by the family. Because the death of a loved one is a stressful event, the family may need to be reminded that they need to call the funeral home so that all final arrangements can be made.

29. Who determines whether an autopsy will be performed?

This decision is usually made by the medical examiner's office, or the patient's attending physician and family if the death is not a coroner's case. Several factors determine whether a patient has an autopsy. First are the events surrounding the death. Any death associated with a known or suspected criminal activity is usually cause for an autopsy. Second, autopsies are done to determine the cause of a sudden, traumatic, or unexpected death. Third, a family member may request an autopsy in certain situations.

Regulations regarding autopsies vary from state to state and among different law enforcement agencies. Medical examiners and private physicians may also have individual preferences regarding autopsy decisions. ED staff should consult with all of the agencies and physicians making autopsy decisions in their area to determine local regulations and preferences.

 Key Points

- Instead of telling families that "there is nothing we can do," tell families what has been done, what is being done, and what can be done.
- Use the sequential notification process to inform families of critical injuries, illness, and death.
- Prepare the family for viewing the body. Explain everything they will see in the room.
- Always ask the family what you can do to help them during this time. Every family is different and may need different things.
- Prepare for deaths and organ donation scenarios in the ED. Understand all legal and ethical requirements related to these areas.
- Keep a staff resource book in an accessible area; this book should include policies, procedures, referrals, and contact telephone numbers for all members of the bereavement response team.
- Establish support systems for the emergency care providers.
- Solicit feedback from families to enhance support programs.

Internet Resources

Association for Death Education and Counseling:
www.adec.org

Coalition on Donation:
www.donatelife.net

Death Notification and Survivor Care Program at the University of California at San Francisco:
www.ucsf.edu/deathnotification

eMedicine, *Grief Support in the ED:*
www.emedicine.com/emerg/topic694.htm

Emergency Nurses Association:
www.ena.org

Medline Plus, Organ Donation:
www.nlm.nih.gov/medlineplus/organdonation.html

National Association of Social Workers:
www.naswdc.org

U.S. Department of Health and Human Services, Donate Life:
www.organdonor.gov

Bibliography

Goldblatt A: Don't ask, don't tell: Practicing minimally invasive resuscitation techniques on the newly dead, *Ann Emerg Med* 25:86-90, 1995.

Iserson K: Postmortem procedures in the emergency department: Using the recently dead to practice and teach, *J Med Ethics* 19:92-98, 1993.

Knapp J, Mulligan-Smith D: Death of a child in the emergency department, *Pediatrics* 115(5):1432-1437, 2005.

Komaromy C: Continuing professional development: Cultural diversity in death and dying, *Nurs Manag (Harrow, London, England)* 11(8):32-36, 2004.

Larson DG: *The helper's journey*, Champaign, Ill, 1993, Research Press.

Meeker MA: A voice for the dying, *Clin Nurs Res* 13(4):326-342, 2004.

Moreland P: Family presence during invasive procedures and resuscitation in the emergency department: A review of the literature, *J Emerg Nurs* 31(1):58-72, 2005.

Oman K: Experiences with practicing procedures on the newly dead. Unpublished thesis. Denver, University of Colorado Health Sciences Center, 1996.

Oman K, Armstrong JA, Stoner M: Perspectives on practicing procedures on the newly dead, *Acad Emerg Med* 9(8):786-790, 2002.

Robinson SM et al: Psychological effect of witnessed resuscitation on bereaved relatives, *Lancet* 352:614-619, 1998.

Ufema J: Insights on death & dying. Hospital visitors: breaking bad news, *Nurs 2005* 35(1):22-23, 2005.

Wakefield A: Nurses' responses to death and dying: A need for relentless self-care, *Int J Palliat Nurs* 6:245-251, 2000.

Self-Care for the Caregiver

Patricia M. Campbell

1. Emergency nursing is a high-stress job. Is this stress necessarily unhealthy?

The emergency department (ED) is a very demanding, high-stress area that requires nurses who are in excellent physical and emotional health. The constant demands of the emergency environment can induce unhealthy amounts of stress that should be managed in a proactive and positive manner.

2. Why is it important to manage stress?

Stress is an essential element to an organism's ability to adapt and exist. The body's ability to respond to stress is achieved through the activation of the "fight or flight" mechanism. This intermittent surge of catecholamines to enable the fight or flight response is an essential component for survival in primitive beings. However, the continuous stress exerted on nurses in the emergency environment exceeds the normal duration and frequency intended for survival. Over time, the continued outpouring of endorphins and catecholamines produces prolonged stress reactions that can result in high blood pressure, headaches, cardiovascular disease, depression, and many other health problems.

3. Does stress affect job performance?

The literature reports that job stress symptoms, which may interfere with job performance, include memory deterioration, increased distractibility, and decreased concentration. Stress can also contribute to maladaptive behavior, chemical dependency, somatic illness (especially cardiovascular disease), and suicide. Job-related stress has also been identified as the primary reason that nurses experience burnout. It may be unrealistic to change or omit the stress in the ED, but learning how to react to it is possible. A person's *reaction* to stress determines the effect the stress has on the person's body and spirit. Therefore, nurses must learn how to manage their *reactions* to stress.

4. What can nurses do during their shift to reduce stress?

Many therapies can be performed with positive results in a short period of time, such as during break or mealtime. It is important that individual nurses discover the stress-reducing modality that works best for them, and then practice the modality on a regular basis. Brief 10-minute stress-reducing treatments such as massage, relaxation techniques, and guided imagery can be performed success-fully on the job in the hospital setting. Humor is also a great stress reducer, but make sure jokes and humor are used at a distance from patients and visitors.

5. What are some therapies an emergency nurse might try? What effects can be expected from the various therapies?

Stress-reducing therapies

Therapy	Benefits
Physical exercise	↓ Stress
	↑ Weight management
	↓ Blood pressure
	↓ Symptoms of depression
Meditation	↓ Oxygen consumption
	↑ Carbon dioxide elimination
	↓ Heart rate, respiratory rate, blood pressure
	↓ Gastric acidity and motility
	↓ Epinephrine level
	↓ Skeletal muscle tension
	↑ Slow alpha waves
	↑ Peripheral blood flow
	↑ Immune system response
Humor (laughter)	↑ Immune system response
	↑ Activated T-lymphocytes, T cells, killer cells
	↓ Cortical levels
Music	↓ Stress
	↓ Anxiety
	↓ Pain
	↑ Relaxation
Touch (acupressure, reflexology, shiatsu, therapeutic massage, therapeutic touch)	↓ Pain
	↓ Anxiety
	↓ Stress
Guided imagery	↓ Blood pressure
	↓ Pain
	↓ Anxiety
	↑ Self-esteem
	↓ Depression
	↓ Cortisol levels
	↓ Fatigue

6. **What stress-reduction therapies have hospitals initiated for employees?**

With the increased awareness of the effects of stress on health and job perform-ance, many hospitals nationwide are instituting stress-reduction modalities for their employees. These therapies have included massage therapy, music therapy, support groups, seminars on alternative therapies, and meditation gardens. Many other modalities could be instituted such as aromatherapy, acupressure, visual imagery, and meditation rooms. Environmental changes can also promote relaxation for staff and patients. Many EDs are adding fish tanks, art, alternative lighting, music, and other design features that promote healing for patients and staff.

7. **How does shift work affect health?**

The importance of stress reduction is especially important for those who work the night shift (permanent or rotating). The human body is governed by circa-dian rhythms that cycle every 24 hours. Generally, the body is programmed to have a 16-hour wake cycle and an 8-hour sleep cycle. When a person works the night shift, the circadian rhythm is disrupted and can cause severe imbalances in psychological and physiological function. These symptoms have been described as follows:
- Sleep disturbances
- Substance abuse
- Chronic fatigue
- Depression and mood disturbances
- Gastrointestinal (GI) problems
- Interpersonal relationship difficulties

A research review by Knutsson (2003) reported that shift work is associated with peptic ulcer disease, coronary heart disease, and adverse outcomes in preg-nancy. Women who work the night shift for more than 6 years have a 70% increase in heart disease compared with women who work during the day. Women who work nights have been shown to have greater menstrual problems, irregular menses, dysmenorrhea, lower rates of normal pregnancy, and increased rates of preterm and low–birth-weight infants.

8. **What steps can emergency nurses and their employers take to reduce personal stress?**

Emergency nurses who want to maintain mental and physical balance and good health should adopt a healthy lifestyle on and off the job. Healthy lifestyles are individual. However, there are guidelines for developing a healthy lifestyle to manage stress.

Healthy lifestyle choices

Choice	Explanation
Practice preventive health	Obtain regular medical checkups and screening exams recommended for your age, gender, medical history, and risk profile.
Stop smoking	Stopping smoking will decrease your risk for many cancers, respiratory illnesses, fetal abnormalities, and erectile dysfunction.
Eliminate or minimize alcohol intake	Research suggests that red wine in moderation may be beneficial in reducing the risk of stroke in males. Recent research, however, suggests that any alcohol intake may increase the risk of breast cancer in women.
Exercise daily	Daily exercise for 30 minutes or more will help reduce blood pressure, weight, risk of heart disease, and some cancers.
Manage your weight	Weight management has been associated with a sense of well-being and improved health.
Follow a healthy diet	Follow a low-fat, high-fiber, plant-based diet. Minimize meat, processed foods, and sweets. Vitamins, mineral, and food supplements may be beneficial to some individuals. Purified water in quantities sufficient to maintain adequate hydration should be consumed.
Maintain healthy relationships	Maintaining healthy relationships is essential to a sense of well-being. Surround yourself with people who have a positive lifestyle and attitude. Seek professional help in eliminating negative relationships that are not salvageable and that have a negative impact on your life.
Overcome addictions	Addictions can be to substances or unhealthy relationships. Seek professional help to overcome addictions.
Practice stress-reduction methods	Individuals often choose the most appropriate method of stress reduction for themselves. Research has demonstrated that meditation, yoga, prayer, massage, guided imagery, music therapy, and other relaxation techniques are effective in restoring balance and harmony.
Take responsibility for your life	Gain control of your life and realize that you created your situation and only you can change it. It is empowering to realize that you are in control of your response and reaction to life events, even during a busy shift in the ED.

Key Points

- Managing stress is key to maintaining health. Stress-reducing therapies include physical exercise, meditation, humor, music, touch therapies, and guided imagery.
- Healthy lifestyle choices include health promotion, smoking cessation, minimizing alcohol intake, daily exercise, weight management, healthy diet, healthy relationships, overcoming addictions, stress-reduction activities, and taking responsibility for your life.
- Reduce stress at work by practicing visual imagery, muscle relaxation, and breathing exercises.
- The adverse health effects of shift work can include sleep disturbances, substance abuse, chronic fatigue, depression and mood disturbances, GI disorders, heart disease, dysmenorrhea, and pregnancy complications.

 Internet Resources

American Heart Association:
www.americanheart.org

American Heart Association, Healthy Lifestyle:
www.americanheart.org/presenter.jhtml?identifier=1200009

American Holistic Nurses Association:
www.ahna.org

Centers for Disease Control and Prevention:
www.cdc.gov

Centers for Disease Control and Prevention, Health Promotion (select area of interest):
www.cdc.gov/node.do/id/0900f3ec80059b1a

National Center for Complementary and Alternative Medicine:
www.nccam.nih.gov

Bibliography

Dossey BM: *Core curriculum for holistic nursing*, Boston, 1997, Jones and Bartlett.

Dossey BM et al: *Holistic nursing: A handbook for practice*, ed 4, Boston, 2005, Jones and Bartlett.

Fitzpatrick MJ, Buevich S, Jones S: The caregivers care shop, *J Nurs Staff Dev* 17:243-247, 2001.

Frisch NC et al: *AHNA standards of holistic nursing practice: Guidelines for caring and healing*, Boston, 2000, Jones and Bartlett.

Keegan L: Alternative and complementary modalities for managing stress and anxiety, *Crit Care Nurs* 23:55-58, 2003.

Knutsson A: Health disorders of shift workers, *Occup Med* 53:103-108, 2003.

Keeping Safe

Patricia M. Campbell

1. What should emergency nurses consider when they think of safety?

Emergency nurses face many risks to their safety and well-being, from slipping on wet floors to being victims of assault. This chapter addresses three areas of risk: violence, infectious diseases, and latex allergy.

2. Is violence in the emergency department (ED) a common experience?

Yes, violence in the ED toward staff and visitors has become an increasing problem throughout the United States. A large majority of emergency nurses have been assaulted during their careers: 82% in one study of 55 emergency nurses by Erikson et al (2000). Violence was defined as verbal or physical assault and contributed to stress, job loss, and poor job performance.

3. Where are the highest risk areas for violence in an emergency nurse's environment?

Violence occurs in a variety of settings in which emergency nurses work, including triage, patient care areas, and during transport to other hospital locations. Trauma room personnel who serve high-risk populations are often exposed to weapons, gang activity, and substance abuse. Parking lots and outdoor hospital campus areas present an element of risk, especially in the evening, late night, and early morning.

4. What precautions can emergency nurses and departments take to prevent being victims of violent acts?

- Become a part of the community. Join community coalitions to work together toward safety, not just for the ED but for the neighborhood that it serves.
- Be observant. If potentially violent patients or visitors are identified, notify hospital police or security for a "standby in the ED." Consider that patients or visitors might have concealed weapons. Communicate to your other team members that there is a potentially violent situation. Be proactive and prepare to protect the staff, visitors, and patients.
- Provide classes for staff on identifying and managing potentially dangerous situations and violent persons.
- Have all visitors sign in, and provide a nametag with the room number of the patient they are visiting. Keep visitors in patients' rooms; do not allow visitors to wander around the department or loiter at the nurses' station. Limit the number of patient visitors according to the staff's ability to monitor them.

- Some believe that staff nametags should show only the first name and credential of the staff member (e.g., John RN). If nurses choose to use their surname, they might consider the risks of having that information readily available to the public. Emergency nurses have been stalked by patients and family members.
- K-9 units in conjunction with well-trained security officers have been highly effective in defusing volatile situations in the ED.
- Do not allow any weapons in the ED, and be observant for potential concealed weapons or objects that could be used as weapons (e.g., bottles). Develop a policy and procedure for searching patients.
- Develop guidelines and policies for the use of restraints, both soft and locking, for combative patients.
- Never put yourself in a situation in which you do not have an escape route. Always ensure that the door is open and clear for a rapid exit. Never allow a violent or hostile patient or visitor to stand between you and the door. Likewise, do not block the exit of a violent person. Avoid making the person feel "trapped."

5. **What safety measures should be considered when renovating or constructing an ED?**

During the initial construction or remodeling of an ED is the ideal time to consider safety issues. A multidisciplinary team should be assembled to evaluate the physical setting and to plan appropriate security measures to be incorporated into the design. A multidisciplinary team might include nurses, physicians, an architect, an engineer, safety/security officers, and a fire official. Certified protection professionals who specialize in the safety and protection of healthcare environments are available for consultation.

The physical layout of the department can assist in creating a safe environment and reducing the risk of violence. Limit access to patient care areas except through security clearance. This can be accomplished by posting a security guard outside the ED to screen and register visitors and by limiting access to all doors by use of a security code or badge swipe. Monitored security cameras are helpful. Metal detectors that are located at all visitor entrances can deter and detect weapons. Handheld metal detectors are useful for identifying weapons carried by visitors or patients. Bulletproof glass is often used to screen the triage and security areas. Non-shatter glass doors on patient rooms for viewing of all activities in the room will assist with monitoring patient activities and is less likely to cause injury or be used as a weapon if damaged. Likewise, framed artwork should have plexiglass instead of real glass.

6. **How can emergency nurses protect themselves from contracting infectious diseases in the ED?**

Nurses must be vigilant. Emergency nurses are at increased risk because they often care for very ill patients who have not yet been diagnosed. Occasionally, the illness is contagious and may have life-threatening consequences (e.g., meningococcal meningitis). Respiratory precautions and standard precautions are essential in the day-to-day practice in the ED. Immunizations against measles, mumps, rubella, varicella, and hepatitis B should be current to prevent disease. Ensure that all staff have been fitted with N95 respiratory masks for protection against tuberculosis (TB), severe acute respiratory syndrome (SARS), and other respiratory pathogens. Hand washing is an important first line of defense against infection for healthcare workers and patients.

7. What are the current guidelines for hand washing?

Hand washing is the first line of defense against contracting infectious diseases and should be done before and after all patient contact, before donning gloves for sterile or nonsterile procedures, and after glove removal. Hand washing should be done before eating and after using the restroom.

Hand washing should be done with nonbactericidal soap, or with bactericidal soap if visible soil or material is present. According to the Centers for Disease Control and Prevention (CDC) guidelines, all types of soap (plain, liquid, bar, leaflet, powdered) are acceptable when washing with water. Avoid hot water because it increases the risk of dry, cracked skin and dermatitis. Alcohol-based hand rubs can be used in between hand washings to decontaminate hands.

The current recommendations for hand washing are as follows:

- Wash hands with soap and running water. Wet hands first and apply the soap as recommended by the manufacturer. Rub hands vigorously together for at least 15 seconds to ensure that all surfaces of the hands and in between the fingers are thoroughly cleansed. Rinse hands under running water. Dry hands with a disposable towel and use the towel to turn off the faucet. Air dryers are not as effective in removing bacteria from the hands as are disposable towels, which use friction. Multiple-use towels are not recommended because of an increase in the risk of cross contamination.

The current recommendations for cleansing hands with an alcohol-based cleanser are as follows:

- Apply the recommended amount of product to the palm of the hand and rub hands together, covering all surfaces of the hands and fingers. Continue to rub the hands together until the hands are dry.

8. Which bloodborne diseases can be contracted from a needlestick injury?

Needlestick injuries present the opportunity for exposure to bloodborne pathogens such as HIV and hepatitis B and C.

9. How often do nurses contract bloodborne pathogens from exposure at work?

The CDC conducts surveillance of occupational exposures to bloodborne pathogens. A 2002 "factsheet" (available at: www.cdc.gov/hiv/pubs/facts/hcwsurv.htm) reported 57 documented cases of occupational transmission of HIV to healthcare workers in the United States through December 2001. An additional 138 cases of possible transmission have been described. Each healthcare worker reported needlestick injuries or mucocutaneous exposure with no other risk factors. Overall, the risk of contracting HIV is relatively low. The estimated risk of contracting HIV from a needlestick or cut is 0.3%; risk from mucocutaneous exposure (eye, nose, mouth) is considered to be 0.1%. In contrast to HIV, hepatitis is 100 times more infectious. The risk of infection with hepatitis B virus in susceptible people (nonimmunized) ranges from 6% to 30%. The average risk for infection after a needlestick injury or cut exposure to hepatitis C virus–infected blood is approximately 1.8%.

10. **What should the emergency nurse do after a needlestick injury or mucocutaneous exposure to blood?**

All institutions should have a postexposure plan in place to assist the nurse in properly managing the situation. The CDC recommends the following action immediately after exposure:

- Wash all needlesticks and cuts with soap and water. Using antiseptics or making the wound bleed does not reduce the chance of infection. Do not use bleach or other caustic substances.
- Flush the nose, mouth, and areas of skin that have been exposed with copious amounts of water. Eye irrigation can be done with saline, lactated Ringer's solution, or clean water.
- Consult a specialist who can evaluate the degree of risk for the exposure. Postexposure antiviral and protease inhibitors are used prophylactically in high-risk cases. Initiation of these medications must begin within a few hours after exposure for maximum effectiveness. CDC guidelines suggest within 24 hours, but many institutions advise initiation within 1 hour.
- Blood samples should be drawn as soon as possible after exposure, followed by testing every 6 months until a final test at 18 months. Blood is tested for the presence of hepatitis B (or antibodies if vaccinated), hepatitis C, and HIV.

11. **Should every nurse who sustains an exposure be treated with prophylactic medications?**

No. Prophylactic medications should be considered only for nurses who sustain significant exposure and in situations in which the patient is judged to be "high risk." These medications are relatively new and their long-term effects and possible toxicities are generally unknown. The possible benefits must be evaluated against the degree of risk. Regular medical follow-up must accompany and guide the therapy. If prophylactic therapy is started, precautions for transmission must be maintained during the follow-up period; that is, abstain from sexual intercourse or use condoms, do not breastfeed, and do not become pregnant.

12. **How does a nurse know if exposure is high risk?**

Healthcare providers trained in infectious disease counseling can evaluate the degree of risk and should be part of the postexposure plan. Many institutions have a 24-hour telephone number to call immediately after exposure to obtain documentation, counseling, and guidance for the recommended course of treatment. If this is not available, consult the CDC or an infectious disease specialist.

13. **Is there any new technology that assists in preventing needlestick injuries?**

Retractable or other safety needles are becoming standard in most EDs. They are designed to immediately retract into the barrel of the syringe after medication injection, thereby eliminating the nurse's exposure to the contaminated needle. Always dispose of sharp objects and instruments in puncture-proof containers. Patient care will continue to evolve to minimize the use of needles.

14. **What is the proper way to dispose of sharps and potentially infectious materials?**

All sharps (e.g., needles, scalpel blades) must be disposed of in the red biohazard sharps containers. Never pick up a needle or scalpel blade with your hands. Use a hemostat or other instrument to prevent injury. All dressings, contaminated linens, and materials must be bagged in a biohazard bag provided by the facility according to facility policy.

15. **Are there any laws or regulations that protect healthcare workers from bloodborne pathogens?**

In 1991, the Occupational Safety and Health Administration (OSHA) wrote a broad public health measure, *The Bloodborne Pathogen Standard* (available at: www.osha.gov/pls/oshaweb/owadisp.show_document?p_table=STAN-DARDS&p_id=10051) to prevent and/or minimize exposure of healthcare workers to bloodborne pathogens. This measure is designed to protect against hepatitis B and C, HIV, and other bloodborne pathogens. The standard defines bloodborne pathogens, contamination, high-risk behaviors (intravenous [IV] drug abuse, multiple sexual partners) and prevention (universal precautions). According to the OSHA standard, it is the responsibility of the employer to provide the necessary equipment for protection from exposure in the workplace. The National Institute for Occupational Safety and Health (NIOSH) monitors the State Needle Safety Legislation. As of 2002, 22 states have enacted legislation related to bloodborne pathogen exposure prevention.

16. **What other pathogen exposures place the emergency nurse at risk?**

The emergency nurse is exposed to many pathogens on a daily basis. Fortunately, most people have a responsive immune system that protects them. Occasionally, exposures may call for prophylactic antibiotics to prevent disease, such as meningococcal meningitis and TB.

17. **What is the risk to the emergency nurse from a terrorist attack using biological weapons?**

The emergency nurse has the potential for significant exposure in the event of a biological warfare attack with pathogens such as smallpox. Triage nurses must have a high index of suspicion for infectious diseases (naturally occurring or weaponized) to prevent the spread of infection and exposure. Removing the patient from the waiting room and isolating the patient in a separate room with negative air flow, masking the patient, and informing staff of the potential risk are all important "first steps" to prevent further exposure and disease transmission.

18. **What precautions should be taken to minimize exposure to radiation in the ED?**

Nurses should adhere to hospital policy regarding precautions during radiation exposure. Ideally, the nurse should leave the room while x-rays are being completed to avoid unnecessary exposure. If more extensive exposures are required or the nurse cannot leave the bedside, protection behind radiation protection screens or lead aprons should be used. Recommendations from the radiology department in the facility should be followed.

19. Why is the use of latex gloves a concern?

Natural latex, which is used in latex gloves, contains natural proteins that have been shown to sensitize and cause allergic reactions in some persons over a period of time with repeated use. During the processing and manufacturing of latex gloves, many impurities are left in the gloves and eventually attach to the cornstarch that is placed in the gloves for ease of donning. When the gloves are removed, the natural proteins, which are attached to the cornstarch, are aerosolized into the air and inhaled by everyone nearby. The person who just took off the gloves may further sensitize himself or herself by touching the nose, eyes, or mucous membranes while the powder is still on the hands.

Latex allergy is an IgE-mediated reaction to the proteins in latex. Persons who are sensitive or allergic to latex may experience a wide variety of symptoms, including rash, asthma, severe food allergies, anaphylaxis, and death. There is a large amount of literature available regarding concerns over the use of latex gloves.

20. What other products containing latex present a risk to patients and healthcare workers?

Numerous products used in healthcare and patient care products contain latex and must be labeled as such. Many of the following items should be suspected of containing latex unless labeled "latex free":

- Catheters (urinary and IV)
- IV products, syringes
- Airway equipment (endotracheal tubes [ETTs], masks, elastic straps)
- Blood pressure cuffs, tourniquets
- Adhesives on devices (electrocardiogram [ECG] leads, tape, dressings)
- Disposable pulse oximeter probes

Many products in everyday use also contain latex, such as latex balloons, hair bands, sneakers, and rubber tires. Many foods are cross-reactive in latex-sensitive persons. Some of the most common foods include bananas, figs, chestnuts, papaya, tomatoes, cherries, celery, peaches, kiwi, and avocado.

21. What measures can be instituted to make the ED safer for latex-sensitive staff and patients?

- Educate staff, physicians, and patients to be proactive in identifying high-risk patients and staff and support measures to reduce the risk. Staff must be educated to identify products with latex.
- Develop a hospital-wide committee that researches the problem and presents solutions. Include key people, such as nurses and physicians who work in high-risk areas, nurse and physician specialists in allergy or latex allergy, and at least one healthcare worker who is latex sensitive.
- Develop policies and procedures for caring for latex-sensitive patients and staff members.
- Develop policies on testing and treatment of latex-sensitive staff.
- Identify products that contain latex and look for replacements that are latex free.

- Develop a latex-free cart with equipment that is latex free to be used when a latex-sensitive patient presents for treatment. Some hospitals have a latex-free exam room. A comprehensive list of contents for a latex-free emergency cart was published in the *Journal of Emergency Nursing* in February 1998.
- Switch to nonlatex exam gloves. Use only powder-free latex when latex is indicated for protection against bloodborne pathogens.
- Ban latex balloons in the hospital. Do not allow children to play with latex gloves or blow them up into balloons. Note that latex balloons and gloves also present a choking hazard to small children and should be discouraged for that reason as well.

22. What should a nurse do if he or she develops an allergy to latex in the workplace?

Latex allergy is a serious, progressive allergy that must be treated and monitored as soon as symptoms develop. If rashes, red or itchy eyes, swelling of the lips, or asthma symptoms develop, consider possible latex allergy. It is important to follow through with an evaluation for two reasons: (1) to obtain medical treatment, and (2) documentation. Documentation may be necessary if the allergy becomes severe enough to prevent the nurse from working. The following steps have been suggested to ensure proper documentation:

- File a claim with worker's compensation.
- Document every event (e.g., doctor visits, hospital visits).
- Obtain copies of progress notes and lab tests.
- Seek medical attention for each event and ensure proper documentation.
- Consult a specialist in latex allergies.
- Consult an attorney to ensure that your rights are being protected.

 Key Points

- Violence in the ED can be minimized through staff training, education, physical design of the ED and hospital campus, as well as strong policies/ procedures for managing violent patients and visitors.
- Prevention of infectious diseases relies on nursing education, immunizations, standard and respiratory precautions, careful hand washing, isolation procedures, and policies/procedures for safety in the workplace as outlined by the CDC and OSHA.
- Needlestick injury prevention relies on education and training, new technology for safety needles, proper disposal of sharps, and policies/procedures.
- After exposure to blood and body fluids, wash the area with soap and water; flush mucous membranes, eyes, or mouth with water; follow policies/procedures; and consult an infectious disease specialist for follow-up care.
- Latex sensitivity poses a serious problem for staff and patients. Measures to reduce exposure include staff education, and policies/procedures for caring for latex-sensitive patients/staff members. Develop policies regarding testing and treatment of latex-sensitive staff. Minimize exposure by reducing latex products and ensuring the availability of latex-free products for sensitive patients.

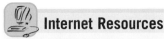
Internet Resources

Centers for Disease Control and Prevention:
www.cdc.gov

Centers for Disease Control and Prevention, Diseases & Conditions:
www.cdc.gov/node.do/id/0900f3ec8000e035

Centers for Disease Control and Prevention, Vaccines & Immunizations:
www.cdc.gov/node.do/id/0900f3ec8000e2f3

Centers for Disease Control and Prevention, Workplace Safety & Health:
www.cdc.gov/node.do/id/0900f3ec8000ec09

Occupational Safety and Health Administration:
www.osha.gov

Occupational Safety and Health Administration, Bloodborne Pathogens and Needlestick Prevention:
www.osha.gov/SLTC/bloodbornepathogens

Occupational Safety and Health Administration, Bloodborne Fact Sheets by Number:
www.osha.gov/OshDoc/data_BloodborneFacts

Occupational Safety and Health Administration, Bloodborne Pathogens, Regulations:
www.osha.gov/pls/oshaweb/owadisp.show_document?p_table=STANDARDS&p_id=10051

World Health Organization:
www.who.int

World Health Organization, Health Topics (hepatitis B, C, HIV):
www.who.int/topics/en

Bibliography

Alabama Nurse: Tips for reducing risk of latex allergy, *Ala Nurse* 27:12, 2000.

Bernstein, ML: Latex-safe emergency care products lists, *J Emerg Nurs* 24:58-61, 1998.

CDC: *Exposure to blood: What healthcare personnel need to know,* July 2003, pp 1-10 (Available at: www.cdc.gov/ncidod/dhqp/pdf/bbp/Exp_to_Blood.pdf).

Erickson L et al: Attitudes of emergency nurses regarding patient assaults, *J Emerg Nurs* 26:210-215, 2000.

Lopes R and Benatti M: Review of latex sensitivity related to the use of latex gloves in hospital, *AORN J* 80(1):64-68, 70-71, 2004.

National Institute for Occupational Safety and Health: *Overview of state needle safety legislation,* 2002.

Case Management

Carolee Whitehill

1. What do case managers do?

Historically, case managers worked in community settings offering long-term social and mental health services to clients. Then, case managers expanded into the acute care setting providing admission and discharge planning, evaluating the appropriate level of care, interfacing with payers, offering clinical expertise, and arranging post–acute care placements and services. Inpatient case managers may coordinate patient care using clinical pathways and monitor trends and variances for groups of patients.

Recently, nurse case managers migrated into emergency departments (EDs). Many are involved with "traditional" admission and discharge planning activities for selected patients. For example, they may evaluate the appropriateness of admission versus alternative placements, arrange home care services, or monitor follow-up compliance. The role may integrate utilization management activities. Various titles may be used such as Case Manager or Clinical Resource Coordinator; the reporting mechanism might be directly to the ED administration or to the hospital case management department. Because of the high volume of patients treated in emergency settings and the number of providers with which the ED staff interfaces, there is a great opportunity to identify patient needs beyond the acute clinical situation; provide resources, education, and assistance with access to care; and improve continuity of care.

2. What are the goals of case management?

Overall goals of case management are to ensure quality of care and efficiency of services, match healthcare needs with access to available resources, improve the health status of patients, and provide for the continuity of care.

3. What does "continuum of care" mean?

Continuum of care is an approach that plans for patients' healthcare needs through an integrated healthcare delivery system. Instead of providers working in isolation, they form partnerships to ensure patients receive appropriate clinical care, psychosocial interventions, education, follow-up, and monitoring. Goals for continuity of care are to ensure quality of care, improve patients' health status, avoid duplication of services, improve communication among all providers, and assist the patient through the complicated delivery system. As the responsibility of managing the cost of care increasingly becomes that of the providers, these linkages are vital to ensure cost-effective use of resources. Systems need to be developed that allow clear communication and planning of care between the ED and other providers of care: primary care physicians, specialists, inpatient units, clinics, healthcare facilities, home health agencies, mental health agencies, and community service organizations.

4. **How is it determined whether a department needs a case manager?**

Answering the following questions about the ED will help identify whether a case management program is needed and what its focus might be.

- Do patients have access to primary care services and specialty care follow-up?
- Does the department have a significant uninsured population?
- Are there smooth communications with inpatient and outpatient specialty services, primary care, and community health services?
- Are admissions at the appropriate level of service?
- Is there a consistent level of care?
- Are there clear expectations among the ED team?
- How does the department compare with available benchmark data such as length of stay, clinical standards, and quality indicators?
- Is the department linked to inpatient clinical pathways?
- Are outcomes of care monitored?
- Are there repeat visitors to the ED?
- Is there a significant chronic care population?

5. **After it has been decided a case manager is needed, what is the best way to start?**

It might help to organize the ED case management program around one or more of the following four categories.

- **Primary care programs.** These programs are helpful for departments that have a significant volume of uninsured patients or patients without primary care providers (PCPs). Programs focus on community resources, low-cost services, patient and staff education regarding use of PCPs, and financial assistance information. Risk assessment screening may assist in targeting patients in need of prevention and resource information, education, and counseling.
- **Admission/discharge planning.** On an individual patient level, the case manager might address hospital admissions with respect to level of care and inpatient versus observational status, expedite the plan for the inpatient case manager or social worker, and initiate insurance notification and out-of-network issues. Discharge planning includes making transfer arrangements; arranging home care, equipment, and community service needs; providing lab and radiology follow-up; and monitoring compliance with discharge instructions. On a system level the case manager might address issues such as compliance with Emergency Medical Treatment and Active Labor Act (EMTALA) regulations, trends with hospital readmissions or return visits to the ED, eligibility criteria for observational status, provisions for continuity of care, or access to specialty care. Case management system issues are often linked to quality or risk indicators.
- **Population-based programs.** Also known as "disease management" or "chronic care management," these programs address patients' clinical, self-management

education, payer source, medications, and resource needs in relation to a specific disease or condition. Although the ED focuses primarily on acute clinical care and expeditious disposition, population-based programs assist in evaluating the patient's needs beyond the ED visit by linking with the continuum of care. Suggestions for population programs are asthma, diabetes, trauma, acute myocardial infarction, sickle cell disease, and stroke. There are two primary approaches to population-based programs in the ED: clinical pathways and risk assessments, which are both described later in the chapter.

- **Individual patient plans.** Designed for patients with special needs, patient plans assist with providing consistent care for patients who are expected to return to the ED. Written in conjunction with the patient's PCP, specialty care provider, and other providers of care, the plan outlines recommendations for care in the department. These plans are guidelines only and are adjusted based on the patient's presentation. Many of these patients have repeat ED visits because of specific clinical needs; others would benefit from access to healthcare resources other than the ED. For those patients, a goal might be to decrease repeat ED visits. Patients with chronic nonmalignant pain who seek care in the ED for acute breakthrough pain can benefit from a patient guideline that reflects the patient's current pain management plan and the PCP's and pain physician's recommendations for breakthrough pain management. Issues regarding narcotic administration may be clarified for the ED staff. These communications will assist in improved consistency in patient care by the ED providers.

6. What are the outcomes of care when implementing an individual patient plan?

- Provide PCP resources and education
- Link to population-based program if indicated
- Develop patient plan for continuity of care
- Refer to social worker or case manager
- Monitor future ED visits
- Decrease ED visits

7. What are clinical pathways?

Clinical pathways are an evolution of standards of care and protocols that incorporate evidence-based practices, include an interdisciplinary approach, contain a time component, and monitor specific outcomes. They assist in clarifying team responsibilities, provide consistent care to a group of patients, allow cost-effective and efficient use of resources, and measure outcomes of care. Types of outcomes are listed in the following table.

8. The clinicians are reluctant to initiate clinical pathways because they fear that the department will be criticized for not meeting outcome criteria. How can the staff get beyond this barrier?

The purpose of pursuing clinical pathways in the ED is to improve quality of care by developing a plan to manage an acute episode of illness or injury of a targeted population. This plan assists in providing consistent care with predefined outcome goals. The term "variance" is used to describe an occurrence in

Clinical pathways: Outcomes of care

Type	Examples
Clinical	Physiological parameter
	Lab value
Functional	Ability to ambulate
	Quality of life indicator
Process	Access to follow-up care
	Length of stay
Financial	Cost of care
	Repeat visits
Patient satisfaction	Regarding care, providers, facility, and education

which outcome goals are not met. Evaluation of variances may assist in the improvement of patient care or system difficulties. The following table gives examples of variances.

Examples of variances

Category	Examples
Patient/family	Patient's response to treatment (peak flow measurement did not meet improvement criteria)
	Patient or family decision to refuse treatment plan
Caregiver	Provider issue: RN, NP, MD, technician
	Clinical care, documentation missing
Internal system	Lab or radiology delay
	Equipment not available
	Length of stay extended because of lack of inpatient bed availability
External system	Discharge or transfer delayed because of slow response of transport company
	Cost of care increased because of pharmaceutical price increase

Many times a variance is not an error but rather an explanation for an event and certainly an opportunity to evaluate the pathway process. Variances may actually support the ED's effort to improve care. For example, a critical trauma pathway identifies a maximum ED length of stay as an outcome goal. If this goal is consistently not being met, an evaluation of the variance may determine that ED efficiency is not the issue, but rather the problem is a delay in obtaining an inpatient ICU bed. Administrative problem-solving focus then shifts from the ED to evaluating ICU staffing, efficiency, and bed control issues.

Evaluating outcomes and variances is an ongoing process aimed at improving quality of care and efficiency of services, maximizing resources, and identifying educational needs of patients, family, and staff. All efforts in these areas may be used as part of the quality management improvement program in the ED.

9. What is meant by the term "risk assessment"?

Risk assessment identifies patients who are at risk for high utilization of health services or in need of access to a PCP, self-management education, medications, medical supplies, and community resources with the goal of improving their over-all health status. Population-based programs that use a risk assessment approach might include asthma, diabetes, congestive heart failure, chronic pain, high blood pressure, HIV/AIDS, or the elderly. The risk assessment may be completed by a stable patient or the nurse as a means of a follow-up referral to the case manager when he or she is not immediately available.

10. How can the issue of repeat visitors to the ED be addressed?

The issue of repeat visitors is controversial. Some people believe that nonurgent and some urgent visits to the ED are inappropriate and costly, and that much of this care should be obtained in the primary care setting instead of in the ED. There are certainly cases in which this is true. However, there are significant issues that lead patients to the ED for care. For example, difficulty locating a PCP, especially for the uninsured; inability to access a PCP for urgent appointments; inflexibility of work or child care responsibilities to allow attending restricted office appointments; and inability to differentiate "emergent" versus "routine" healthcare needs. For many patients, the ED addresses a healthcare need that is not being met elsewhere. Some would argue that because the ED is staffed 24 hours a day, it is not that costly to quickly treat nonurgent and urgent patients. Nevertheless, it is difficult to approach the issue of repeat visitors as a whole because the reasons for the visits vary. It is recommended that repeat visitors be addressed in relation to specific case management programs. For example, do patients need information to locate a PCP? Do they fit a population-based program? Do they need an individual patient plan? As case management programs evolve, overall visits by repeat visitors tend to decrease.

It may also be helpful to complete an audit on patients returning to the ED within a defined time frame (e.g., 72 hours) and categorize the reasons for the return visits. Categories may include but are not limited to:

- The patient was asked to return (e.g., a patient with cellulitus was asked to return to evaluate effectiveness of outpatient antibiotic treatment).
- The patient was advised to follow up with primary care, but the patient does not have a PCP or is unable to gain access in a timely manner.
- The patient's conditioned worsened, and the patient returned to the ED per discharge instructions. If the patient required admission to the hospital with the return visit, a quality review for appropriate care during the first visit is recommended.

Each of the categories identified may help in clarifying needed resources and realistic discharge instructions regarding follow-up care.

11. How can a new case management position be funded?

Because case management positions are not revenue generating, it is helpful to build financial outcomes into the programs to justify the position. For example, a population-based risk assessment program designed to screen asthma patients for education and resource needs would have as a goal to decrease repeat ED visits as a result of a decrease in the number of asthma exacerbations by identifying the previous 12-month ED visit history and monitoring the 12-month visit history following program implementation. Calculating the average cost of an asthma visit multiplied by the decreased number of visits identifies the "cost avoidance." Because the ED generally operates on a fixed budget, actual cost savings may be minimal until a significant decrease in patient volume occurs. Diverting staff to more critical patients, decreasing wait time, and improving patient satisfaction are commendable goals. In addition, decreasing hospital admissions quickly results in actual cost savings. Developing partnerships with or integrating with existing hospital departments such as case management, utilization management, and social services offers the opportunity to develop programs to improve the continuum and efficiency of care. These trends demonstrate what case management programs can accomplish.

 Key Points

- ED case management programs vary based on the needs of the population, the healthcare system, and the available community resources. Conduct a needs assessment to identify issues appropriate for the specific ED.

- Develop linkages to related healthcare agendas, such as public health issues, needs of the chronic care population, access to care for the medically underserved, quality and risk issues to incorporate established benchmarks, and health-related goals.

- Develop partnerships with PCPs, specialty providers, social workers, case managers, utilization managers, pharmacy, quality and risk, other EDs, and community resources.

Internet Resources

American Academy of Pain Medicine:
www.painmed.org

American Diabetes Association:
www.diabetes.org

American Heart Association:
www.americanheart.org

American Pain Society:
www.ampainsoc.org

American Society of Addiction Medicine:
www.asam.org

Centers for Disease Control and Prevention, Chronic Disease Prevention:
www.cdc.gov/nccdphp

Healthy People 2010:
www.healthypeople.gov

The Henry J. Kaiser Family Foundation:
www.kff.org

Improving Chronic Illness Care:
www.improvingchroniccare.org

Institute of Medicine of the National Academies:
www.iom.edu

National Heart, Lung, and Blood Institute:
www.nhlbi.nih.gov

National Institutes of Health:
www.nih.gov

Bibliography

Bristow D, Herrick C: Emergency department case management: The dyad team of nurse case manager and social worker improve discharge planning and patient and staff satisfaction while decreasing inappropriate admissions and costs: A literature review, *Lippincotts Case Manag* 7(6):243-251, 2002.

Gautney L et al: The emergency department case manager: Effect on selected outcomes, *Lippincotts Case Manag* 9(3):121-129, 2004.

McCaig L, Burt C: *National hospital ambulatory medical care survey: 2001 emergency department summary, Advance data,* Washington, DC, 2001, US Department of Health and Human Services, National Center for Health Statistics, Vital and Health Statistics.

McCusker J et al: Prediction of hospital utilization among elderly patients in the 6 months after an emergency department visit, *Ann Emerg Med* 36(5):438-445, 2000.

Meldon S et al: A brief risk-stratefication tool to predict repeat emergency department visits and hospitalizations in older patients discharged from the emergency department, *Acad Emerg Med* 10(3):224-232, 2003.

Okin R et al: The effects of clinical case management on hospital service use among ED frequent users, *Am J Emerg Med* 18(5):603-608, 2000.

Walsh K: ED case managers: One large teaching hospital's experience, *J Emerg Nurs* 25:17-29, 1999.

Whitehill C: A model of emergency department case management: Developing strategies and outcomes. In Cohen E and Cesta T, editors: *Nursing case management: From concept to evaluation,* ed 4, St Louis, 2005, Mosby.

Chapter 8

Risk Management

Lorna K. Prutzman

1. What is risk management?

Risk management is proactive intervention and behavior to decrease the likelihood of injury and loss. In healthcare, the goal of risk management is to prevent injury to patients and avoid professional liability. High-quality nursing care and sound delivery systems are key to effective risk management in emergency nursing. The majority of injuries to patients can be traced to flawed systems that either primarily cause the injury or set up the nurse to make a mistake that results in injury to a patient. After an injury has occurred, risk management focuses on mitigation to decrease the likelihood of legal action against the provider.

2. What is malpractice?

Malpractice is professional misconduct or lack of reasonable skill. Negligence is the most common legal theory used to sue nurses for malpractice. Nursing negligence is an act or failure to act that causes injury to a patient. This theory encompasses four distinct requirements: (1) duty, (2) breach of duty (failure to meet one's duty), (3) causation, and (4) injury. All four elements must be met for the nurse to be successfully sued for negligence.

3. How is "standard of care" or "degree of care" determined?

Duty and breach of duty are measured by the standard of care. The legal standard of care is the degree of care that a reasonably prudent nurse would exercise in the same or similar circumstances. "Degree of care" requires that the professional standards of practice (such as those published by the Emergency Nurses Association [ENA]) be compared with the nurse's actual behavior. In addition, institutional policies, procedures, and protocols, as well as standards set by accrediting organizations such as the Joint Commission on Accreditation of Healthcare Organizations (JCAHO), are used to assess the requisite degree of care. At trial, expert nurse witnesses offer their testimony as evidence of the degree of care a reasonably prudent nurse would exercise under the circumstances in which the defendant nurse was laboring.

4. How does the law apply to circumstances a nurse cannot control?

The law recognizes that a nurse cannot control certain circumstances and may be prevented from fulfilling his or her duty. In the emergency setting, circumstances that commonly invoke forgiveness for failing to meet professional duty are noncompliant behavior of the patient and violent or abusive behavior of the patient toward the nurse or others. These are circumstances the patient creates.

5. **What happens in situations in which the nurse has control?**

The law does not forgive circumstances created by the nurse. A good example of this is failure of the nurse to be present when the patient is in need of care, such as if a nurse leaves the patient to tend to personal needs. In a busy emergency department (ED) it is not uncommon for hours to go by without an opportunity to take a break. If a patient in need of care is left without being formally handed over to another nurse and the patient is injured during the absence of the responsible nurse, the law is likely to find the nurse negligent. The fact that the nurse is entitled to a break is no defense for abandonment of the patient.

6. **Is a nurse negligent if he or she leaves a patient to give urgent care to another patient?**

A legal "catch-22" for emergency nurses is the conflict created when multiple patients are in need of immediate care. Unfortunately, if a patient is injured because of the absence of a nurse, even if that nurse is caring for another patient, the law could find the nurse negligent for abandonment of the patient in need of care. The risk management approach to this conundrum is solid teamwork and communication among all emergency nurses and staff on duty. A guiding principle of emergency nursing is that "all patients are everyone's patients." The delicate but necessary ballet of shifting team priorities in emergency nursing and conscientious resource management is the cure for this potential legal exposure.

7. **How do causation and injury relate to negligence?**

That a nurse has failed to fulfill professional duty is not enough to satisfy the theory of negligence. The breach of duty must cause an injury or damage to the patient. As the third necessary element of negligence theory, causation means that the nurse's act or failure to act *directly* harmed the patient. The fourth requirement of negligence theory is injury. The patient must demonstrate either physical harm or emotional pain and suffering as a result of the nurse's behavior.

8. **Besides negligence, what other legal theories are used to prove malpractice?**

Although negligence is the most common legal theory under which nurses are successfully sued, breach of confidentiality and intentional or negligent infliction of emotional harm also constitute professional malpractice. The duty of confidentiality requires the nurse to maintain the privacy of a patient's medical information. Imprudent disclosure, even if unintentional, is a violation of the trust relationship between the patient and the nurse. Infliction of emotional harm can be unintentional, or in the more rare instance, intentional or negligent. These legal theories recognize the emotional vulnerability of a patient and impose liability on a nurse whose outrageous conduct inflicts mental pain and anguish.

9. Can an emergency nurse be sued if a mistake is made?

Not necessarily. For a nurse to be successfully sued, the nurse's mistake must constitute a failure of professional duty to the patient that results in injury. For example, a medication error (a failure of duty) in and of itself may not be lawfully negligent. The medication error must directly injure the patient. Many medication errors do not result in actual harm. Without causing harm, the medication error cannot stand alone as professional negligence. However, medication errors are always a call for the nurse to reevaluate his or her professional practice and make adjustments in behavior for the future.

American society is highly litigious and mistakes can be viewed as an enrichment opportunity. Frivolous lawsuits (meaning those that will not succeed) comprise the majority of legal actions brought against nurses. Although it is unlikely that a patient will prevail in a lawsuit in which all the elements of negligence are not met, all Americans are entitled to bring their legal complaints to court. Most frivolous lawsuits are recognized early on and resolved relatively quickly through a series of pretrial motions, thus sparing the nurse the anguish of trial.

10. If an error is made, should the patient be told?

The traditional approach has been to avoid disclosure of harmless error. The rationale for this approach was that a patient's confidence in the provider and in the healthcare system would be unnecessarily diminished and that disclosure is an invitation for a lawsuit. Recent publications contradict this reasoning. Regulatory agencies including the JCAHO recommend that even harmless error be revealed to the patient. Rather than undermining a patient's confidence, disclosure actually enhances the trust relationship and decreases the likelihood of legal action. Patients who discover that an error was made and that the provider did not disclose the mistake feel betrayed and may respond with anger. Angry patients become litigious patients. *In situations in which harm has occurred, it is wise for disclosure to be made to the patient and significant others as soon as possible.* Under no circumstances should patients be deceived or lied to if they directly question whether a mistake has occurred. When an error results in serious injury, notify the facility's administration and the risk management, quality, or legal department as soon as possible. In addition, the malpractice liability insurance carrier may require timely notification of the event to preserve coverage.

11. What are some tips about disclosure and apologies for errors?

- *Always apologize at the time of disclosure.* Disclosure accompanied by a *sincere* apology is often enough to prevent the patient from taking further steps. Most patients have a large capacity to forgive and will respect the honesty and ethics of organizations and providers who disclose mistakes as routine practice.
- *One person should be the initial emissary for disclosure and apology.* A patient can be overwhelmed and confused by a barrage of providers who all feel the need to disclose and apologize. Remember that it is the patient who was the recipient of substandard care and the patient's needs get first consideration. Providers who make an error, especially one that results in injury to a patient, can be panicked and self-recriminating. They too are needy and this need can be displaced to the

patient with very negative results. Support for the responsible provider should be solid and immediate. Everyone will make a mistake at some time in practice. It is particularly painful for nurses to make mistakes because of the values of human caring and the ethos "do no harm" that are inherent in their training and value system.

- *As a general rule, a provider with whom the patient has a strong relationship should be the person to disclose a harmful error.* This is often the same person who makes the error. If it is not, then the provider who made the mistake should offer his or her own apology after the initial disclosure and apology.
- *If more than one provider is involved with the error, discuss the situation and organize a thoughtful, timely response to the patient.* Again, the danger of an unorganized disclosure is further confusion for the patient. Each involved provider may have her or his own view of the events, and a fragmented approach leaves the patient in the position of putting the pieces together. This may result in the patient arriving at an erroneous conclusion about what truly occurred.
- *Be prepared for an emotional reaction from the patient and anticipate questions.* It is normal for a patient to be upset when a mistake has occurred. Be present for the patient's process of understanding the mistake and accept the patient's reaction. Telling a patient he or she should not be upset may inflame the situation. What patients need is information about the possible consequences of the error, how the error occurred, and what will be done in the future to prevent such errors from happening to the patient or others (the latter two points may not be evident immediately). Stay available to the patient for any further questions he or she may have after the initial conversation.
- *Do not disclose the error of another provider without first discussing the event with that provider.* What may seem like an error to one person may in fact be something very different. Pointing fingers without all the facts is legally dangerous and unwarranted. In addition, the responsible provider generally should be the one to offer the apology and disclosure.
- *When offering an apology, do not make an admission of fault for yourself or another.* Most mistakes stem from a malfunctioning system. It is premature to admit fault before all the contributing factors to an event are understood. Although disclosure and apology should not be delayed pending conclusions of an investigation, admission of liability is unnecessarily gratuitous. Providers, especially nurses, have a propensity for blaming themselves for an error when in fact their actions were the natural outcome of a series of system flaws.

12. Why do some patients sue and others don't?

Patients expect courteous, dignified, compassionate, and supportive relationships with their nurses. When a strong relationship is lacking and an error occurs, patients are more likely to sue. Conversely, patients who have enjoyed a caring relationship with their providers are less likely to sue and are able to forgive the mistake, even when they are injured. As a general rule, people do not sue those they care about. The one exception to this rule is for large medical bills caused by the injurious error. In conjunction with disclosure and apology, the institution should be notified of the error and given the opportunity to dissolve medical bills. At the very least, bills can be put on hold until after an investigation is concluded.

The majority of lawsuits are frivolous and resolved by either being thrown out of court before trial or judged in favor of the defendant provider. Nonetheless, enmeshment in a legal action is one experience most nurses want to avoid. It is costly both emotionally and financially. The three biggest reasons patients bring frivolous lawsuits are:

- Poor communication with healthcare providers
- Negative bedside manner from healthcare providers
- Large medical bills for patient-perceived poor care

13. What can be done to decrease the risk of being sued?

- Develop a strong relationship with the patient and significant others. Relationships are the foremost mitigator of legal action against healthcare providers. It is well known that patients do not sue those they feel connected with in a strong, caring relationship. In addition, juries are less likely to adversely judge a caring nurse. Emergency nurses rarely have the luxury of time to develop relationships because of the episodic and intense nature of contact with patients and their significant others during emergency encounters. *Use every opportunity to impart compassion and caring.*
- Protect the patient's privacy and dignity. Do not discuss highly confidential information in the presence of non-healthcare providers. Do not leave a patient physically exposed.
- Listen to what the patient is saying and respond to his or her concerns.
- Answer questions as completely as possible or find the person who can.
- Whenever possible, give the patient the power of choice.
- Use nonverbal expressions of caring, such as eye contact, appropriate touch, and tone of voice. Appearing rushed and stressed can cause a patient to lose confidence in the clinician's ability to provide adequate care.
- Anticipate the patient's needs for comfort, and intervene. This can be as simple as a warm blanket or as sophisticated as pain control.
- Explain what is happening and why. Whenever possible, prepare patients for the experience of pain or discomfort.
- Respond promptly to nurse call bells and patient requests.
- Apologize for any inconvenience, delay, or mistake.
- Create opportunities to extend the caring relationship past the ED encounter through follow-up phone calls (for patients who are discharged from the ED) or personal visits (for those patients who are admitted).
- Document care in the medical record. As a close second to the relationship with the patient, thorough and professional medical record documentation is a key mitigator of risk. A properly composed medical record can dissuade an attorney from filing suit on behalf of the patient. When suit is filed, the medical record becomes the chief source of information for both the patient's case against the clinician and the clinician's defense. Ultimately, the jury views the medical record as the most persuasive objective evidence on which to decide the case.
- Follow institutional policy, procedure, and protocols. As a general rule, anything written that dictates precise action in particular circumstances must be followed. Failure to follow written direction raises a presumption that something was done incorrectly or negligently. Although it is not possible to memorize every word in a policy and procedure manual, review the table of contents and have knowledge of the policies that are most relevant.

When a situation arises that is confusing or contentious, refer to the written guidelines for direction. On a rare occasion and as an exception to the general rule, an extraordinary situation may arise in which it is not reasonable to follow a written policy, procedure, or protocol. Because this is an extremely unusual circumstance, confer with others and clearly document both the consultation and rationale for the action taken that contradicts any written guideline. An institutional review and revision of policy, procedure, or protocol should be requested whenever stepping outside written guidelines.

- Act in accordance with professional standards of practice. In addition to institutional written guidelines, professional standards of practice dictate a clinician's actions. Often, but not always, written institutional guidelines embody professional standards of practice. Professional organizations and accrediting bodies set standards of practice that clinicians are expected to know and follow. The ENA publishes standards of practice that should be reflected in nursing care.
- Employ professional behavior at all times. Patients are sensitive to unprofessional behavior and equate such behavior with poor care, disregard, personal insult, and misconduct. Inappropriate use of humor, labeling the patient with subjective terms or acronyms (e.g., "dirtball"; "FLK" for "funny looking kid"; "LOL" for "little old lady"), or making jokes at the expense of the patient's dignity are invitations for lawsuits. Socializing among staff away from the patient's bedside, but within sight or hearing, imparts a message that the patient is not a priority. These types of behaviors negate any positive relationship the patient has with the clinician or the rest of the healthcare team. Without a positive relationship, the risk of being sued increases substantially. If the patient can show an ethical transgression, the chances of the hospital winning a lawsuit are greatly decreased.
- Communicate with the healthcare team, the patient, and the patient's significant others. Whether it is a professional duty of notification to a physician or giving information to the patient and those significant to the patient, communication is an integral part of decreasing risk. Clear, thoughtful communication negates the possibility of misperception and can relieve anxiety. Failure to notify is one of the top three reasons for lawsuits against nurses.
- Emergency nurses have an important safety net role for the patient and the healthcare team. A nurse's professional duty may require questioning a physician order or the course of treatment. Although this often is an uncomfortable situation because it causes conflict, communication is a part of professional duty. Do not do something just because it is ordered, even when the physician says, "Go ahead, I'll cover you." Nurses hold independent professional licenses and are responsible for their own actions; a physician cannot "cover" a nurse.

14. Why is documentation so important?

Proper documentation provides the best defense in a legal action. Emergency nurses are limited in their ability to establish relationships with patients and this further emphasizes the need for proper documentation. Strong long-term relationships rank as the primary deterrent to legal action. The emergency environment is not conducive to fostering relationships. Documentation, on the other hand, is fully within the nurse's control. Documentation can prevent legal action altogether; or, in the event of legal action, provide the necessary tool for resolution in the clinician's favor.

15. What should be documented?

Document the care provided so that the events of care can be precisely recreated many years (and many patients) later. Documentation should cover the full spectrum of the nursing process, including gathering subjective (what was reported) and objective information, assessment (information gathered about the patient using professional knowledge and skill), any interventions initiated, the result of those interventions, and the involvement of others in the patient's care. Create a professional product that is concise, to the point, and thorough. Electronic documentation systems are aimed at achieving that outcome. The rules listed in the following table are critical elements in the composition of successful documentation.

Documentation rules

Rule	Reason
Write in blue or black nonerasable ink.	This enables document reproduction to be clear and complete.
Never leave blank spaces other than traditional, expected margins.	This prevents alteration of the medical record.
Line through areas of flow sheets not used.	Areas left unmarked can be viewed as failure to gather required information.
Use proper grammar and spelling.	The ability to deliver competent nursing care is called into question with poor use of the English language. Also, imprecise use of language can create the opportunity for multiple interpretations of the meaning.
Write legibly and do not squeeze words between lines or margins.	Sloppy handwriting and sloppy form decrease the appearance of professionalism in the eyes of the jury. They may also invite a different interpretation of the words used, to the clinician's detriment. Writing in unnatural places can be construed as intentional alteration of the medical record. Chart alteration is a serious legal offense that can result in criminal penalties.
Make changes to the record obvious and allow what was changed to be clearly viewed.	No obliterations (Sharpie pen, scratch outs, or "white out") are allowed that prevent viewing what is underneath. Courts have judged obliterations to be part of a fraudulent scheme to hide the truth.
Properly document notification.	The time of notification The name and title (or relationship to the patient) of the person notified What was reported The response you received from the person notified

Documentation rules—cont'd

Rule	Reason
Accurately and precisely time events.	The time the event occurs is the time to place an event in the medical record (not when there is finally time to write during a busy shift). Use specially created flow sheets, such as cardiac arrest or major trauma records, when caring for a patient in these situations. Flow sheets are usually designed to facilitate efficient, thorough documentation during a rapidly occurring event in which predictable activities occur. If merely recording an event and not participating in care, put "Recorder" after your name. Keep crib notes from which to construct an accurate medical record if events are happening so rapidly that thorough documentation and nursing care cannot happen contemporaneously. Avoid relying on memory alone.
Put date and patient name on each page of documentation.	Mystery pages that appear in the record can be used against you.
Avoid late entries.	Make late entries only if you can say yes to the following three criteria: (1) Is it new information that is not already documented? (2) Is the information significant and patient focused? (3) Can the entry be made in a timely manner (the next time you are on duty)? Late entries are acceptable but far from optimal. Never make a late entry to explain actions or an injury in retrospect or after legal action is commenced. This appears as self-serving and suspicious. If uncertain whether to make a late entry, consult the institution's legal department or risk manager. How to make a late entry is as important as whether to make a late entry. The goal is to make the late entry as obvious and straightforward as possible. Write on a separate sheet of paper, labeling the entry as late with the date of the entry and the date to which the information pertains.
Use abbreviations reasonably.	Medical records are not the place to demonstrate creative skills. Nor are they the place to try out a foreign language or secret code. Abbreviations must be approved by institutional policy and be well known and used within the medical community in which you practice. Abbreviated medical language is dangerous to legal health when more than three abbreviations are used in succession or the abbreviation used is a trendy, new creation.

Continued

Documentation rules—cont'd

Rule	Reason
Thoroughly document medication administration.	Include date, time, and your initials. If the medication is given by injection, note the site, size of needle, and method (intramuscular [IM], subcutaneous, intravenous [IV], or intradermal). For extended IV administration, chart any amount of fluid mixed with the medication and the rate of administration. "As needed" medication requires justification for administration by documenting the malady for which the medication is given and a description of the effect. If a medication is omitted, state the reason. It also may be necessary to notify the physician when medications are omitted.
Provide written discharge instructions.	This is particularly important for emergency nursing because most patients are sent home to care for themselves after their visit. Any and all instruction needs to be noted in the record and given to the patient in writing. Include the following: Medication dosage, frequency, reason for administration, and side effects Treatments the patient is to perform at home with appropriate patient or family teaching on how to perform the treatment Reasons for a return to the ED Follow-up appointments or contact with the primary care physician Activity Diet restrictions or suggestions Preventive self-care for the future
Document the use of both professional and lay translators by name and other identifying data.	A professional translator will usually be sponsored by an outside agency. Lay translators (including family or friends) should be used as a last resort. Clearly note the translator's name, relationship to patient (if any), and translator's phone number and address for possible future contact should questions arise. Any unsuccessful attempts to obtain a translator should be noted with a statement explaining why one could not be found and any alternative communication mode used.
Avoid words such as "somehow," "inadvertently," or "unfortunately."	These kinds of words allude to fault and give the impression that not everything that happened is in the record.
Document patient noncompliance or failure to follow medical direction.	This shows that the patient chose to disregard advice or treatment intended to improve his or her health. Therefore, it is evidence of why improvement was not attained and can explain health decline or further complications.
Document any abusive language or behavior.	Place the exact language in quotes and describe any abusive behavior without elaborate explanation. This is powerful because it shows the adverse circumstances under which you were laboring. Nurses are generally held in high esteem by the public and a jury can be sympathetic when nurses are treated poorly.

16. **What are critical charting errors?**

Failure to document and vague, uncertain documentation top the list. Other common errors are:
- Advance entries
- Charting for someone else
- Labeling the patient
- Alterations to the medical record (or *anything* that can be construed as an alteration whether or not intended to be an alteration)
- Illegible handwriting

17. **Should an adverse event be documented?**

Always document an adverse event and any unusual occurrences. The most important purpose of documentation is communication to other providers. An adverse event often has ongoing implications for care and, if it is not documented, others may not be aware of the patient's true status. The result can be injurious to the patient. Failure to document an adverse event can be viewed as a deceitful and calculated cover-up.

Document the event objectively, recording only what you witnessed. Place descriptive statements made by the patient or others in quotations and attribute the statement to the speaker. Do not explain why the event happened, attribute fault to anyone (including yourself), or make speculations or conclusions about the event. Assessment of the patient after the event and any interventions (including physician notification) also need to be recorded. An organization's risk management program may require completion of an "occurrence report" for all events. If such reporting is requested either on paper or electronically, do not mention this in the patient's record. Mentioning an incident report in the patient's medical record may make that report "discoverable" by attorneys even if it would normally be protected from such discovery by law. Event reporting is an essential component in the management of risk issues. Completing an event report and notifying risk management or the legal office represent comprehensive and responsible reporting and are considered "privileged."

18. **Do nurses really need malpractice insurance?**

Yes. If a nurse provides care to anyone (including gratuitous care in the form of advice to neighbors and friends), professional duty is invoked. Where there is professional duty, there is a chance of being sued. The cost of defense can easily reach six figures. If the jury does not decide in a nurse's favor, a monetary award is usually made to the person suing. Without insurance, these costs become the nurse's individual responsibility. This can mean wage garnishment into the indefinite future and/or confiscation of any assets.

19. **Can a nurse's hospital sue the nurse?**

Under the legal doctrine of contribution, it is possible for the hospital or employer to sue the nurse to recover legal expenses it incurred because of the nurse's malpractice. However, it is rare for institutions to exercise this legal right against employees.

20. What is the Emergency Medical Treatment and Active Labor Act (EMTALA)?

The EMTALA is a federal statute that imposes a duty on hospitals and physicians who are reimbursed for their services with federal money through Medicare. The name of this law was recently changed to the Emergency Medical Treatment and Women in Labor Act to more closely match the current requirements. Other nicknames include the "anti-dumping law" because its original intent was to prevent non paying patients, especially women in labor, from being "dumped" on public hospitals only and "COBRA" because EMTALA is part of the Consolidated Omnibus Budget Reconcilitation Act of 1986. EMTALA is concerned with preventing discrimination against those unable to pay for medical care and is best viewed as a safety net for the uninsured, underinsured, and poor.

21. What does EMTALA require?

For the ED setting, EMTALA requires that any person requesting medical examination while on hospital property be given a medical screening examination (MSE) to determine if an emergency medical condition exists. "Any person" means the person needing the examination or someone requesting the examination on the person's behalf. "Hospital property" is broadly defined to go beyond the physical boundaries of the property to any contiguous property within 250 yards. The request for care can be made to any hospital personnel for the law to be triggered. MSE does not mean triage; it is much more expansive and requires a thorough examination by a qualified provider to rule out an emergency medical condition. The hospital must define "qualified provider" for purposes of an MSE in its medical bylaws as well as policy and procedure. Usually physicians, physician assistants, and/or nurse practitioners are the identified qualified providers. If an emergency medical condition is identified, EMTALA requires that treatment be given until the condition is stabilized. If patient stabilization requires services the hospital does not provide, then the patient may be transferred to another facility that does provide the needed services. The risks and benefits of such a transfer must be explained to the patient and informed consent documented when possible.

EMTALA absolutely forbids inquiry into method of payment, including insurance coverage, before the MSE is completed. Managed care primary physician authorization is irrelevant to EMTALA requirements. Discouraging a patient from receiving services by disclosing cost is viewed as duress and coercion. The law wants to prevent delay in care and to ensure all patients receive needed medical services based on their medical condition and not their pocketbooks. EMTALA does provide for patient refusal of an MSE when the refusal is initiated and desired by the patient. An explanation about the risks of refusal and the benefits of examination must be given to the patient. The patient should sign a form acknowledging the offer of examination, the explanation of risks and benefits, and the voluntary refusal. If a patient leaves before signing, thorough documentation of the encounter to demonstrate the provider's attempt to comply with the law must be done.

22. What are EMTALA requirements for transfer to another facility?

A transfer can be made in only two situations: (1) The patient requests transfer in writing, or (2) A physician certifies that the medical benefits outweigh the risks of transfer and the transfer is necessary for treatment.

23. What are the duties of the transferring facility and the receiving facility?

The transferring facility must provide care within either its capacity or capability, identify and notify an accepting facility and physician, ensure safe transfer by qualified personnel with the necessary equipment to care for the patient en route, and provide copies of pertinent medical records and diagnostic tests. Condition of the patient upon departure must be clearly documented on a transfer form, to include departure vital signs. The receiving facility must have space and qualified personnel to care for the patient and agree to the transfer. Hospitals with specialized capabilities, such as level I trauma designation, burn units, and neonatal ICUs, are obligated to accept a patient requiring their specialized services unless space (capacity) or qualified personnel (capability) are not available.

24. What happens if EMTALA is violated?

Both the physician and the hospital can be penalized with fines as high as $50,000 for each violation; a single episode may include many separate violations. In addition, Medicare licensing can be revoked, which would make it impossible to receive reimbursement for services under Medicare. This effectively puts the institution out of business. Although the individual nurse is not penalized by EMTALA for violations, nursing has an important responsibility by way of institutional policy and procedure for executing EMTALA requirements or ensuring they are met.

25. What is the Health Insurance Portability and Accountability Act (HIPAA)?

HIPAA was enacted by Congress in 1996. It is designed to provide for improved access to health insurance, reduce fraud and abuse, and lower overall healthcare costs.

26. What are the components of HIPAA?

Title I protects the portability of insurance for workers and their families when they change or lose their jobs. Title II (also known as the Administrative Simplification provision) requires that the U.S. Department of Health and Human Services (HHS) establish national standards for electronic healthcare transactions and identifiers for providers, health plans, and employers. Additionally, it provides for the security and privacy of personal health data. Title II includes the following three rules that require further explanation:
- Privacy Rule (effective April 15, 2003). This provides for federal protection for the privacy of broad forms of health information.
- Transactions and Code Set Standard (effective October 16, 2003). This mandates the use of predefined transaction standards and code set for communication in the healthcare industry.

- Security Rule (effective April 21, 2005). This is specific to the protection of electronic health information.

27. How do HIPAA's Title II rules apply to the ED?

There are many challenges to HIPAA compliance in the emergency setting. Communication in the emergency setting includes both verbal and visual methods for managing the delivery of care expeditiously. Tracking boards are typically visible throughout the department to document patients' progress; they must not reveal patient-specific data. Incoming calls inquiring about a specific person being in the department, whether from frantic family members or others, may not be acknowledged without the patient's consent. Visitors to a patient may not be allowed without the patient's consent. Computer screens with patient-specific data must not be visible to the general public. Paper charts may not be left open where the contents may be viewed by persons not directly involved with the care of the patient. Compliance with HIPAA requires very specific training and facility planning.

28. How can an ED record be shared with another provider or health plan?

EDs routinely share a patient's record with a healthcare provider who is a specialist and may not be the primary care provider for the patient. According to HHS, healthcare providers can share information as necessary to provide treatment. This means information may be shared with clinics or other hospitals when referring patients for treatment or coordinating care with others who may help in finding patients appropriate health services. Providers can also share information to the extent necessary to seek payment for healthcare services.

29. Can the nurse notify a patient's family if the patient's condition is serious?

Healthcare providers should get verbal permission from the patient whenever possible, but if the patient is incapacitated, then HHS expects healthcare providers to use their professional judgment and do what they believe to be in the patient's best interest. Special provisions are made for mass casualty situations. In that case the hospital may disclose whether an individual is listed on the facility directory if someone calls to inquire.

30. What level of security exists in ED information systems (EDISs)?

Vendors in today's markets are well versed in the regulatory requirements hospitals must meet. Reputable vendors focus on ensuring the security of the information while it is being created, maintained, transmitted, stored, and accessed in its electronic format.

31. What are important elements to look for in a HIPAA-compliant EDIS?

- Double-level password protection; logon to electronic medical records must prevent unauthorized access to patient information
- Reduction in fraud through the use of standardized forms and identifiers
- Time- and date-stamped audit trails documenting who has accessed and updated a record

- Support of standardized medical data code sets such as ICD-9 and CPT-4
- Standardization of content and interfaces that help to improve compliance with department and hospital protocols and minimize billing irregularities
- HIPAA-compliant report capability that may be requested from local, state, and/or federal health agencies

 Key Points

- The majority of injuries to patients can be traced to flawed systems that either primarily cause the injury or set up the nurse to make a mistake that results in injury to a patient.
- The legal standard of care is the degree of care that a reasonably prudent nurse would exercise in the same or similar circumstances.
- A guiding principle of emergency nursing is that "all patients are everyone's patients."
- Medication errors are always a call for the nurse to reevaluate his or her professional practice and make adjustments in behavior for the future.
- When harm has occurred, it is wise for disclosure to be made as soon as possible to both the patient and significant others.
- Develop a strong relationship with the patient and significant others. Relationships are the foremost mitigator of legal action against healthcare providers.
- Documentation should cover the full spectrum of the nursing process, including gathering subjective (what was reported) and objective information, assessment (information gathered about the patient using professional knowledge and skill), any interventions initiated, the result of those interventions, and the involvement of others in the patient's care.
- EMTALA requires that any person requesting medical examination while on hospital property be given an MSE to determine if an emergency medical condition exists.
- The HIPAA Privacy Rule provides federal protection for the privacy of health information.

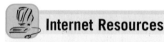

Internet Resources

American Nurses Association, The Nursing Risk Management Series:
www.nursingworld.org/mods/archive/mod311/cerm2abs.htm

Armed Forces Institute of Pathology, The Journal of Nursing Risk Management:
www.afip.org/Departments/legalmed/jnrm.html

Emergency Nurses Association, EMTALA Information:
www.ena.org/government/emtala

Health Privacy Project:
www.healthprivacy.org

Institute of Medicine, Identifying and Preventing Medication Errors:
www.iom.edu/project.asp?id=22526

U.S. Department of Health and Human Services, Office for Civil Rights—HIPAA, Medical PrivacyNational Standards to Protect the Privacy of Personal Health Information:
www.hhs.gov/ocr/hipaa

Bibliography

Hobgood C, Hevia A, Hinchey P: Profiles in patient safety: When an error occurs, *Acad Emerg Med* 11(7):766-769, 2004.

Kohn LT, Corrigan JM, Donaldson MS, editors: *To err is human: Building a safer health system*, Washington, DC, 2000, Committee on Quality of Health Care in America, Institute of Medicine, The National Academies Press.

Laurant LS: Risk management. In Oman K, Koziol-McLain J, Scheetz, editors: *Emergency nursing secrets*, Philadelphia, 2001, Hanley & Belfus.

Mazor KM, Simon SR, Gurwitz JH: Communicating with patients about medical errors: A review of the literature, *Arch Intern Med* 164(15):1690-1697, 2004.

Saville MK, Barker E: Emergency nursing malpractice issues. In Iyer PW: *Nursing malpractice*, ed 2, Tucson, 2001, Lawyers & Judges Publishing.

Summers K: Casting your net wide: An innovative process for closing the loop on risk management reporting, *Nurs Risk Manage 2004*, pp 7-16.

White AA et al: Cause-and-effect analysis of risk management files to assess patient care in the emergency department, *Acad Emerg Med* 11(10):1035-1041, 2004.

Section II

Chief Complaints

Chapter 9

Resuscitation Issues

Reneé Semonin Holleran

1. What is one of the earliest records of human resuscitation?

There is a record of resuscitation in the Old Testament in the Bible. It describes how Elijah laid himself upon a stricken child and prayed to the Lord. Some people speculate that the pressure of Elijah's body may have caused compression and his beard tickling the child's nose may have caused him to sneeze and begin breathing.

In early times, fear and religion forbade interference with death. During the Renaissance, people began to challenge death. Vesalius conducted dissection on animals that uncovered how the heart worked and blood circulated through the body and responded to asphyxiation. He also demonstrated resuscitation by intratracheal mouth-to-tube positive pressure ventilation.

2. What are some past methods used to resuscitate patients?

In 1767 the Society for the Recovery of Drowned Persons was formed in Amsterdam. This was a group of people (early EMS) who responded to sudden deaths—particularly drowning. These societies were formed all over the world, including the United States. In mid-1770, the components of cardiopulmonary resuscitation (CPR)—respiration, compressions, and electricity—began to come together. In 1788, a scientist named Kite first began to discuss how to identify apparent death, also known as "suspended animation" or "real death." He proposed applying an electric shock to the patient to determine death. He further stated that successful resuscitation too frequently depended on circumstances wholly out of one's power to prevent. He proposed that equipment be taken to patients for resuscitation or patients be transported to "houses" where trained individuals could work on them.

Some of the recommended methods for resuscitation included:
- Warming the victim
- Removing swallowed or aspirated water by positioning the patient's head lower than the feet and applying manual pressure to the abdomen and tickling the victim's throat
- Stimulating the victim by such means as rectal and oral fumigation with tobacco smoke
- Yelling at the patient or making loud noises
- Using a bellows or mouth-to-mouth or mouth-to-nostril breathing for the patient
- Blood letting

Kite developed a "spreadsheet" to document all of the information related to the resuscitation, as well as the patient's response. He also analyzed near-drowning resuscitations and found that successful cases resulted most often in a time period of 13.5 minutes. Longer than 30 minutes of resuscitation usually did not produce a positive outcome.

3. **How did modern CPR evolve?**

History of modern CPR

Step	Source	Year
A—Airway: Found that to open the airway, the head should be tilted back and the jaw-thrust maneuver applied.	Safar P, Aguto-Escarraga L, Chang F: Upper airway obstruction in the unconscious patient, *J Appl Physiol* 14:760-764, 1959.	1959
B—Breathing: Demonstrated that direct mouth-to-mouth or mouth-to-nose ventilation effectively oxygenated nonbreathing patients. It is interesting to note that curarized and sedated volunteers were used for this research.	Safar P: Ventilatory efficacy of mouth-to-mouth artificial respiration: Airway obstruction during manual and mouth-to-mouth artificial respiration, *JAMA* 167:335-341, 1958.	1958
C—Circulation: Found with defibrillation when paddles were applied to a dog's chest, the pressure produced an arterial pulse wave.	Kouwenhoven WB, Jude JR, Knickerbocker GG: Closed cardiac massage, *JAMA* 173:1064-1067, 1960.	1960
Basic Life Support (BLS): Combination of A, B, and C.	Safar P: Ventilatory efficacy of mouth-to-mouth artificial respiration: Airway obstruction during manual and mouth-to-mouth artificial respiration, *JAMA* 167(3):335-341, 1958.	1958

4. **What are some of the common causes of cardiopulmonary arrest?**

In adult patients, the common causes include:
- Sudden cardiac death: cardiac arrhythmia, especially ventricular fibrillation
- Drug induced
- Hypoxia
- Trauma (e.g., aortic rupture, atlantooccipital dislocation [AOD], head trauma)
   In pediatric patients, the common causes include:
- Respiratory failure
- Poisoning
- Drowning
- Head trauma

5. **What are some of the current guidelines used for CPR?**

- Basic Life Support (BLS)
- Advanced Cardiac Life Support (ACLS)
- Pediatric Advanced Life Support (PALS)

   Most emergency departments (EDs) require that the nursing staff have ACLS verification or its equivalency. For example, specific scenarios may be used to test the emergency nurse's ability to manage a ventricular fibrillation arrest.

6. **When should CPR be started?**

Using the American Heart Association (AHA) comprehensive electrocardiogram (ECG) algorithm, CPR should be initiated when:
- A person collapses, is found "down," or is unresponsive

and
- An assessment of the airway, breathing, and circulation finds that the person is not breathing and/or does not have a palpable pulse

7. **When should CPR be stopped?**

Evidence continues to demonstrate that if there is no return of spontaneous circulation in the prehospital environment, the chance of morbidity (anoxic brain injury) and mortality increases. Each local EMS service and each ED should have guidelines in place as to when resuscitation may be stopped. The AHA states that CPR should be stopped when:
- The patient responds, has a perfusing pulse, and begins to breath
- A trained professional responder arrives at the scene of the resuscitation and assumes patient care
- The rescuers are too exhausted to continue
- Continued resuscitation of the patient could pose a threat to the rescuers

8. **When should CPR not be performed?**

The AHA states that CPR should not be initiated when:
- There are valid Do Not Attempt Resuscitation (DNAR) orders
- There are obvious signs of death, such as dependent lividity, rigor mortis, algo mortis (continued decrease in body temperature), or injuries incompatible with life (e.g., decapitation)

   In 2003, the National Association of EMS Physicians (NAEMSP) published guidelines to withhold resuscitation for the following traumatically injured patients:
- Blunt trauma patients who are found apneic, pulseless, and without any organized ECG activity
- Victims of penetrating trauma found apneic and pulseless
- Victims with decapitation or hemicorporectomy
- EMS-witnessed cardiopulmonary arrest and 15 minutes of unsuccessful resuscitation

   All these decisions should be based on guidelines and when in doubt with medical direction.

9. **What are advance directives?**

Advance directives such as a living will or medical durable power of attorney are documents that patients create to direct their medical care in the event they lose decision-making capacity. A living will, usually used when the patient's condition is terminal, stipulates the type of medical care the individual desires if he or she becomes unable to make such decisions. Medical durable power of attorney states who the patient wishes to make medical care decisions if he or she is unable to do so. Advance directives are available for both medical and mental healthcare.

10. What are DNAR orders?

Another type of advance directive, a DNAR order (also known as Do Not Resuscitate [DNR]), is a physician order that directs EMS and healthcare providers as to the patient's wishes related to specific resuscitation measures. DNAR orders generally outline what type of resuscitation procedures the patient may or may not desire. These orders may be written for the hospitalized patient; many states also have statutes allowing for DNAR orders in the home setting. In addition to the written copy of the order, patients may have bracelets or necklaces that identify their wishes. Orders should be made accessible in case they are needed. Patients are often told to hang the DNAR form on the kitchen refrigerator for easy access in an emergency. It is important for patients to let their families and healthcare providers know of their wishes.

11. What role does the family play in resuscitation?

Many studies have documented that families want to have a role in the resuscitation of their loved ones. Despite previous myths that family members may not be able to tolerate watching as their family members are resuscitated, there is no evidence to support this belief. The advantages of allowing family members to witness resuscitation include:
- The family member can witness the efforts of the resuscitation team
- The family member can express the wishes of the patient as to whether the patient would want "futile" resuscitation to continue
- The family is provided an opportunity to say good-bye to the patient

12. What are the current survival rates from CPR?

Survival rates continue to remain low (ranging from 0% to 16 %), particularly depending on the cause of the arrest. One problem is related to the definition of survival from cardiac arrest. Is survival defined as from the field to the ED, or as discharge from the hospital? There is also the issue of the quality of survival. Unfortunately, many people who survive to discharge have some type of neurological injury.

In one published series of 161 resuscitation attempts for traumatic cardiac arrest in a level I trauma center in North Carolina, 53 (33%) survived out of ED and 15 (9%) survived to be discharged from the hospital. No patient with agonal rhythm or ventricular fibrillation/tachycardia survived in the study, and 14 out of the 15 hospital survivors had reactive pupils on arrival in the ED.

13. What factors improve out-of-hospital survival rates?

Out-of-hospital cardiac arrest survival is increased by early CPR and use of automated external defibrillators (AEDs). Suggestions for improving survival include:
- Public access defibrillation: Place AEDs in public access areas.
- Home AED: Place AEDs in homes of high-risk patients.

- Correcting the weak link (length of time to resuscitation) in the chain of survival, such as unwitnessed cardiac arrests (unable to determine how long the patient has been down, which makes it difficult to determine the time interval from collapse to the start of resuscitation), absence of trained bystanders, dispatch time, first responder and Advanced Life Support (ALS) provider not rapidly available, and absence of information about the exact time of collapse and the subsequent steps during the resuscitation effort.
- Development of a device that can minimize time between collapse and the need for resuscitation. This device would measure vital signs and transmit the need for help with an AED or other method of resuscitation depending on the cause of the arrest.

14. **What medication has been shown to produce better blood flow to vital organs during resuscitation?**

Small clinical trials found vasopressin (an antidiuretic hormone that functions as a vasoconstrictor when given at supraphysiological dose) to improve blood flow to vital organs, enhance delivery of cerebral oxygen, improve chances of resuscitation, and contribute to better neurological outcomes compared with epinephrine. ACLS recommendations reflected this finding in 2000 revisions, advising a one-time 40 IU dose, replacing epinephrine 1 mg every 3 to 5 minutes. A recent metaanalysis, however, stated that there is "no clear advantage of vasopressin over epinephrine in the treatment of cardiac arrest." The resuscitation polypharmacy regimen is continually being examined, reflecting new drugs, new drug combinations, and new research evidence.

15. **What are some of the complications related to resuscitation?**

Complications from resuscitation include:
- Sternal fractures
- Rib fractures
- Pneumothorax
- Pulmonary barotraumas
- Liver and splenic lacerations
- Anoxic brain injury

Complications such as rib and sternal fractures can be avoided by monitoring the amount of pressure that is being used by the person performing chest compressions. Liver and splenic lacerations may be avoided by proper hand placement. Anoxic brain injury can be avoided by initiating CPR in a timely manner or discontinuing it when resuscitation is found to be futile.

16. **What are some current investigational methods of resuscitation?**

In 1961 the first cardiopulmonary cerebral resuscitation (CPCR) system was proposed. The focus was not only on restarting the heart but also on protecting the heart and brain from the ischemic anoxia that occurs from the causes of the arrest and the resuscitation that follows. Experimental work in resuscitation has evolved to include some of the following:
- **Pharmacological strategies.** For example, fibrinolysis during CPR to prevent the microemboli that occur in the brain, heparin to decrease risk of microemboli in the brain, vasopressin, and antiapoptic strategies (medications to stop programmed cell destruction).

- **Hypothermic cerebral resuscitation.** This strategy's use is time dependent and needs to be induced generally within 15 minutes of return of spontaneous circulation (ROSC).
- **Suspended animation.** Keeping the patient in suspended animation for as long as 2 hours during cardiac arrest so the patient can be transported to a facility that can manage the cause of the cardiac arrest. This is accomplished by lowering the patient's body temperature. A catheter is inserted in the aorta and the patient is cooled. The purpose of cooling the brain is to delay energy failure and reduce ion refluxes, glutamate release, lactic acidosis, free radical reactions, cerebral edema, intracranial pressure (ICP), and tightening of the membranes.
- **Impedance valves.** Impedance valves in the respiratory circuit are currently being studied and may play a role in improving oxygenation and cerebral outcomes. A small disposable plastic valve is attached to the endotracheal tube (ETT) or a face mask and works by impeding inspiratory air flow during the decompression phase of CPR when the patient is not being actively ventilated. This creates a small vacuum within the chest that enhances venous return.

17. What lies ahead in the future of resuscitation?

- Develop uniform data points related to the definitions of "cardiac arrest" and "survival." The Utstein model was developed as a method of collecting data based on when the arrest occurred, how the patient was resuscitated (BLS versus ACLS), time to care from time of arrest, and other related variables. It was revised in 2004 but is still not uniformly used because data collection is cumbersome. The National Registry of CardioPulmonary Resuscitation (NRCPR) was started by the AHA based on the Utstein definitions.
- Develop core time events to be recorded (e.g., date of death, time when call received, time of first rhythm analysis/assessment of need for CPR, time of first CPR attempt, time of first defibrillation attempt if shockable rhythm).
- Ensure consistent delivery of cardiac compressions to maintain perfusion pressure; increase the rate of chest compressions.
- Development of a portable cardiopulmonary bypass (CBP) machine that can be placed in the field to support the patient in cardiac arrest.
- Initiation of ultra-ALS physician-led mobile critical units.
- Switching earlier to open-chest CPR.
- Using aortic flush to induce hypothermia in the field or as early as possible.
- Development of medications to prevent the "programmed" destruction of neuron and cardiac cells.
- Focus on prevention of cardiac arrest (e.g., diet, exercise).
- Determining "when dead is dead."

Safar is quoted with saying, "Death is not the enemy, but occasionally needs help with timing."

Key Points

- The best method of managing a cardiac arrest is prevention (never having one in the first place) through a healthy lifestyle. Diet and exercise contribute greatly to this.

- Electricity saves lives. AEDs need to be available in places where people are, and the public should be educated as to their use.

- The best way to manage a cardiac arrest is to use practice scenarios so that staff feel comfortable with equipment and medications.

- Use tools that provide weight-based medications, ETT sizes, defibrillation joules, and general arrhythmia management. Many monitor companies will provide these.

- Emergency care providers need to have guidelines for the initiation and ceasing of resuscitation. These guidelines should be communicated to all who may need to use them (prehospital care providers, ED personnel) and periodically evaluated based on clinical evidence.

- Emergency care providers need to be aware of DNR orders for the patients they care for and respect their patients' wishes.

- States, counties, cities, and hospitals need to participate in DNR legislation and public education.

- Emergency care providers should discuss how they would like to be managed if they sustain a cardiac arrest and are not able to make end-of-life decisions on their own.

- The occurrence of cardiac arrests and survival rates are not well defined. Research must continue in that area.

- Emergency care providers must keep an open mind about resuscitation and its future.

Internet Resources

American Heart Association:
www.americanheart.org

National Registry of CardioPulmonary Resuscitation:
www.nrcpr.org

Society of Critical Care Medicine:
www.sccm.org

Bibliography

Casner M, Anderson D, Isaacs M: The impact of a new CPR assist device on rate of return of spontaneous circulation in out-of-hospital cardiac arrest, *Prehosp Emerg Care* 9:61-67, 2005.

Cera SM et al: Physiologic predictors of survival in post-traumatic arrest, *Am Surg* 69:140-144, 2003.

Cummins R, editor: *ACLS provider manual*, Dallas, Tex, 2001, American Heart Association.

Ewy G: Cardiocerebral resuscitation: The new cardiopulmonary resuscitation, *Circulation* 111:2134-2142, 2005.

Jacobs I, Nadkarmi V, and the ILCOR Task Force on Cardiac Arrest and Cardiopulmonary Resuscitation Outcomes: Cardiac arrest and cardiopulmonary resuscitation outcome reports, *Circulation* 110:3385-3397, 2004.

Levy M et al: Outcomes of patient with do-not-intubate orders treated with noninvasive ventilation, *Crit Care Med* 32:2002-2007, 2004.

National Association of EMS Physicians (NAEMSP) Standards and Clinical Practice Committee and the American College of Surgeons Committee on Trauma: Guidelines for withholding or termination of resuscitation in prehospital traumatic cardiopulmonary arrest, *J Am Coll Surg* 196:475-481, 2003.

Nozari A et al: Mild hypothermia during prolonged cerebral resuscitation increases conscious survival in dogs, *Crit Care Med* 32:2110-2116, 2004.

Safar P: The future of reanimatology, *Acad Emerg Med* 7:75-89, 2000.

Safar P et al: Cerebral resuscitation potentials for cardiac arrest, *Crit Care Med* 30:S140-144, 2002.

Safar P, Fink B, McGoldrick K, editors: From Vienna to Pittsburgh for anesthesiology and acute medicine. In *Careers in anesthesiology*, vol V, Park Ridge, Ill, 2000, Wood Library-Museum of Anesthesiology, 2000:343.

Sayre MR et al: Measuring survival rates from sudden cardiac arrest: The elusive definition, *Resuscitation* 62:25-34, 2004.

Wellens H, Gorgels AP, de Munter H: Cardiac arrest outside of the hospital: How can we improve results of resuscitation? *Circulation* 107:1948-1950, 2003.

Wenzel V et al: A comparison of vasopressin and epinephrine for out-of-hospital cardiopulmonary resuscitation, *N Engl J Med* 350:105-113, 2004.

Wenzel V, Linder K: Arginine vasopressin during cardiopulmonary resuscitation: Laboratory evidence, clinical experience and recommendations and a view to the future, *Crit Care Med* 30:S157-161, 2002.

Headache

Lois Schick

1. What are the different classifications of headache?

The International Headache Society (IHS) classifies headache into primary and secondary disorders. Primary headache disorders include migraine, tension, and cluster. Secondary headache disorders result from a pathological process such as head or neck trauma, cranial or cervical vascular disorder, nonvascular intracranial disorder, substance use or withdrawal, infection, disturbance of homeostasis (e.g., hypoxia, hypercapnia, arterial hypertension, fasting, dialysis), facial or cranial structure disorder, or psychiatric disorders.

2. What are migraine headaches and how are they described?

Migraine headaches are divided into those without an aura (the common migraine) and those with an aura (the classic migraine). Patients with migraines usually have a family history of migraines. Migraine attacks can last from 4 to 72 hours, are usually unilateral, have a pulsating quality, are moderate or severe in pain intensity, and are aggravated by or cause avoidance of routine physical activity such as walking or climbing stairs. Other symptoms commonly associated with migraine headaches include nausea, vomiting, photophobia, and phonophobia.

Migraines often begin in childhood and are more frequent during adolescence. Before puberty, boys are more affected than girls. Parents become concerned that a more serious condition is present when their child complains of a headache. Children with serious underlying conditions such as intracranial hemorrhage, brain tumor, and meningitis have one or more objective findings on their neurological examination. These findings include altered level of consciousness, nuchal rigidity, papilledema, abnormal eye movements, ataxia, and hemiparesis. If these abnormalities occur, further neurological imaging is indicated. For the child with a migraine, treatment is usually divided into general measures and pharmacological treatment. General measures include reassuring the patient and caregiver of the cause of the headache if known, removing triggers, and instituting behavioral therapies such as analgesics and adequate sleep. Pharmacological treatment of pediatric migraines includes intermittent use of oral analgesics and antiemetics.

3. Do migraines increase with the menstrual cycle in women?

Women suffer migraines more frequently than men and these headaches occur before, during, and immediately after the female period or during ovulation. Migraines are primarily caused by estrogens that regulate the menstrual cycle fluctuations. Women on birth control pills that influence estrogen levels may experience more menstrual headaches. Medications for treating females with menstrual migraines include nonsteroidal antiinflammatory drugs (NSAIDs), ergotamines, beta blockers, and selective serotonin reuptake inhibitors (SSRIs). Pregnancy seems to protect women against migraines because of the estrogen and progesterone levels being fairly consistent. If women do suffer migraines during pregnancy, they usually disappear after the first trimester. When migraines occur during the first trimester, medications are avoided because the fetus is susceptible to drug-induced deformities.

4. What are tension headaches?

Tension headaches are the most common type of primary headache. They can last from 30 minutes to 7 days. Common characteristics of tension headaches include pressing/tightening (nonpulsating) pain of mild or moderate intensity, bilateral location, and not being aggravated by or causing avoidance of routine physical activity such as walking or climbing stairs. Nausea, vomiting, photophobia, and phonophobia are usually absent with tension headaches.

5. What are cluster headaches?

Cluster headaches can last from 15 to 180 minutes. Cluster headaches are more frequent in men, and patients usually do not have a positive family history. Cluster headaches typically occur multiple times per day for weeks, followed by pain-free intervals. Cluster headaches frequently are associated with one of the following signs: conjunctivae injection, lacrimation, nasal congestion, forehead and facial sweating, miosis, ptosis, and eyelid edema. The following table summarizes the clinical features of the three primary types of headache.

Clinical features of primary headache

	Tension	Migraine	Cluster
Common features	Depression Anxiety	Aura in 20%	Occurs in clusters Seasonal
Length of headache	30 min-7 days	4-72 hrs	15-180 min if untreated
Types of pain	Dull Persistent Tightening Pressing	Severe Pulsatile Throbbing	Excruciating
Location of pain	Bilateral Band around head	Unilateral or bilateral	Unilateral Behind one eye Radiates to temple, jaw, nose, chin, or teeth
Physical activity	Not aggravated	Aggravated	Restlessness/agitation Incapacitating

From McCaffery M, Pasero C: *Pain: Clinical manual*, ed 2, St Louis, 1999, Mosby.

Clinical features of primary headache—cont'd

	Tension	Migraine	Cluster
Accompanying symptoms	None	Phonophobia	Facial flushing
		Photophobia	Nasal congestion
		Facial paleness	Drooping eyelid
		Nausea and vomiting	Pupillary changes

---

6. **What are the triage priorities for a person complaining of a severe headache?**

    A diagnosis of the headache type is based on the patient's history and the presenting symptoms. Important assessment parameters include:
    - Vital signs
    - Onset of pain (sudden or gradual? how long ago?)
    - Neurological assessment, including evaluation for facial droop by asking patient to smile; evaluation for arm weakness by holding arms outstretched with eyes closed; and evaluation of speech for slurring, inappropriate words, and inability to speak
    - Quality of pain
    - Intensity of pain
    - History of trauma
    - Vision problems or photophobia
    - Presence of nausea or vomiting
    - Medications taken

7. **In patients presenting with a headache, what signs and symptoms indicate a possible life-threatening situation?**

    The patient's history and presenting symptoms are essential in diagnosing underlying disease. Considerations in the history include sudden headache onset without similar headaches in the past, concomitant infection, altered mental status, headache precipitated by vigorous exercise, and pain radiating into the neck and between the shoulders. The physical examination may show nuchal rigidity, a toxic appearance, decreased level of consciousness, neurological abnormalities, and papilledema.

8. **What is the significance of the chief complaint, "This is the worst headache of my life"?**

    Patients who complain of having the worst headache of their life may be having a subarachnoid hemorrhage. Subarachnoid hemorrhage is the most common cause of intense and incapacitating headache of abrupt onset (thunderhead headache). Loss of consciousness along with nuchal rigidity, nausea, and vomiting may accompany the headache. Physical findings are focal neurological deficits, low-grade fever, meningeal irritation, and altered level of consciousness. Subarachnoid hemorrhage is associated with polycystic kidney disease, fibromuscular dysplasia, and coarctation of the aorta. Subarachnoid hemorrhage is a neurosurgical emergency. Aneurysm rupture is most common in patients 35 to 65 years of age, and multiple aneurysms may occur in 10% to 15% of patients.

9. Is there a way to distinguish legitimate headache sufferers from the drug-seeking patient?

The National Headache Foundation (NHF) has identified a guide for distinguishing between the drug seeker and the legitimate headache patient. These differences are listed in the following box.

Differences between the drug-seeking patient and legitimate headache sufferer

Drug-Abuse/Drug-Seeking Patient
Makes frequent emergency department (ED) visits
States multiple allergies to non-narcotic interventions
Has extensive knowledge of drug action
Requests specific medications and dosages
Has multiple prescriptions for analgesic medications
Requests large number of pills and refills
Relays unusual or irrational stories
Pain requirement is inconsistent with drug requirement
Sees multiple physicians and/or multiple treatment sites
Does not make provision for follow-up care

Legitimate Headache Sufferer
Has a physician who can confirm diagnosis and give reliable patient information
Medical history is consistent with diagnosis of headache
Has had prior diagnostic work-up
Is nondemanding regarding medication necessity
Is deemed reliable by emergency staff

Possible Headache Sufferer
May experience depression
May exhibit feelings of low self-esteem
May indicate feelings of frustration with home or work
Feels loss of control over situation
May feel headache encompasses entire life
May exhibit hostility over physician's inability to control or alleviate headache

Modified from National Headache Foundation,
www.headaches.org/professional/educationresources/erprotocol.html.

10. **What comfort measures can be effective for patients with headaches?**

Provide the patient with cold compresses and a darkened, quiet environment.

11. **What are the expected pharmaceutical treatments for headaches? How do they work?**

Palliative medications include analgesics, antiemetics, ergotamine preparations, and NSAIDs. For prophylactic drug therapy, the physician may order serotonin agonists (triptans), beta-adrenergic blockers, calcium channel blockers, monoamine oxidase inhibitors (MAOIs), or tricyclic antidepressants. Diuretics, antihistamines, anticonvulsants, and short courses of steroids may be used. Female patients with migraines should avoid oral contraceptives. The following table identifies medications that are frequently used to treat headaches. Refer to other sources for appropriate dosing amounts.

Headache medications

Type	Medication
Antiemetics	Metoclopramide (Reglan)
	Prochlorperazine (Compazine)
	Promethazine (Phenergan)
Beta blockers	Atenolol
	Metoprolol
	Nadolol
	Propranolol
Calcium channel blockers	Diltiazem
	Verapamil (Verelan)
Cyclooxygenase-2 (COX-2) inhibitors	Celecoxib (Celebrex)
Ergot alkaloids	Dihydroergotamine (DHE)
	Ergotamine and caffeine
Narcotics	Butorphanol spray (Stadol)
	Butorphanol IV (Stadol)
	Meperidine (Demerol)
	Oxycodone (Percodan)
	Propoxyphene (Darvon)
	Tramadol (Ultram)
NSAIDs	Diclofenac K (Cataflam)
	Flurbiprofen (Ansaid)
	Ibuprofen (Advil, Motrin, Nuprin)
	Ketoprofen (Orudis)
	Naproxen (Aleve, Anaprox DS, Naprosyn)
	Piroxicam (Feldene)

Data from Markovchick V, Pons P, editors: *Emergency medicine secrets*, ed 3, Philadelphia, 2003, Hanley & Belfus; Tauro J: Clinical diagnosis and treatment of headache. In Miller R, Abram S, editors: *Atlas of anesthesia, vol VI: Pain management*, Philadelphia, 1998, Churchill Livingstone; and American Council for Headache Education: *Understanding your medicines*, www.achenet.org.

Continued

Headache medications—cont'd

Type	Medication
Serotonin agonists	Almotriptan (Axert)
	Eletriptan oral tabs (Relpax)
	Frovatriptan (Frova)
	Naratriptan (Amerge)
	Rizatriptan (Maxalt tabs)
	Sumatriptan (Imitrex)
	Zolmitriptan (Zomig)
Tricyclic antidepressants	Amitriptyline
	Doxepin
	Imipramine
	Nortriptyline

12. **When should a lumbar puncture (LP) be performed?**

Computed tomography (CT) scan and magnetic resonance imaging (MRI) may miss infection in a small percentage of subarachnoid bleeds. An LP is indicated to diagnose or rule out meningitis and subarachnoid bleed. Usually LP will not be performed until the CT scan has ruled out a major bleed or intracranial mass lesion.

13. **What kind of discharge instructions should be given to the patient diagnosed with a tension headache?**

Symptoms for a tension headache may be the same as those for a migraine or cluster headache. After diagnosis of a tension headache, teaching is the key intervention for patients. Offer reassurance and education about the use of non-addictive analgesics such as NSAIDs, acetaminophen, enteric-coated aspirin, tricyclic antidepressants, and SSRIs (e.g., fluoxetine, trazodone). Biofeedback, acupuncture, and cervical spine manipulation performed by experts may benefit the patient with tension headaches. Include information about foods (see the following question), activity, and stress reduction.

14. **What specific foods can trigger headaches?**

Any type of ethanol can trigger a headache, but red wines and other foods containing tyramines (e.g., beer; aged cheeses such as cheddar, Gruyere, Brie, and Camembert) seem to be the worst. Caffeinated beverages and nuts may trigger many types of headaches. Nitrates and nitrites in hot dogs, salami, processed meats, ham, and bacon, as well as yeast in sourdough bread, pizza, and raised doughnuts have been implicated. Monosodium glutamate (MSG) in packaged soups, chocolate, beer, and ale also have triggered headaches.

15. Other than foods, are there other triggers for headaches?

Other triggers for headaches include hormones in both men and women; sensory stimuli including flickering or strong lights, odors, and noise; and changes in the environment including weather, seasons, altitude, sleeping patterns, dieting, and irregular physical activity. Stress can also be a trigger for patients, such as occurs with losses or life changes involving death, separation, divorce, job changes, moving, and times of intense activity.

16. What is a rebound headache?

Rebound headaches are caused by withdrawal from an excessive use of over-the-counter or prescription medications. Many patients with rebound headaches have been treated over a long period for migraines or have had a previous head injury. Rebound headaches are more intense on awakening because usually the patient has slept through the night drug-free. Patients with rebound headaches frequently suffer depression because of the chronicity of their pain. Clinical experience has shown that opioid or nonopioid analgesic or ergotamine use for more than 2 days per week can lead to rebound headache after the medication is discontinued.

17. How are rebound headaches treated?

Treatment consists of detoxifying the patient by tapering medications slowly. This is a difficult time for the patient, and it may take 3 to 5 days before the withdrawal headache, with associated nausea and vomiting, subsides. If patients can tolerate 3 to 5 days of discomfort, the rebound headache will disappear. NSAIDs have proven to be effective in treating rebound headaches and do not cause rebound. Dihydroergotamine and metoclopramide also do not cause rebound headaches.

Key Points

- There are two classifications of headaches: primary and secondary.
- Primary headaches include migraine, tension, and cluster, none of which are considered life threatening, but may be temporarily disabling.
- Secondary headache disorders result from a pathological process, so assessment and making the differential diagnosis are essential when evaluating patients in the ED.
- Secondary headaches associated with subarachnoid hemorrhage, meningitis, and brain tumors with increased intracranial pressure (ICP) can be life threatening. Other secondary headaches accompanying sinusitis, hypertension, and LP are generally benign and reversible.
- A patient who complains of the "worst headache of my life" and describes a sudden, thunderclap onset, may have a potentially life-threatening subarachnoid bleed.
- During triage and treatment of patients with headaches, consider the differences between legitimate headache sufferers and drug-seeking patients.
- Pharmaceutical treatments for headaches range from mild to moderate to severe. Antiemetics and rescue medications may be used in conjunction with pain relievers.
- There are multiple triggers for patients developing headaches, including diet, hormones, sensory stimuli, stress, and changes in one's environment or habits.
- When assessing the patient presenting with a headache, consider the possibility of a rebound headache.

 Internet Resources

Aetna InteliHealth, Diseases & Conditions, Headache:
www.intelihealth.com/headache

American Council for Headache Education:
http://achenet.org

American Headache Society:
http://ahsnet.org

International Headache Society:
www.i-h-s.org

National Headache Foundation, Educational Resources, The Emergency Room Guide to Distinguishing the Legitimate Headache Sufferer from the Drug Seeking Patient:
www.headaches.org/professional/educationresources/erprotocol.html

Bibliography

Headache Classification Subcommittee of the International Headache Society: The international classification of headache disorders, ed 2, *Cephalagia* 24(suppl 1):1-160, 2004.

Markovchick V, Pons P, editors: *Emergency medicine secrets*, ed 3, Philadelphia, 2003, Hanley & Belfus.

McCaffery M, Pasero C: *Pain: Clinical manual*, ed 2, St Louis, 1999, Mosby.

Newberry L: *Sheehy's emergency nursing principles and practice*, ed 5, St. Louis, 2003, Mosby.

Pathophysiology: A 2-in-1 reference for nurses, Philadelphia, 2005, Lippincott Williams & Wilkins.

Schick L: Headache. In Oman K, Koziol-McLain J, Scheetz L, editors: *Emergency nursing secrets*, Philadelphia, 2001, Hanley & Belfus.

Schull M: Headache and Facial Pain. In Tintinalli J, editor: *Emergency medicine: A comprehensive study guide*, ed 5, New York, 2000, McGraw-Hill.

Skillmasters: *3-Minute assessment*, Springhouse, PA, 2003, Lippincott Williams & Wilkins.

Snyder J: Neurological emergencies. In Jordan K, editor: *Emergency nursing core curriculum*, ed 5, Philadelphia, 2000, WB Saunders.

St Marie B: *Core curriculum for pain management nursing*, Philadelphia, 2002, WB Saunders.

Stone CK, Antonacci NJ: Headache. In Stone CK, Humphries RL, editors: *Current emergency diagnosis and treatment*, ed 5, New York, 2004, McGraw-Hill.

Tauro J: Clinical diagnosis and treatment of headache. In Miller R, Abram S, editors: *Atlas of anesthesia, vol VI: Pain management*, Philadelphia, 1998, Churchill Livingstone.

Waldman S: *Atlas of interventional pain management*, Philadelphia, 2004, WB Saunders.

Seizures

Barbara A. Overby

1. What is a seizure? How does it differ from epilepsy?

A seizure is an electrical storm inside the brain consisting of abnormal or excessive discharge from neurons. The brain is overwhelmed by this chaotic, disorganized activity and a seizure ensues. Therefore, a seizure is a symptom rather than a disease. In contrast, epilepsy is a clinical condition characterized by recurrent seizures. The term "epilepsy" comes from the Greek word "epilambanein," which means to seize or to attack. Approximately 1% to 2% of the U.S. population has a seizure disorder. However, one seizure does not constitute a diagnosis of epilepsy.

2. What can cause seizures?

- Infections (meningitis)
- Fever in children
- Head trauma or hemorrhage
- Brain tumor
- Drug overdoses
- Drug toxicities
- Alcohol or benzodiazepine withdrawal
- Cocaine
- Stroke
- Metabolic imbalances (e.g., hypoglycemia and hyperglycemia, hypoxia, hyponatremia and hypernatremia, hypocalcemia, hypomagnesemia)

3. How are seizures classified?

Seizure classifications

Generalized (Involving Entire Body)
Tonic-clonic (grand mal)
Absence (petit mal)

Partial or Focal (Specific Part of the Body)
Simple partial
Complex partial
Partial with secondary generalization

4. **What first-line medications are used to treat seizures?**

TONIC-CLONIC SEIZURES
Carbamazepine (Tegretol, Carbatrol)
Phenytoin (Dilantin)
Valproate (Depakene, Valproic acid)

PARTIAL SEIZURES
Carbamazepine (Tegretol, Carbatrol) in children
Phenytoin (Dilantin) in adults
Valproate (Depakene, Valproic acid)

ABSENCE SEIZURES
Ethosuximide (Zarontin)
Valproate

5. **How do healthcare providers select a medication for epilepsy treatment?**

The selection of a seizure medication is based on seizure type. The healthcare provider's goal is for medication monotherapy with as low a dose as possible to prevent side effects while controlling the seizures. From the patient's perspective, the cost of the medication and resulting side effects will play a role in compliance. About 75% of people diagnosed with epilepsy will be able to achieve seizure control with antiepileptic medicines.

6. **What type of activity should one expect during a seizure?**

The activity depends on the type of seizure. The tonic-clonic seizure (formerly known as grand mal) is the most common seizure in the emergency department (ED)—and the most dramatic. The patient experiences an abrupt loss of consciousness and loses organized muscle tone. The patient may fall, causing injuries. In the tonic phase, the patient becomes rigid with extensor muscle spasms affecting the trunk, arms, and legs. Many patients experience apnea during this phase. Bladder and bowel control may be affected with resulting incontinence. During the clonic phase, the patient experiences strenuous, rhythmic muscle contractions accompanied by hyperventilation, sweating, tachycardia, and excessive salivation. At the conclusion of the seizure, the patient experiences muscle relaxation and deep breathing. Tonic-clonic seizures usually last for less than 2 minutes, even though bystanders frequently overestimate the duration.

The classic absence seizure occurs in children (4 to 12 years old). The seizure involves the child appearing to stare off into space. It is brief (less than 15 seconds), beginning and ceasing abruptly, and then the child resumes his or her prior activity without awareness of the event.

Partial or focal seizures are classified as "simple" if there is no alteration in consciousness or awareness of environment and "complex" if such a change occurs. Partial seizures may involve focal motor activity, somatic sensory symptoms, or disturbances in the patient's senses. Partial seizures (simple or complex) with secondary generalization originate in one part of the body and then progress until the entire body is involved.

7. What is a jacksonian march?

A jacksonian march is a partial seizure that may begin in a finger and progress—or "march through"—in an organized fashion to involve the rest of the arm. It also may spread to the face, other arm, or legs.

8. Do people see lights or experience unusual sensations before seizing?

Some patients experience an "aura" immediately before the physical manifestation of the seizure. Auras have been described as a "funny" or "sick" feeling, or as disturbances in the senses—lights, odd smell, strange taste, or sound (crying out).

9. Why is glucose measurement important for seizure patients?

Hypoglycemia is an easily corrected cause of seizures, saving the patient from unnecessary and expensive lab work and tests. Because the act of seizing requires large amounts of glucose, a patient can experience hypoglycemia as the result of a seizure.

10. What are the treatment priorities for a seizing patient?

Ensure the safety of the patient and remember your own safety. The goal is to prevent injuries; therefore, pad or remove objects around the patient. Although the patient's physical movements cannot be stopped, they can be guided during the seizure. Turn the patient to one side, and have suction and airway equipment readily available. Attempting to force an airway in an actively seizing patient can cause tooth avulsion, oral injuries, respiratory distress, vomiting, aspiration for the patient, and bitten fingers for the nurse. To prevent bite injuries place nothing in the patient's mouth. If an airway adjunct is needed, remember the nasal airway.

At the conclusion of the seizure, assess pulse oximetry, and place the patient on oxygen (if not already done). Obtain a blood sample as soon as possible to test for hypoglycemia, initiate an intravenous (IV) line, and collect a blood specimen to measure anticonvulsant medication levels. Observe for more seizures, and monitor the patient's return to baseline neurological function. Make sure that the bed is in a low position with upright, padded siderails. Because most seizures are self-limiting, keen observation skills and supportive care are usually enough. As always, reassure and reorient the patient frequently.

11. What should be documented after witnessing a patient having a seizure?

- Document what you saw: body parts involved, motor activity, and seizure progression. Pay special attention to the head, eyes, and extremity movements. This information may lead to finding the focus of the seizure.
- Estimate the duration, or (preferably) time the various components of the seizure.
- Note whether the patient experienced incontinence (urine or stool) with the seizure.
- Note whether the patient experienced any trauma during the seizure.
- Monitor and make chart entries about the patient's recovery during the postictal phase.

12. **What is considered normal during the postictal phase?**

Patients feel like they have run a marathon. A seizure, like a marathon, requires large amounts of oxygen and glucose. The patient is fatigued and may sleep for many hours after the seizure. The patient is usually amnesic to the event and may be confused or combative. It is normal for the postictal patient to have a depressed level of consciousness during recovery. The postictal phase varies in length from minutes to hours, depending on what is normal for each patient.

13. **What is status epilepticus? Why is it life threatening?**

Status epilepticus is prolonged seizure activity for 15 to 30 minutes or two or more seizures without full recovery between seizures. Repetitive or prolonged seizures require increased muscle activity associated with periods of decreased or absent ventilation. These actions cause hypoxia and a switch from aerobic to anaerobic metabolism. Prolonged hypoxia results in lactic and metabolic acidosis. The patient's temperature, blood pressure, and pulse are increased, and there is a potential for hypoglycemia. The real danger is interruption of the oxygen supply to brain cells and the metabolic demands on the brain. The patient needs definitive airway management, and control of the seizures is critical.

14. **What medications are used to control seizures emergently?**

Uncomplicated seizures generally do not require emergent treatment with IV medications. For management of acute recurrent or prolonged seizures, benzodiazepines are the treatment of choice and are usually given via IV line. The most commonly used medications are lorazepam (Ativan), diazepam (Valium), and midazolam (Versed).

15. **What are the second-line medications?**

Anticipate an order for an IV loading dose of either phenytoin (Dilantin) or fosphenytoin (Cerebyx). Phenytoin is the "old timer" and fosphenytoin is rather new on the market. Both can be given in an IV loading dose requiring cardiac monitoring and observation. Phenytoin can be mixed only in 0.9% normal saline; it precipitates when mixed with 5% dextrose. Administer a loading dose of 10 to 15 mg/kg at a rate not to exceed 50 mg/min.

Fosphenytoin is converted to phenytoin rapidly in the body after administration. Fosphenytoin orders must be written in phenytoin equivalents (PE). The dosage for fosphenytoin is 15 to 20 mg PE/kg at a rate of 100 to 150 mg PE/min. An advantage of fosphenytoin is markedly less venous irritation, allowing faster infusion rates with an IV loading dose. Fosphenytoin also can be mixed with 5% dextrose or 0.9% normal saline or given in an intramuscular (IM) injection. The major disadvantage of fosphenytoin is cost; it is much more expensive than phenytoin.

16. **Are alcohol withdrawal seizures managed differently?**

Yes. The management of the generalized seizure is no different; benzodiazepines are used as needed to treat the acute seizure. Management may differ, however, because the person who experiences an alcohol withdrawal seizure is also at high risk for metabolic abnormalities, subdural hematoma, and central nervous system infections.

17. EMS just delivered a lethargic patient who had several seizures before arrival at the emergency department (ED). The paramedic reported that she was unable to establish an IV line but gave the patient a benzodiazepine medication to stop the seizure activity. How was this done?

The paramedic may have given the benzodiazepine via IM injection. Even more common in EMS systems (although not particularly popular among paramedics) is rectal administration of diazepam. Some EMS systems have protocols that allow rectal administration in both pediatric and adult patients. Wolfe and Bernstone (2004) report that several studies have investigated intranasally administered benzodiazepines in treating acutely seizing patients. They concluded that intranasal midazolam is more effective than rectal administration and as effective as IV administration. Scott et al (1999) investigated buccal (between cheek and teeth) administration of midazolam for management of seizures by nonmedical caregivers at home and concluded that buccal midazolam is as effective as rectal diazepam and involves a more acceptable route. Some of these methods may soon be common.

18. A patient exhibiting unilateral paralysis and speech problems 30 minutes before arrival in the ED was initially assessed and treated according to the ED stroke pathway but was then diagnosed with Todd's paralysis. What is Todd's paralysis, and is treatment different than for stroke?

Todd's paralysis is a neurological condition characterized by a period of temporary paralysis after a seizure. The paralysis is usually unilateral and also may affect speech or vision. The cause of Todd's paralysis is unknown and the treatment is supportive because the paralysis resolves quickly. It is important to distinguish the condition from a stroke, which requires different care and treatment.

19. What is a "breakthrough" seizure?

A breakthrough seizure occurs when a patient has a seizure despite a therapeutic level of medication. The therapeutic level may be different for each patient depending on the optimal drug level needed to control seizures. Dosing adjustments may be necessary based on the patient's seizure and medication history.

20. What is special about new-onset or first-time seizures?

The patient who has a first-time seizure causes more concern because seizures are sometimes the initial presentation of serious conditions such as brain tumor, intracranial hemorrhage, or drug overdose. The acute treatment is the same regardless of whether the seizure is new or recurrent. However, the first-time seizure patient should receive a computed tomography (CT) scan; extensive laboratory tests, including a sepsis work-up; and a neurological evaluation. Depending on the results of the CT scan, the patient may undergo a lumbar puncture (LP) and an electroencephalogram (EEG), either in the ED or after admission to the hospital.

21. **What observational clues, other than witnessing a seizure, support the suspicion of a seizure?**

First look for medical alert tags, usually a bracelet or necklace. Then look for medication bottles (possibly empty) or prescriptions. Inspect the patient's mouth for intraoral injuries, which may be indicative of biting during the seizure. Note if the patient was incontinent of urine or stool. After a seizure, the patient usually cannot recall the event and is confused. A patient who experienced a generalized seizure exhibits an anion gap that resolves quickly, usually within the first hour after the seizure.

22. **What are febrile seizures?**

A febrile seizure is a generalized tonic-clonic seizure associated with fever; the source of the fever is outside the central nervous system. Febrile seizures typically are seen in children (6 months to 5 years of age) with a rapidly rising temperature greater than 102° F (39° C). Febrile seizures usually consist of a single, brief episode with a short postictal phase. Beyond the ABCs (airway, breathing, circulation), treatment should include checking for hypoglycemia and administering antipyretic medications. The cause of febrile seizures is uncertain. They are usually benign, but parents need a lot of reassurance. Children who experience a febrile seizure are at greater risk of having a similar seizure in the future.

23. **Is there a clear method for determining when a patient is experiencing a pseudoseizure (psychogenic seizure)?**

Patients with pseudoseizures have no postictal phase and frequently recall events during the seizure activity. They do not experience incontinence or sustain injuries as a result of the seizure. Inconsistent motor manifestations are common, and the seizure activity may occur only in the presence of bystanders. Only an EEG can distinguish a pseudoseizure from a true seizure. The patient with known pseudoseizures most likely has a treatment protocol; coordinate care with the patient and primary care provider (PCP).

24. **What is the most likely cause of a seizure during pregnancy?**

Eclampsia. Pregnancy-induced hypertension includes preeclampsia and eclampsia. Both are characterized by hypertension, proteinuria, and edema. The progression from preeclampsia to eclampsia occurs when the patient has a seizure. Eclampsia usually occurs during the third trimester and is a life-threatening emergency. Treatment is with IV magnesium sulfate and may require emergent delivery of the fetus. Preeclampsia and eclampsia can also both occur postpartum.

25. **Is everyone susceptible to having a seizure?**

Yes. The brain is a sensitive organ, and given the right circumstances, anyone can have a seizure. For example, a college student with a remote history of significant head trauma with brief loss of consciousness, under the stress of college exams and lack of sleep, might have a one-time tonic-clonic seizure. Approximately 10% of the American population will experience a seizure during their lifetime.

26. What is a vagal nerve stimulator (VNS)?

The VNS was approved by the Food and Drug Administration (FDA) in 1997 for use in patients with intractable epilepsy. The VNS can be used in adults and adolescents over 12 years of age with partial onset seizures who have failed to respond adequately to multiple antiepileptic medications. The pacemaker-like device is placed in the left anterior chest wall and a stimulating electrode is wrapped around the left vagus nerve in the neck. The pulse generator of the VNS can be programmed through the skin using a magnetic wand. After implantation, it usually takes several weeks to program the pulse parameters to effective settings.

The exact mechanism of action of the VNS is unknown. In theory, the VNS can directly activate inhibitory circuits in relevant cortical regions to abort the seizure activity. A major advantage of the VNS is that it allows a patient's medications to be reduced, thus decreasing the side effects that are common with seizure medications. The most common reported side effects of the VNS are hoarseness, throat pain, dyspnea, coughing, and skin tingling when the stimulation is on.

27. What is the link between tuberculosis (TB) and seizures?

Isoniazid (INH) is a first-line drug for tuberculosis, and INH toxicity can cause intractable (refractory) seizures that do not respond to standard therapy. Consider INH toxicity in patients who have access to the medication, prescribed for themselves or for someone in their household.

28. The family of a patient who experienced a generalized seizure states that he has no medical problems and takes no medications. They deny alcohol or illicit drug use and report that he recently arrived from Latin America. What could be the problem?

Cysticercosis, which is caused by the pork tapeworm *Taenia solium*. Humans acquire the tapeworm by eating inadequately cooked pork that contains the tapeworm cysts. After ingestion, larval cysts are formed in the brain. A seizure, either generalized or focal, is a common initial presentation. The disease occurs worldwide but is prevalent in Latin America. Antiparasitic treatment is generally recommended (see the Centers for Disease Control and Prevention [CDC] Cysticercosis fact sheet available at www.cdc.gov/ncidod/dpd/parasites/cysticercosis/factsht_cysticercosis.htm).

29. A patient who has not taken his seizure medication for a week has a seizure. Shouldn't the discharge instructions read, "Take your seizure medication"?

The leading cause of recurrent seizures in the patient with epilepsy is a lapse in taking medication. Because most seizure medications require a serum therapeutic level to be effective, patients must take them continually. But for many patients, medication side effects (lethargy, drowsiness, confusion, and inappropriate sleep) are worse than the risk of a seizure. Before judging, ask the patient for his or her thoughts about taking seizure medicine; focus the education accordingly. Advocate for the patient who cannot afford his or her medications, and consider referral to an emergency case manager or social services.

30. During an ED visit, what can the nurse teach a patient who was recently diagnosed with a seizure disorder?

Talk to the patient about obtaining a medical alert tag or a wallet card. Also stress the need to wear identification at all times. Instruct the family and significant others about seizure first aid and providing a safe environment at home. Patients who have seizures should shower rather than tub bathe and should swim with a friend or in the presence of a lifeguard to prevent drowning. They also should avoid heights and working with heavy or dangerous machinery. Excellent information about these topics is available from the Epilepsy Foundation (www.efa.org). Also discuss medication side effects and signs of toxicity. The patient should avoid stress when possible and be encouraged to have routine appointments with a healthcare provider. Continuity of care is important, because medication choices need to be made over time.

31. Are clinicians mandated by law to report patients with epilepsy to the department of motor vehicles?

Regulations vary from state to state; check the local ordinances. However, it is the clinician's responsibility to warn the patient with epilepsy about the risks of driving. Being unable to drive is a major barrier to independent living (employment, social, school) for epilepsy patients. Many states require a patient to be seizure-free for a period of time (6 months to 2 years) to obtain driving privileges.

32. Should all seizure patients be admitted to the hospital?

If the seizure activity is terminated and a known cause is identified and treated, the patient is discharged home. When the cause is undetermined, seizure activity continues, or the seizure is new-onset, hospitalization is usually required.

 Key Points

- One seizure does not constitute a diagnosis of epilepsy.
- Hypoglycemia is an easily corrected cause of seizures, so always check the glucose level in a seizing patient.
- The tonic-clonic seizure is the most common seizure in the ED and the most dramatic.
- In an actively seizing patient, the goal is to ensure the safety of the patient. Also remember your own safety.
- Status epilepticus is prolonged seizure activity for 15 to 30 minutes or two or more seizures without full recovery between seizures. This condition is life threatening, and controlling the seizures is critical.
- IV benzodiazepine is the drug treatment of choice in managing acute or prolonged seizures.
- Patients who experience an alcohol withdrawal seizure are also at high risk of metabolic abnormalities, subdural hematoma, and central nervous system infections.

Internet Resources

American Academy of Neurology Foundation, The Brain Matters:
www.thebrainmatters.org

American Epilepsy Society:
www.aesnet.org

Centers for Disease Control and Prevention:
www.cdc.gov

Epilepsy Foundation:
www.epilepsyfoundation.org

Epilepsy Therapy Development Project, Epilepsy.com:
www.epilepsy.com

International League Against Epilepsy:
www.ilae-epilepsy.org

National Institute of Neurological Disorders and Stroke:
www.ninds.nih.gov

Vagus Nerve Stimulation Therapy:
www.vnstherapy.com

Bibliography

Catlett CL: Seizures and status epilepticus in adults. In Tintinalli JE, Kelen GD, Stapczynski JS, editors: *Emergency medicine: A comprehensive study guide*, New York, 2004, McGraw-Hill.

Cosby C: Pediatric emergencies. In Newberry L, editor: *Sheehy's emergency nursing: Principles and practice*, St Louis, 2003, Mosby.

Dean P: The treatment of pediatric epilepsies, *Clin Nurs Pract Epilepsy* 1(2):1-7, 2000.

Gambrell M, Flynn N: Seizures 101, *Nursing* 34:36-41, 2004.

Jacobs MP, Shafer PO: Care versus cure of epilepsy: The paradigm shift, *Clin Nurs Pract Epilepsy* 1(3): 1-7, 2000.

Jeffries EM, Ting TY, Buelow J: Newly diagnosed epilepsy: Initial considerations and medical management, *Profiles Seizure Manag* 2(1):9-16, 2003.

Newberry L, Barrett DT: Neurologic emergencies. In Newberry L, editor: *Sheehy's emergency nursing: Principles and practice*, St Louis, 2003, Mosby.

Ong S et al: Neurocysticercosis in radiographically imaged seizure patients in U.S. Emergency Departments, *Emerg Infect Dis* 8:608-613, 2002.

Scott RC et al: Buccal midazolam and rectal diazepam for treatment of prolonged seizures in childhood and adolescence: A randomised trial. *Lancet* 353:623-626, 1999.

Shinnar S, O'Dell C: Evaluation and treatment of febrile seizures, *Profiles Seizure Manag* 2(4):4-9, 2003.

Steinmann R, Rickel M: A 23-year-old with refractory seizures following an isoniazid overdose, *J Emerg Nurs* 28:7-10, 2002.

Talbert S: Neurologic conditions. In Fultz J, Sturt P, editors: *Mosby's emergency nursing reference*, St Louis, 2005, Mosby.

Wolfe TR, Bernstone T: Intranasal drug delivery: An alternative to intravenous administration in selected emergency cases, *J Emerg Nurs* 30:141-147, 2004.

Chapter 12

Stroke

Barbara A. Overby

1. **Why does so much healthcare information focus on stroke?**

   Although hemorrhagic stroke has always been considered an emergency, ischemic stroke treatment formerly included only supportive care and prevention of future strokes. However, treatment attitudes toward ischemic stroke have changed dramatically in the past few years because ischemic strokes can now be treated with thrombolytic therapy within a narrow time window. Ischemic strokes should be viewed as true neurological emergencies requiring rapid assessment, accurate diagnosis, and appropriate interventions.

2. **Hospitals may now apply for certification as a primary stroke center. What does this mean?**

   The aim of primary stroke center certification is to improve the care of stroke patients. This process is similar to trauma center certification. The Brain Attack Coalition developed recommendations for patient care and support services for certification as a primary stroke center: stroke team, written protocols, integrated EMS and emergency department (ED) response, stroke unit, neurosurgical services, lab and radiology services, medical education, quality improvement, and organizational commitment. This certification will affect treatment in the ED, with the intended goal of ensuring rapid and consistent treatment.

3. **What is a stroke?**

   A stroke is an intracranial vascular event involving the sudden interruption of blood flow to the brain. Lack of blood flow leads to infarction in the affected area, which results in neurological deficits. The neurological deficits vary according to the location and duration of the ischemia. Strokes are classified as ischemic or hemorrhagic.
   - **Ischemic strokes** are caused by a thrombus or an embolism occluding blood flow in the cerebral vessels. Approximately 80% to 85% of all strokes are ischemic.
   - **Hemorrhagic strokes** involve bleeding into the parenchyma of the brain and are caused by vascular disorders such as ruptured aneurysms or arteriovenous malformation (AVM), or chronic hypertension in which blood leaks from small intracerebral arterioles. Approximately 15% to 20% of all strokes are hemorrhagic.

4. **Are strokes common?**

   Yes. Stroke is the third leading cause of death in the United States, and the leading cause of disability in adults. These statistics translate to 700,000 patients who experience stroke yearly. Presidents Woodrow Wilson, Franklin Roosevelt, and Richard Nixon each suffered a stroke.

5. **Is the proper terminology stroke or cerebrovascular accident (CVA)?**

Both terms are acceptable. However, the latest trend is to speak of stroke as a "brain attack." Especially for the lay public, this term conveys the same sense of urgency to pursue help and treatment as "heart attack." One of the major limitations in stroke treatment is failure of patients or family members to recognize the need to act quickly.

6. **What are the signs and symptoms of stroke?**

Signs and symptoms depend on which area of the brain is affected. A stroke may affect mental ability, motor function, or speech. All stroke symptoms occur with sudden onset. The Brain Attack Coalition of the National Institute of Neurological Disorders and Stroke (NINDS) agreed on the following defining stroke symptoms:
- Sudden numbness or weakness of the face, arm, or leg, especially unilateral
- Sudden confusion, difficulty with speaking or understanding speech
- Sudden difficulty with seeing in one or both eyes
- Sudden difficulty with walking, dizziness, loss of balance or coordination
- Sudden, severe headache with no known cause

7. **How is the severity of stroke assessed?**

A standardized stroke assessment commonly used in the ED is the National Institutes of Health Stroke Scale (NIHSS). The scale assesses five major areas: (1) level of consciousness, (2) visual assessment, (3) motor function, (4) sensation and neglect, and (5) speech and language. The scale is available from the Brain Attack Coalition at www.brainattackcoalition.org.

8. **What are some of the medical terms for describing stroke symptoms?**

Use plain English whenever possible in describing a patient's symptoms. Common stroke terms include:
- Aphasia: impaired or absent communication
- Ataxia: problems with motor coordination
- Broca's aphasia: expressive aphasia
- Dysarthria: imperfect speech articulation, slurred speech
- Dysphagia: difficulty in swallowing
- Hemiparesis: muscle weakness or partial paralysis on one side of the body
- Unilateral neglect: the patient tends not to pay attention to one side of the body
- Wernicke's aphasia: receptive aphasia
  The following terms are used less frequently:
- Agnosia: loss of the ability to recognize an object
- Agraphia: inability to write
- Alexia: inability to read
- Apraxia: inability to carry out familiar, purposeful movements
- Hemianopia: loss of vision in one eye
- Prosopagnosia: inability to recognize familiar faces

9. A patient experienced sudden onset of slurred speech and right hemiparesis 40 minutes before arrival at the ED. What are the treatment priorities?

Reassess the ABCs (airway, breathing, circulation) and vital signs. Continue oxygen therapy, cardiac monitoring, and pulse oximetry. A 12-lead electrocardiogram (ECG) and chest radiograph should be performed. Glucose should be measured if not already done by EMS. Hypoglycemia can give the appearance of a stroke in some patients. Place an intravenous (IV) line, or ensure patency of the IV line established by EMS. Laboratory tests should include complete blood count, serum chemistries, prothrombin time (PT), and partial thromboplastin time (PTT), and a sample should be sent to the blood bank. Immediately alert radiology of the need for a computed tomography (CT) scan of the head (noncontrast) to determine whether the stroke is hemorrhagic or ischemic. Rapid identification of the stroke type is critical to successful treatment and management.

10. Many patients with stroke arrive with an elevated blood pressure, but many practitioners are reluctant to reduce blood pressure in the ED. Why?

Lowering blood pressure abruptly does not allow the body time to autoregulate and can increase cerebral ischemia. The brain may be depending on the elevated pressure to perfuse tissue. Hypertension in a stroke patient is not treated unless the blood pressure is higher than 220 mmHg systolic or higher than 120 mmHg diastolic; even in those situations, rapid reduction of blood pressure is avoided.

11. What is tissue plasminogen activator (TPA)? Is it effective in treating stroke?

TPA is a naturally occurring substance involved in the body's intrinsic mechanism for dissolving clots. Activase (Alteplase) was produced by recombinant DNA technology and is a synthetic form of TPA. It has been used in patients with myocardial infarction to dissolve clots in the coronary arteries. Since 1996, it has proved effective in treating acute ischemic stroke if administered within 3 hours of onset of symptoms in selected patients.

12. What does a nurse need to know to administer TPA safely?

- **Selection criteria.** The patient must be an adult (older than 18 years) with a clinical diagnosis of ischemic stroke, and the onset of symptoms must be less than 3 hours. Patients with recent head trauma, a history of intracranial hemorrhage, recent or current bleeding, recent surgery or invasive procedures, or uncontrolled hypertension must be excluded.
- **Dosage.** The dose is 0.9 mg/kg IV with a maximum total dose of 90 mg. Ten percent of the total dose should be administered as an IV bolus over 1 minute with the remainder given over 60 minutes.
- **Monitoring.** Vital signs and neurological checks should be assessed every 15 minutes for 2 hours. Even after completion of the infusion, assessment should continue every 30 minutes for 6 hours, then every hour for 18 hours. A deterioration in neurological status may herald an intracranial hemorrhage; notify the physician immediately and prepare for repeat CT scan.

- **Complications.** Bleeding is the most common complication. Avoid unnecessary intramuscular (IM) injections, venipunctures, arterial sticks, or insertion of tubes (nasogastric tube, urinary catheter) before, during, and after the infusion of TPA. All potential bleeding sites should be monitored, including puncture sites and all orifices. The patient also should be monitored for signs of internal bleeding. The patient should not receive any additional antiplatelet or anticoagulant therapy (e.g., aspirin, heparin, warfarin, ticlopidine) for 24 hours. If serious bleeding occurs and the TPA is infusing, discontinue the TPA and notify the physician.

13. Is the 3-hour TPA rule flexible? If a patient wakes up in the morning with symptoms of a stroke, is he or she a candidate for TPA?

Probably not. The onset of symptoms is defined as the time since the patient was last known to be symptom free. In the case of someone who wakes up with symptoms, the time the patient went to sleep is considered to be the time of onset. Accurate identification of the exact time of stroke onset is important and often difficult.

14. What is a transient ischemic attack (TIA)? What is its significance?

A TIA is a sudden but temporary interruption in the brain's blood supply. Most TIAs resolve within minutes but can continue for as long as 24 hours and still be considered a TIA. The symptoms are the same as for stroke but disappear with resolution of the TIA.

TIAs have been referred to as "mini-strokes," and rightly so. Approximately 10% to 30% of strokes are preceded by a TIA, and approximately 5% of patients with TIA experience a stroke within 30 days. TIAs are warning signs of an underlying problem, and the patient should receive further evaluation to determine the cause.

15. When considering thrombolytic therapy, how can a clinician know whether the patient is experiencing a stroke rather than a TIA?

A contraindication to receiving TPA is a minor neurological deficit or rapidly improving symptoms, which suggest a TIA. The majority of TIAs last only a few minutes. But it is difficult to know for sure.

16. If a patient is not a candidate for TPA, are there other treatment options?

There has been research examining other thrombolytic medications, intraarterial thrombolysis, or a combination therapy of IV TPA plus intraarterial thrombolysis. Although none of these treatments have yet been approved by the Food and Drug Administration (FDA), studies continue with the hope of providing more treatment options or increasing the treatment window.

17. What is the "corkscrew" device for treating brain clots?

The "corkscrew" is Concentric Medical's Merci Retriever, which was approved by the FDA in 2004 for removal of blood clots in patients experiencing an ischemic stroke. The device is guided into a blood vessel in the patient's groin and threaded to the brain artery, and the clot is then snared with a coil and removed. The use of this device potentially increases the treatment time window beyond the 3-hour limit with TPA. During the Phase 1 Mechanical Embolus Removal in Cerebral Ischemia (MERCI) trial, the device successfully recannulated arteries in 12 of 28 patients (43%) treated as long as 8 hours after their stroke.

18. Do rural patients have access to stroke care?

Providing access to thrombolytic therapy for patients in rural areas is a challenge. Most hospitals can initiate IV TPA and arrange for transfer to a tertiary center for further care. Many hospitals are promoting helicopter transport either from the field or from the rural hospital to the stroke center to provide thrombolytic therapy access during the 3-hour treatment window.

19. What are neuroprotective agents?

In ischemic stroke an area of marginally perfused tissue, called the ischemic penumbra, surrounds the infarcted tissue. The goal of a neuroprotective agent is to stop or slow the ischemia cascade and minimize the damage in the penumbra. Although no effective neuroprotective agent has yet been developed, studies continue with the hope of administering these agents in the field by EMS personnel or in the ED in the future.

20. Can young people have a stroke?

Yes. The chapter author had a stroke at age 39. Two thirds of strokes occur in patients older than age 65, but the next most common group is young to middle-age adults. Stroke is rare in children. When an ischemic stroke occurs in a child, sickle cell anemia is a common cause. In sickle cell anemia, red blood cells with abnormal hemoglobin "sickle" and become stiff and sticky, leading to vasocclusion in cerebral arteries and cerebral infarction.

21. Can people recover from a stroke?

Emergency nurses typically witness patients in the acute phase, rarely seeing patients 1 year after their stroke. Patients can recover some or all of their neurological function. Recovery depends on several factors: age, severity of the stroke, resulting disabilities, motivation of the patient, and early therapy in a qualified rehabilitation program.

22. Should family, significant others, and friends be present at the bedside of a stroke patient?

It is reassuring for patients to see or hear familiar faces or voices. If possible, allow visitors.

23. How can a clinician communicate with a patient who has had a stroke?

First, remember that a stroke affects every patient differently; communication may not be an issue. If the patient's speech is affected, ask questions in a format that can be answered with a simple "yes," "no," or nod of the head. If concerned about the patient's ability to understand, establish eye contact and speak slowly in simple terms. Because the patient's vision may be affected, approach the patient from one side. Limit distractions such as multiple conversations at the same time, multiple people talking to the patient, and noises (e.g., television, alarms).

24. A 45-year-old woman has an obvious facial droop but no other associated symptoms. Could other conditions mimic stroke?

Yes. Bell's palsy involves the seventh cranial nerve (facial nerve). Patients experience facial paralysis without extremity involvement. Although the cause of the condition is unknown, symptoms usually resolve within 3 weeks, and steroids have been found to be helpful. If unsure, treat the patient as experiencing a stroke until proved otherwise. Other conditions that can mimic stroke include hypoglycemia, atypical migraine, trauma, and tumor.

25. Many ED patients take aspirin. Should everyone take an aspirin a day to prevent stroke?

Many practitioners think that aspirin may be beneficial in preventing stroke, and some recommend a daily aspirin to all seniors. The antiplatelet action of aspirin is thought to prevent the formation of blood clots and thus prevent strokes. The dose is still debated, ranging from 80 to 325 mg daily. Aspirin usually is recommended in the prevention of stroke after the occurrence of a TIA and in the prevention of recurrent strokes.

26. Because time is so critical to treatment of ischemic strokes, what can be done to avoid time delays in the ED?

First, assess the role of the EMS system. Are the paramedics aware of the therapeutic window for thrombolytic treatment, the need for rapid evaluation and transport, and the importance of communication with the ED? If the answer is no, offer education. Establish a stroke protocol or clinical pathway to streamline the process of alerting key team members (ED physician, radiologist, neurologist) and to allow nurses to initiate an IV line and collect blood for lab tests without an order. According to NINDS, every stroke protocol or plan should have the following ideal time frames in treating patients with ischemic strokes:
- Door to physician within 10 minutes
- Door to CT scan within 25 minutes
- Door to CT interpretation within 45 minutes
- Door to drug infusion within 60 minutes
- Door to monitored bed within 3 hours

However, the most important part of this plan is the nurse, who is instrumental in its initiation.

27. What is an emergency nurse's role in stroke prevention?

As always, talk to patients about risk factors that predispose them to stroke occurrence: smoking, diet, lack of exercise, hypertension. Educate the public, patients, and family members about stroke warning signs and the need to perceive these signs as an emergency and to call 911 immediately.

Key Points

- Stroke is the third leading cause of death, with approximately 80% to 85% being ischemic strokes.

- TIAs are warning signs of an underlying problem and further evaluation is needed to determine the cause.

- Rapid reduction of blood pressure in stroke patients should be avoided.

- Ischemic strokes are viewed as neurological emergencies requiring rapid assessment, diagnosis, and interventions.

- To avoid treatment delays of patients with stroke, establish a stroke protocol or clinical pathway to streamline processes.

- TPA administration for ischemic stroke must be initiated within 3 hours from the onset of stroke symptoms.

- TPA dose is 0.9 mg/kg IV with a maximum dose of 90 mg. Ten percent of the total dose should be administered as an IV bolus over 1 minute with the remainder given over 60 minutes.

- The Merci Retriever device was approved by the FDA in 2004 as an option for treating ischemic stroke patients.

- The ED environment is anxiety producing for all patients, but communication with the stroke patient can be a challenge. Limit distractions, establish eye contact, and speak slowly with simple yes/no questions.

- Educate patients and family members about the signs and symptoms of stroke, and emphasize the need to call 911 immediately.

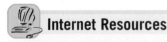

Internet Resources

American Stroke Association:
www.strokeassociation.org

Brain Attack Coalition:
www.brainattackcoalition.org

Concentric Medical, Merci Retriever:
www.concentric-medical.com

Genentech:
www.gene.com

Internet Stroke Center at Washington University in St. Louis:
www.strokecenter.org

National Aphasia Association:
www.aphasia.org

National Institute of Neurological Disorders and Stroke:
www.ninds.nih.gov

National Stroke Association:
www.stroke.org

Stroke Information Directory:
www.stroke-info.com

Bibliography

Adams H et al: Guidelines for the early management of patients with ischemic stroke, *Stroke* 34:1056-1083, 2003.

Alberts M et al: Recommendations for the establishment of primary stroke centers, *JAMA* 283:3102-3109, 2000.

American Heart Association: Acute ischemic stroke. In Cummins RO, editor: *Advanced cardiac life support provider manual,* Dallas, 2001, American Heart Association.

Blank FSJ, Keyes M: Thrombolytic therapy for patients with acute stroke in the ED setting, *J Emerg Nurs* 26:24-30, 2000.

Bonnono C et al: Emergi-paths and stroke teams: An emergency department approach to acute ischemic stroke, *J Neurosci Nurs* 32:298-305, 2000.

Brandt L: Code stroke: Rapid diagnosis and treatment of stroke in the ED, *Adv Nurs* 7:21-22, 26, 2005.

Criddle LM, Bonnono C, Fisher SK: Standardizing stroke assessment using the National Institutes of Health Stroke Scale, *J Emerg Nurs* 29:541-546, 2003.

Gobin YP et al: MERCI 1: A phase 1 study of mechanical embolus removal in cerebral ischemia, *Stroke* 35(12):2848-2854, 2004.

Hinkle JL, Bowman L: Pharmacology update: Neuroprotection for ischemic stroke, *J Neurosci Nurs* 35: 114-118, 2003.

Jahnke HK et al: Stroke teams and acute stroke pathways: One emergency department's two-year experience, *J Emerg Nurs* 29:133-139, 2003.

Jovin T, Gebel JM, Wechsler LR: Intra-arterial thrombolysis for acute ischemic stroke, *J Stroke Cerebrovasc Dis* 11:148-161, 2002.

Kalafut MA, Saver JL: The acute stroke patient: The first six hours. In Cohen SN, editor: *Management of ischemic stroke*, New York, 2000, McGraw-Hill.

Kuether TA, Nesbit GM, Barnwell SL: Mechanical thrombolysis of acute ischemic stroke, *J Stroke Cerebrovasc Dis* 11:162-173, 2002.

Meschia JF, Brott TG: Thrombolysis for acute ischemic stroke: Future directions, *J Stroke Cerebrovasc Dis* 11:183-196, 2002.

Miller J, Elmore S: Call a stroke code, *Nursing* 35:58-63, 2005.

Newberry L, Barrett DT: Neurologic emergencies. In Newberry L, editor: *Sheehy's emergency nursing: Principles and practice*, St Louis, 2003, Mosby.

Scott PA, Timmerman CA: Stroke, transient ischemic attack, and other central focal conditions. In Tintinalli JE, Kelen GD, and Stapczynski JS, editors: *Emergency medicine: A comprehensive study guide*, New York, 2004, McGraw-Hill.

Silliman SL et al: Use of a field-to-stroke center helicopter transport program to extend thrombolytic therapy to rural residents, *Stroke* 34:729-733, 2003.

Eye Problems

Gretta J. Edwards

1. Are there any true eye emergencies?

Although eye problems are not life threatening, a delay in care can result in permanent loss of vision, so any eye problem that threatens visual acuity must be treated as an emergency. Two emergent eye conditions requiring immediate treatment are chemical burns to the eye and central retinal artery occlusion (CRAO). Additional eye problems that must be treated emergently include acute angle closure glaucoma, open globe, and retrobulbar hemorrhage.

2. How should a patient with an eye complaint be assessed?

As always, assessment of the patient with an eye complaint starts with the ABCs (airway, breathing, circulation), as well as C-spine precautions. In patients with an isolated eye complaint, the primary survey can be brief. Trauma patients need a more complete assessment to rule out any additional injuries. Obtain a medical history, including allergies, tetanus status, and any history of previous eye problems or surgery. Ask about the onset and duration of symptoms such as pain, itching, burning, tearing, photophobia, and visual changes. If the patient complains of pain, determine the type and degree of pain and any aggravating or relieving factors. For trauma-related complaints, document the time and mechanism of injury and whether the patient was using eye protection. For patients involved in motor vehicle collisions, ask if the air bag deployed.

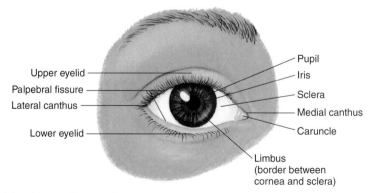

Frontal view of the eye. (*From Jarvis* C: Physical examination and health assessment, *ed 4, St Louis, 2004, Mosby.*)

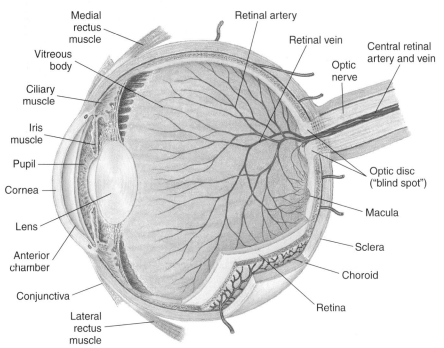

Lateral view of the structures of the eye. (*From Seidel HM et al:* Mosby's guide to physical examination, *ed 5, St Louis, 2003, Mosby.*)

Assessment of the eye should be done systematically, moving from the area surrounding the eye toward the center. Examine the periorbital area for redness, swelling, or signs of trauma, and palpate for crepitus or step-offs. Look for symmetry and observe whether the eyes appear to be bulging or sunken. Ask the patient to follow your hand as you move it through the six cardinal positions of gaze, in which one muscle is responsible for each movement (see figure). Both eyes should move symmetrically to all positions without turning the head. Check the lids for redness, swelling, or lacerations. Examine the conjunctiva for foreign bodies, redness, or swelling and look for discharge or tearing. If the conjunctiva is red, observe if the redness appears in a specific pattern (e.g., surrounding the iris) because this can provide an important clue to the diagnosis. If the patient gives a history of trauma, examine the sclera carefully for any areas of black tissue caused by extrusion of the choroid through a break in the sclera, indicating that the eye has been punctured. The cornea should be clear with a smooth, glistening surface. Look for any irregularities or haziness. The anterior chamber is normally clear, deep, and free of blood or other debris. In examining the iris, ensure that it is intact and there are no irregularities. Shimmering or quivering of the iris may indicate that the lens is missing or displaced. Pupils should be equal, round, and reactive to light and accommodation (PERRLA). The lens is usually not visible without a slit lamp but may appear white or cloudy if a significant cataract is present.

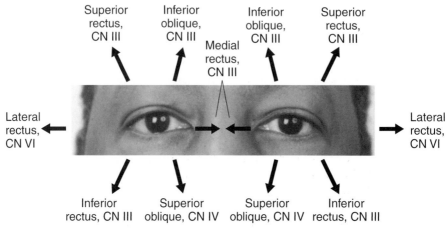

Superior rectus, CN III | Inferior oblique, CN III | Medial rectus, CN III | Inferior oblique, CN III | Superior rectus, CN III

Lateral rectus, CN VI

Lateral rectus, CN VI

Inferior rectus, CN III   Superior oblique, CN IV   Superior oblique, CN IV   Inferior rectus, CN III

Cranial nerves and extraocular muscles associated with the six cardinal fields of gaze. (*From Seidel HM et al:* Mosby's guide to physical examination, *ed 5, St Louis, 2003, Mosby.*)

3. **What is the most important point about caring for the patient with an eye emergency?**

    An accurate assessment of visual acuity is essential for both diagnostic and legal purposes. Visual acuity is the vital sign for the eye and should be obtained as soon as possible. Except in the case of chemical burns to the eye, visual acuity must be assessed before treatment is administered. If the patient is unable to open the eye because of pain or lid spasm, topical anesthetic can be used to decrease discomfort. If the lids are swollen, it may be necessary to gently hold them open although this should not be attempted if there is a possibility that the eye is not intact.

4. **What is the correct way to assess visual acuity?**

    Visual acuity is usually checked with a Snellen chart. The E chart can be used for nonreaders. If available, always check the visual acuity with the patient's corrective lenses. Instruct the patient to stand facing the eye chart at a distance of 20 feet. Ask the patient to cover one eye (the covered eye should remain open) with an eye occluder or hand. Record the last line in which more than half of the letters are read correctly. Subtract the number read incorrectly and add any figures read on the next smaller line. For example, if the patient reads all but one of the letters on line six (20/30) correctly plus two letters on line seven (20/25) with the right eye, the visual acuity is recorded as OD (right eye) 20/30 −1 +2. Repeat the visual acuity with the left eye (OS). If the patient is wearing glasses or contact lenses, note on the chart that visual acuity was assessed with corrective lenses. In the emergency department (ED), there is no need to check the visual acuity in both eyes together or to repeat the visual acuity without the patient's corrective lenses. Checking visual acuity is a time-consuming but essential part of the assessment of patients with eye complaints.

5. **What is the best way to check the visual acuity of a patient who is immobile or cannot read the chart?**

There are several simple ways to check visual acuity for the patient who has limited vision or who is immobile. A Rosenbaum pocket screener or a newspaper, held at reading distance, can be used if the patient is immobile. If the patient wears glasses for reading, near visual acuity should be checked with corrective lenses. Record the size of type and the reading distance. The following box describes alternative methods for determining visual acuity when the patient's visual acuity is not sufficient to read the Snellen chart.

Alternative methods for determining visual acuity

Ask the patient to stand closer to the Snellen chart and record the visual acuity as the number of feet the patient is standing from the chart over the smallest line read. For example, if the patient is standing 10 feet from the chart instead of 20 feet and reads the top letter (20/200), record the visual acuity as 10/200. Stand 5 feet in front of the patient and move forward slowly while waving your hand. When the patient can see your moving hand, record the visual acuity as HM (hand motion) @ _____ (distance). Shine a light in front of the eye. If the patient can see the light, record the visual acuity as LP (light perception). If no light can be seen, record the visual acuity as NLP (no light perception).

---

6. **Is there an accurate way to test visual acuity in patients who wear corrective lenses if the lenses are not available?**

It is important to determine if poor visual acuity is related to trauma or disease or simply the result of a refractive error. A pinhole occluder provides a good estimate of the patient's corrected visual acuity. This method works because the light rays hitting the retina from an angle are blocked and only light rays that hit the retina directly, and that don't need to be focused, are allowed to reach the retina. Visual acuity obtained using this method corrects most refractive errors to approximately 20/30. In general, a pinhole occluder should be used if visual acuity is less than 20/30, even if the patient is wearing corrective lenses. If there is not a pinhole occluder available, a suitable substitute can be made by piercing a sheet of stiff paper with an 18-gauge needle. While the opposite eye is covered, ask the patient to hold the paper close to the eye and read the eye chart while looking through the hole. Be sure to document that the visual acuity was obtained by using a pinhole.

7. **What is the treatment for a chemical burn?**

Chemical burns to the eye require the most urgent treatment of all eye emergencies. The key to treating chemical exposure of the eye is to flush the material out of the eye as quickly as possible. Ideally the treatment for chemical burns starts in the field by flushing the eyes with copious amounts of clean tap water. Irrigation in the ED must be started immediately on arrival and continued for

20 to 30 minutes, using 2 to 3 liters of fluid for each eye. Check the pH in the inferior conjunctival sac with pH (litmus) paper before starting the irrigation and again 5 to 10 minutes after the irrigation has been completed. If the pH is outside the 7.3 to 7.7 range, resume irrigation until the pH falls within those parameters. It is important to determine the type of substance that caused the burn. Both acid and alkaline substances can cause significant, irreversible damage to the eye. However, most acids bind with surface proteins, coagulating the tissue and preventing further penetration. Alkalis continue to damage eye tissues until they are flushed out. Common causes of alkali burns include drain and oven cleaners, hair neutralizers, concrete, plaster, industrial solvents, and fertilizers.

Although labor intensive, intravenous (IV) bags and tubing work well for eye irrigations. Lactated Ringer's solution is less irritating to the eye than normal saline and warm fluids are more comfortable for the patient. Morgan irrigating lenses are efficient but not tolerated well by some patients. Do not use a Morgan lens if any foreign bodies are present in the eye. Instill topical anesthetic before starting the irrigation because eye irrigations are uncomfortable. Care must be taken to ensure that the entire conjunctiva has been irrigated. The following box describes the procedure for eye irrigation. Treatment for chemical burns will also include artificial tears, antibiotic ointment, cycloplegic drops to prevent painful spasms of the ciliary muscle, and, for more severe burns, topical corticosteroids to reduce inflammation.

Eye irrigation

- Thoroughly clean the lids and the area around the eye. Remove any particulate matter with a moist cotton-tipped swab. Evert the lid and remove any remaining foreign bodies.
- Position the patient supine on a gurney with the head turned toward the affected side.
- Place towels under the head. A plastic sheet or shower board (used for washing hair) can be used to direct irrigation fluid into a waste container on the floor. An emesis basin placed next to the face can also be used to catch fluid.
- Instill topical anesthetic and repeat as needed during long irrigations. Insert a lid retractor if the patient has difficulty keeping the eye open, or hold the lids open with gauze pads to keep the fingers from slipping.
- Direct the stream of fluid at the conjunctiva and corners of the eye, avoiding the cornea. Ask the patient to blink frequently and look in all directions so that the entire surface of the eye can be irrigated.

8. What is CRAO?

CRAO is one of two eye conditions requiring emergency treatment. CRAO occurs when the main artery to the eye becomes occluded by a thrombus or embolus. The patient will complain of sudden, painless loss of vision in one eye. The visual loss may be almost total, with most patients having visual acuity ranging from being able to count the number of fingers held up to being able to perceive light and dark. Risk factors include age older than 60, hypertension, diabetes, and carotid and cardiovascular disease. Treatment to restore retinal blood flow must begin immediately to prevent permanent visual loss. The goal of treatment is to dislodge the embolus by increasing the intravascular pressure in the artery and by decreasing the intraocular pressure. Treatment may include massaging the eye, giving IV acetazolamide, or withdrawing small amounts of aqueous humor from the anterior chamber to decrease intraocular pressure. Having the patient breathe into a paper bag for 10 minutes will elevate blood levels of carbon dioxide and may cause dilation of the retinal artery, allowing the obstruction to pass. Treatment is frequently not successful, even if started soon after the event.

9. **How is a corneal abrasion diagnosed and treated?**

Corneal abrasions are commonly seen in the ED. The patient with a corneal abrasion may or may not give a history of foreign body exposure. The chief complaints are pain and foreign body sensation accompanied by tearing, redness, and photophobia. Visual acuity may be decreased if the central cornea is involved. Even if the foreign body is no longer in the eye, residual scratches on the cornea can still cause a foreign body sensation. *Patients with a history of pounding or grinding metal or stone must also be evaluated for a penetrating foreign body (see question 15).* Because foreign bodies frequently lodge on the inner surface of the upper lid, the lid must be everted for inspection (see figure). When fluorescein stain is applied to the cornea, damaged areas appear green under a cobalt blue light. Any remaining foreign bodies can be removed by the physician with a cotton swab or needle. Metallic foreign bodies may leave a rust ring that must be removed by an ophthalmologist in several days. Multiple foreign bodies can be flushed out of the eye with normal saline. Antibiotic drops or ointment may be applied but ointments are preferred because of their lubricating properties. Cycloplegics are no longer recommended for the treatment of corneal abrasions. Corneal abrasions are painful, so oral or topical analgesics may be prescribed. If the patient receives prescriptions for both ophthalmic drops and ointment, instruct the patient to use the drop before the ointment to maximize absorption.

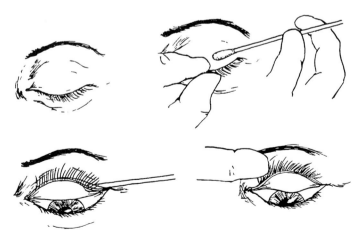

Steps in everting the eyelid. (*From Egging D: Ocular emergencies. In Newberry L, editor:* Sheehy's emergency nursing: Principles and practice, *ed 4, St Louis, 1998, Mosby.*)

10. When should eye patches be applied?

This issue is controversial. Traditionally, all patients with superficial corneal injuries were patched because it was believed that patching reduced pain and sped healing by reducing blinking. Recent studies have indicated that patients are more comfortable without an eye patch and that eye patches can actually delay healing and increase the risk of infection. In addition, patching decreases depth perception, which may make the patient more prone to falls and motor vehicle crashes.

11. What should be known about topical ophthalmic anesthetics?

Pain is a protective response for the eye. When the eye has been anesthetized, the patient can inadvertently damage the eye, causing further damage. The patient should be cautioned not to rub the eye for at least 1 hour after topical anesthetic has been applied. Patients often obtain so much pain relief with topical anesthetics that they want to continue using them at home. When used frequently, topical anesthetics are toxic to the eye and prevent the cornea from healing. *Topical anesthetics should never be prescribed for or given to patients.*

12. How is hyphema diagnosed?

The tissues of the iris and ciliary body are fragile and highly vascular. When the vessels in this area are damaged, blood escapes into the anterior chamber causing hyphema (see figure). Most hyphema results from trauma although it may occur spontaneously in some eye diseases or in patients with clotting disorders. Because red blood cells must first settle to the bottom of the anterior chamber for hyphema to be visible, hyphema may not be apparent at first, especially if the patient is supine. The severity of the bleeding can be accurately assessed only after the patient has been quiet and sitting upright for 5 to 10 minutes and the "layering out" has occurred. The amount of blood in the anterior chamber varies from microscopic amounts to bleeding that fills the entire anterior chamber. Hyphema may be difficult to detect in dark-eyed patients. Deficits in visual acuity depend on the amount of bleeding and any associated trauma. Patients with hyphema are often lethargic or sleepy, although the exact mechanism is not known. These symptoms can be confusing, especially if hyphema has occurred in conjunction with a head injury.

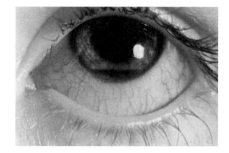

Small hyphema layering out in the inferior portion of the anterior chamber. (*From Brunette D: Ophthalmology. In Marx J: Rosen's emergency medicine: Concepts and clinical practice, ed 5, St Louis, 2002, Mosby.*)

13. What is the treatment for the patient with hyphema?

The treatment goals for the patient with hyphema are to control intraocular pressure and to prevent rebleeding. Complication rates from hyphema are related directly to the amount of blood in the anterior chamber. Patients who have less than one third of the anterior chamber filled with blood are at low risk for complications. This amount of blood is resorbed within a few days. If more than one third of the anterior chamber is filled with blood, the risk of complications and permanent damage to the eye is increased. These patients must be followed by an ophthalmologist. Acute glaucoma can occur if the trabecular meshwork becomes clogged with fibrin or blood clots and aqueous humor can no longer drain from the anterior chamber. Surgical evacuation of the clot may be necessary. Rebleeding is also a major complication and usually occurs 2 to 5 days after the initial injury when the clot begins to lyse. Hyphema is generally treated on an outpatient basis, but the patient may be hospitalized if the hyphema is extensive, or if the patient is at high risk for rebleed or is noncompliant. Treatment includes cycloplegics, medications such as topical beta blockers to control intraocular pressure, and possibly aminocaproic acid (Amicar) to prevent rebleeding. The patient should be medicated for pain and nausea as needed. Activity is restricted to quiet ambulation and bed rest with the head of the bed elevated at least 30 degrees. Instruct the patient to avoid medications that contain aspirin or nonsteroidal antiinflammatory drugs (NSAIDs). The eye must be covered with a metal shield to protect it from further damage. Notify the doctor immediately if the patient complains of increased pain, which may indicate that intraocular pressure is rising to dangerous levels.

14. What is the difference between hyphema and a subconjunctival hemorrhage?

As described in question 12, hyphema occurs when blood collects inside the anterior chamber of the eye. A subconjunctival hemorrhage results when vessels of the conjunctiva rupture and blood is trapped between the subconjunctiva and the sclera. There is no such thing as a "scleral hemorrhage" because the sclera is avascular and cannot bleed. Subconjunctival hemorrhages are frightening to the patient but rarely serious. The hemorrhages appear suddenly, frequently after straining, coughing, or rubbing the eye. They can occur in any area on the conjunctiva and are bright red with a flat, smooth surface. The patient is usually asymptomatic or complains only of mild discomfort. There is no effective treatment, but cold packs may be used. The blood may take 2 to 4 weeks to dissolve. Patients who are taking anticoagulants or have coagulopathies require a more extensive evaluation.

15. What is an open eye?

"Open eye" is a general term that applies to both rupture of the globe and penetrating ocular trauma. Patients with penetrating trauma frequently complain of a foreign body sensation after pounding or grinding metal or stone. The entrance wound can be difficult to detect, so an accurate history is key to making the diagnosis. A computed tomography (CT) scan or ultrasound can be used to confirm the diagnosis. Magnetic resonance imaging (MRI) is contraindicated if a metallic foreign body is suspected. A ruptured globe is a more serious injury that usually occurs with blunt trauma and results in significant disruption of orbital tissues from acceleration and deceleration forces. Suspect an open eye if the patient has a significant decrease in visual acuity, severe pain, an abnormally shaped pupil, hyphema, hemorrhage, extrusion of intraocular tissue, or a soft or asymmetrical globe. *A rigid eye shield should be placed over the eye as soon as an open eye is suspected.* Do not use an eye pad because it may apply pressure to the eye. If the lids are swollen, do not attempt to open them; such attempts may cause further damage to the eye. Medicate for pain and nausea and keep the patient NPO in anticipation of surgery. Topical medications in the eye should be avoided since they may be toxic to the internal structures.

16. What causes ultraviolet (UV) keratitis? How should it be treated?

UV keratitis is a type of corneal burn caused by exposure to UV light. The patient gives a history of snow skiing in bright sunlight, use of a sun lamp or tanning beds, or exposure to a welder's arc (often referred to as a "flash burn" in this instance). The presenting symptoms are the same as those for corneal abrasion but involve both eyes, and the onset of symptoms is delayed until 6 to 10 hours after exposure. Corneal burns of this type are quite painful. Cycloplegic drops may help to decrease discomfort. The patient should be discharged with a prescription for oral narcotics. *Topical anesthetics should not be used repeatedly as they ultimately delay healing.*

17. At triage, how can a patient with acute angle closure glaucoma be recognized?

Acute angle closure glaucoma occurs when the iris blocks the drainage of aqueous humor from the eye. The pressure increases rapidly, causing severe pain. Acute angle closure glaucoma is more common in women, diabetics, the elderly, Inuits, and Asians. Use of anticholinergic drugs also can trigger acute closure of the angles in patients who are anatomically susceptible. The patient will often give a history of sudden onset of pain while in an area of semidarkness such as a movie theater because the dilated iris blocks the canal of Schlemm and the outflow of aqueous humor. Early recognition of acute angle closure glaucoma is essential to prevent damage to the optic nerve, but the symptoms of angle closure glaucoma may be similar to those of other emergencies commonly seen in the ED, especially migraine headache. Patients with both acute angle closure glaucoma and migraine headaches often complain of a severe unilateral headache, nausea, vomiting, photophobia, blurred vision, and halos around lights. Some patients may be asymptomatic or complain only of nausea and vomiting. Additional signs of acute angle closure glaucoma include redness of the affected eye, corneal haziness, and a pupil that is fixed and dilated to midpoint. The anterior chamber will appear shallow with the iris appearing just below the cornea. Assessment of the eye helps to differentiate between acute angle closure glaucoma and migraine headache. The quickest screening method is to gently palpate both eyes with the lids closed. If the intraocular pressure in one eye is elevated, the eye will feel firm.

18. What is the treatment for acute angle closure glaucoma?

Treatment to lower the intraocular pressure must be started immediately to prevent permanent damage to the optic nerve. Treatment includes oral or IV acetazolamide (Diamox), mannitol, topical beta blockers (timolol), pilocarpine, and topical corticosteroids. After the pressure is controlled, a surgical or laser procedure is needed to provide definitive treatment and to prevent further episodes.

19. **What is a retrobulbar hemorrhage?**

A retrobulbar hemorrhage can occur after blunt trauma when blood accumulates in the potential space surrounding the eye. If the bleeding is significant, pressure inside the eye can rise to dangerous levels and occlusion of the central retinal artery may occur. Unfortunately, the bleeding is hidden and may not be recognized before permanent damage has occurred. Because retrobulbar hemorrhage is frequently associated with head and facial trauma, the patient may not be alert enough to complain of pain or visual changes. Monitor patients with head and facial trauma carefully for signs of retrobulbar hemorrhage, including unilateral bulging of the eye, severe subconjunctival hemorrhage, restriction of eye movements, and increased firmness of the eye to palpation. The treatment is similar to that for angle closure glaucoma but also may include cutting the lateral canthus to relieve the pressure. Immediate recognition is essential to prevent permanent visual loss.

20. **What are floaters? What is their significance?**

Floaters are caused by debris in the vitreous of the eye. They are very common and are usually not significant. A good rule of thumb is to ask the patient how many floaters he or she can see. If the patient can count the number of floaters, they are usually benign and do not require treatment. However, if the patient reports a sudden onset of "hundreds" of floaters or "too many to count," this is an indication of the presence of blood in the vitreous. Such bleeding can result from a retinal detachment. Ask the patient about risk factors for retinal detachment: cataract surgery, severe myopia (nearsightedness), or recent trauma. Other symptoms of retinal detachment, such as flashing lights, visual changes, and the presence of a "curtain" or "veil" in the visual field, may be present. Retinal detachments require repair by either laser treatment or a scleral buckle within 24 to 48 hours of the detachment to avoid permanent damage to vision.

21. **What is a "blowout" fracture?**

A blowout fracture occurs when force is applied to the front of the eye. The eye becomes deformed and the pressure to the top and bottom of the orbit is increased. If the applied force is strong enough, the orbit may fracture, usually at the floor, where the bone is the weakest. Some of the orbital contents (muscle, nerves, fat) are then forced into the maxillary sinus (see figure). The patient will give a history of a blow to the eye, often from a ball or fist. Signs and symptoms include double vision when looking upward, limitation of upward gaze in the affected eye, a sunken-appearing eye, crepitus in the periorbital area, and numbness of the cheek and lip on the affected side. Surgical repair may be delayed as long as 2 weeks because symptoms frequently resolve as the swelling decreases. The patient should be cautioned against blowing the nose, which can force more air and nasal secretions into subcutaneous tissues. Swelling can be minimized by keeping the head of the bed elevated and applying ice packs. Nasal decongestants and oral antibiotics may also be prescribed.

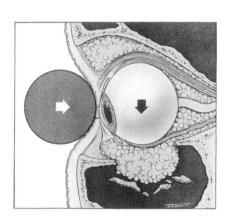

Blow out fracture caused by the impact of a ball.
(*From Ragge NK, Easty DL:* Immediate eye care,
St Louis, 1990, Mosby.)

22. What should patients be taught about eye safety?

Most eye injuries seen in the ED are preventable. Protective eyewear is easily accessible, but people frequently do not wear goggles or masks while engaged in hazardous activities. Sports, including paintball, are a major source of serious eye injuries, as are pounding, grinding, or drilling metal. Always encourage patients to wear eye protection whenever there is a risk of damage from flying objects or direct blow to the eye.

23. What are the special needs of a patient who experiences sudden loss of vision?

The patient with sudden visual loss has significant anxiety and fear related to the treatment and outcome of the emergency. Patients may experience extreme anxiety about the potential for blindness. In addition, many patients require a surgical procedure within a matter of hours. This allows little time to prepare themselves and their families. Encourage the patient to talk about fears regarding the possibility of vision loss. Providing the patient with information about the surgery and postoperative process helps to decrease anxiety. Patients with significant loss of sight have lost a large portion of their sensory input. Using touch communicates concern and helps reassure a frightened patient. The patient's family or significant others may fear that the patient's loss of sight will be permanent; therefore, they also need support.

24. What are the nurse's responsibilities if a patient is a potential eye donor?

ED staff have an ethical and legal responsibility to determine the deceased patient's wishes about organ and tissue donation. Before contacting the family, check with the local eye bank or organ procurement agency to determine eligibility. There are few exclusions for eye donation, and the eyes generally are acceptable as long as 12 hours after death.

Proper care of the eyes in the ED ensures that the tissue is still usable and that the body is maintained in a condition suitable for viewing. After death, tear production stops and the cornea dries out. The eyes must be kept moist to maintain the corneal epithelium in optimal condition. Flush the eyes with normal saline. Gently close the lids with clean fingers but do not tape the lids shut. Tape may cause tears in the delicate skin of the lids that may be difficult for the mortician to repair. Cover the eyes with gauze 4 × 4s saturated with normal saline. Do not use ice packs because the weight may cause damage to the cornea. Elevating the head on a towel roll or pillow will allow fluids to drain and minimize bruising from the tissue retrieval process.

 Key Points

- Two eye emergencies require immediate initiation of treatment: chemical burns and CRAO. Open eyes, acute angle closure glaucoma, and retrobulbar hemorrhage also need to be treated emergently.
- Visual acuity is the vital sign for the eye. An accurate assessment of visual acuity is essential for diagnosis and treatment.
- If a penetrating eye injury or open globe from blunt trauma is suspected, a rigid eye shield should be placed immediately after obtaining the visual acuity. Care must be taken to ensure that no pressure is applied to the eye, because this can increase the extent of damage.
- Pain is a common complaint in patients with eye emergencies. Topical anesthetics should be used only with the initial exam. Oral analgesics, narcotics, and topical analgesics can be prescribed for outpatient pain control.
- Proper care of donor eyes is essential to prevent damage to the corneas and to maintain the body in optimal viewing condition.

 Internet Resources

American Academy of Ophthalmology:
www.aao.org

Doctor's Guide:
www.docguide.com

Prevent Blindness America:
www.preventblindness.org

Review of Optometry Online:
www.revoptom.com

Rocky Mountain Lions Eye Bank, Critical Insight:
www.corneas.org/eyecare

St. Luke's Cataract & Laser Institute:
www.stlukeseye.com

Bibliography

Brunette D: Ophthalmology. In Marx J: *Rosen's emergency medicine: Concepts and clinical practice,* ed 5, St Louis, 2002, Mosby.

Carley F, Carley S: Mydriatics in corneal abrasion, *J Emerg Med* 41:134-140, 2001.

Egging D: Ocular emergencies. In Newberry L, editor: *Sheehy's emergency nursing,* ed 5, St Louis, 2003, Mosby.

Egging D: Ocular emergencies. In Newberry L, editor: *Sheehy's emergency nursing: Principles and practice,* ed 4, St Louis, 1998, Mosby.

Gillett P, Goldblum K: Ophthalmic patient assessment, *Insight* October-December, 2004.

Jarvis C: *Physical examination and health assessment,* ed 4, St Louis, 2004, Mosby.

Kaiser PK, Friedman NJ, Pineda R: *The Massachusetts eye and ear infirmary illustrated manual of ophthalmology,* ed 2, Philadelphia, 2004, WB Saunders.

Knoop KJ, Dennis WR, Hedges JR: Ophthalmic procedures. In Roberts JR, Hedges JR, editors: *Clinical procedures in emergency medicine,* ed 4, Philadelphia, 2003, WB Saunders.

Le Sage N, Verreault R, Rochette L: Efficacy of eye patching in traumatic corneal abrasions: A controlled clinical trial, *Ann Emerg Med* 38:129-134, 2001.

Mitchell JD: Ocular emergencies. In Tintinalli JE, Ruiz E, Krome RL, editors: *Emergency medicine: A comprehensive study guide,* ed 5, New York, 2000, McGraw-Hill.

Ragge NK, Easty DL: *Immediate eye care,* St Louis, 1990, Mosby.

Seidel HM et al: *Mosby's guide to physical examination,* ed 5, St Louis, 2003, Mosby.

Smith SC: Ocular injuries. In McQuillen KA et al: *Trauma nursing: From resuscitation through rehabilitation,* Philadelphia, 2002, WB Saunders.

Trauma nursing core course, ed 5, 2000, Emergency Nurses Association.

Traverso CE, Bagnis A, Bricola G: Angle-closure glaucoma. In Yanoff M, Duker J, editors: *Ophthmology,* ed 2, St Louis, 2004, Mosby.

Walton W et al: Management of traumatic hyphema, *Surv Ophthalmol* 47:4, 2002.

Chest Pain

Jean A. Proehl

1. **Should clinicians mainly worry about cardiac disease in men older than age 40 who complain of chest pain?**

   No. Cardiovascular disease is the leading cause of death in American women. Young people may also present with chest pain caused by myocardial infarction (MI), especially after using cocaine. In addition, not all patients experiencing life-threatening cardiac problems have chest pain. Misdiagnosing a patient who is having an MI can have fatal consequences and is a leading cause of emergency department (ED) medical malpractice suits. It is better to be safe than sorry when triaging patients who have any suggestion of cardiac disease.

2. **If a patient is not having chest pain, when should MI be suspected?**

   Some patients, particularly elderly, female, and diabetic patients, may experience little or no pain associated with MI. Other patients at risk for MI without chest pain include patients who have previously had some type of invasive coronary intervention such as surgery or angioplasty. Some patients have symptoms described as "indigestion," and in others the pain is mild and ignored (or denied). Instead of chest pain, the patient may have pain in the jaw, shoulder, neck, or arms. Other symptoms may include dyspnea, diaphoresis, nausea and vomiting, dizziness, syncope, or fatigue and malaise.

3. **How quickly should a patient exhibiting signs and symptoms of MI receive a 12-lead electrocardiogram (ECG)?**

   The American Heart Association (AHA) guidelines state that a 12-lead ECG should be performed and shown to an experienced emergency physician within 10 minutes of ED arrival. Other treatment goals from the AHA include door-to-needle time for fibrinolytic therapy within 30 minutes and door-to-balloon time for percutaneous coronary intervention (PCI) within 90 minutes. These are aggressive goals intended to ensure rapid diagnosis and treatment of MI to decrease subsequent morbidity and mortality. To achieve these goals, an efficient and coordinated response is needed. Some hospitals now have a special team that is paged and responds immediately to the ED in this situation. The team may include nurses, physicians, ECG technicians, laboratory personnel, x-ray technologists, and pharmacists.

4. What is acute coronary syndrome (ACS)?

ACS includes a spectrum of conditions caused by ruptured or eroded atheroma-
tous plaque in the coronary arteries. ACS diagnoses include unstable angina,
non–Q-wave MI, and Q-wave MI. Sudden cardiac death is a risk for all types of ACS.

5. What are the similarities and differences between angina and MI?

Both angina and MI are caused by coronary artery disease (CAD). When a
patient suffers MI (commonly referred to as a "heart attack"), blood flow through
one or more coronary arteries is decreased or stopped. This decrease in blood
flow leads to ischemia and infarction of the myocardium and will cause necrosis
if perfusion is not reestablished. Angina can be caused by a narrowing of one or
more coronary arteries or by vasospasm. In either case, the narrowing causes
decreased blood flow, leading to ischemia but *not* to infarct or necrosis. Beware
if a patient with CAD suffers more frequent anginal episodes or if the episodes
become more intense or occur at rest; such changes may signal unstable angina
and impending MI.

6. How do patients describe the pain of angina versus the pain of MI?

The signs and symptoms may be similar. Patients with stable angina usually
present for emergency care only if something about their pain and other symptoms
is different from their normal pain. The pain associated with an MI is typically
described as heaviness, burning, aching, squeezing, severe crushing, or the feeling
that "an elephant is sitting on my chest." It may be mistaken for "indigestion."
The pain may or may not radiate to the neck, jaw, arms, or back. Other reported
signs and symptoms may include:
- Pallor
- Diaphoresis
- Nausea and vomiting
- A sense of impending doom (known as "angor animi")
- Weakness
- Anxiety
- Shortness of breath

Some patients deny that their pain and other symptoms are significant and
therefore delay seeking care. This is a risky situation as evidenced by the fact that
most people who die from MI do so before ever reaching the hospital.

7. If the symptoms are similar, how can a patient suffering from MI be
differentiated from a patient suffering from angina?

In both cases, cardiac tissue is deprived of oxygen (ischemia). The ischemia
causes chest pain. Anginal pain typically lasts 2 to 15 minutes and is usually
relieved with rest or nitroglycerin. However, if the pain is not relieved by rest
or nitroglycerin, the cause may be MI. *Patients should be instructed to access
emergency medical care if their pain is not improved within 5 minutes of one dose
of nitroglycerin.*

In addition to the patient's clinical presentation, a 12-lead ECG and
biochemical cardiac markers are used to make the diagnosis. If the diagnosis
remains uncertain, treat the patient as suffering from MI. Definitive diagnosis is

based on clinical presentation, presence of risk factors, ECG changes, and levels of biochemical cardiac markers.

8. What does the 12-lead ECG show in patients with MI?

A 12-lead ECG may be normal during the first few hours after MI. Heart muscle is composed of three layers. Extension of the damage across these layers accounts for the ECG changes. Look specifically for the following indicators:

- **ST segment.** If a coronary artery is occluded, the ST segment elevates and the T wave inverts in the leads at the area of infarction (see the following table). ST depression (or reciprocal changes) may be seen in the leads opposite the area of infarction. ST-segment depression also may be present in subendocardial infarctions.
- **Q wave.** A Q wave appears when all three layers of heart muscle are infarcted (also known as a transmural infarct). A non–Q-wave MI (sometimes referred to as a subendocardial infarct) involves only one or two layers. (*Reminder: A Q wave is the first negative deflection following the PR segment.*)

ECG changes in acute MI

Type of MI	Leads
Inferior wall	II, III, aV_F
Anterior wall	V_3, V_4
Septal wall	V_1, V_2
Lateral wall	I, aV_L, V_5, V_6
Anterolateral wall	I, aV_L, V_3-V_6

9. What is an ST-elevation MI (STEMI)?

STEMI diagnosis is made in the presence of ST elevation greater than 0.1 mV (one small box on the ECG paper), in at least two contiguous leads, or new left bundle branch block. Most of these patients will develop Q-wave MI if reperfusion is not achieved rapidly.

10. How is non–Q-wave MI diagnosed?

When non–Q-wave MI occurs, only the innermost layer of the myocardium (subendocardium) is injured. Therefore, an ECG diagnosis is not possible; cardiac biomarkers make the definitive diagnosis.

11. What are cardiac biomarkers?

Cardiac biomarkers are substances that indicate cardiac muscle damage. The biomarkers most commonly used in the diagnosis of ACS are the troponins; troponin I, troponin T, and troponin C are highly cardiac-specific. They are released into the bloodstream during MI and levels rise within 2 to 4 hours of the onset of infarction. Troponins remain elevated for as long as a week; therefore they are useful for patients who delay seeking care. Others biomarkers for cardiac disease include creatine kinase (CK; CK-MB), lactate dehydrogenase (LD or LDH), and myoglobin. These have largely been replaced by troponin.

12. Are there any new diagnostic tests for cardiac disease?

B-type natriuretic peptide (BNP) and N-terminal proBNP (NT-proBNP) measure a hormone secreted by the myocardium in response to stretching. If the pumping capability of the heart deteriorates, these hormone levels increase. It is useful in diagnosing heart failure and may be useful in addition to troponin when assessing patients for ACS.

High sensitivity C-reactive protein (hs-CRP) is a marker of inflammation and cardiovascular disease. Inflammation contributes to plaque instability and rupture. Measuring hs-CRP may be useful for risk assessment for cardiovascular disease in symptomatic and asymptomatic patients.

13. If the pain is not relieved with nitroglycerin tablets or spray, what will help with pain relief?

Improved oxygenation may decrease pain and ischemia. Patients with suspicious chest pain should receive oxygen; if STEMI is diagnosed, oxygen is administered for the first 6 hours–even in the presence of normal SpO_2. Additional medications that are administered for pain relief include morphine sulfate and/or nitroglycerin via intravenous (IV) infusion.

14. How does nitroglycerin relieve chest pain? Why does a headache sometimes develop?

The heart receives its oxygen supply via the coronary arteries during diastole. Nitroglycerin dilates the smooth muscle of the venous system, decreasing venous return to the heart, ventricular filling, and wall tension (preload). This leads to improved coronary perfusion. In addition, nitroglycerin dilates the coronary arteries, increases coronary collateral circulation, and retards vasospasm. Simply put, nitroglycerin improves coronary blood flow to meet cardiac oxygen demand and thus decreases chest pain.

Headache is the most common side effect associated with the use of nitroglycerin and is related to vasodilation of blood vessels in the head. Usually headache is self-limited or can be reduced and/or eliminated with aspirin, acetaminophen, or another mild analgesic. The patient's blood pressure may also drop because of the decrease in systemic vascular resistance as a result of systemic vasodilation. For this reason, *nitroglycerin should not be given to patients with a systolic blood pressure less than 90 mmHg.*

15. Why is pain relief important?

Pain relief isn't just a "nice thing to do." Pain causes catecholamine release. Catecholamines increase heart rate and cause vasoconstriction, both of which increase the workload of the heart and may cause further damage to the already ischemic myocardium.

16. **Can aspirin really save a person's life if suffering a heart attack?**

Yes. Low-dose aspirin (162 to 325 mg) suppresses platelet aggregation. Aspirin should be given immediately after the onset of symptoms and may be self-administered by the patient or given by prehospital care providers before arrival in the ED. It is important that the aspirin be chewed to speed absorption; enteric coated preparations should not be used. If the patient is experiencing MI, he or she will probably be instructed to take aspirin every day to reduce the risk of reinfarction, stroke, and death.

17. **What medications should be on hand to administer to the patient suffering from MI?**

First-line medications include morphine, oxygen, nitroglycerin, and aspirin. These are easily remembered with the mnemonic "MONA." In addition, anticipate giving heparin or low–molecular-weight heparin and an IV beta blocker (e.g., metoprolol). Beta blockers appear to decrease the size of the infarction and complications associated with MI. Clopidogrel reduces platelet aggregation through a different mechanism than aspirin and may be prescribed in addition to aspirin or for patients who are allergic to aspirin. A glycoprotein IIb/IIIa platelet inhibitor such as abciximab, eptifibatide, or tirofiban may also be prescribed, especially if the patient is going to the cardiac catheterization lab. If rapid access to a cardiac catheterization lab for PCI is not available, fibrinolytics such as alteplase (TPA), tenecteplase (TNKase), or reteplase may be used to reperfuse the artery.

18. **What is PCI?**

PCI refers to invasive techniques that are used to open the artery and keep it open. Techniques include balloon angioplasty and the insertion of stents.

19. **Which is better, fibrinolytic therapy or PCI?**

Many studies have demonstrated improved outcomes with PCI over fibrinolytic therapy as long as the procedure is performed in a timely fashion by experienced personnel in high-volume centers. However, not all hospitals have this capability or, if they do have the capability, they may not be able to provide it in a timely fashion 24 hours per day, 7 days a week. If PCI cannot be performed in a timely manner, fibrinolytic therapy is probably just as effective as delayed PCI and is used as long as there are no contraindications.

20. **How is a right ventricle infarct diagnosed, and how should treatment be different?**

Right ventricle infarctions occur in about 50% of patients with an inferior MI. When ST elevation is present in leads II, III, and aV_F, indicating an inferior MI, right-sided ECG leads are assessed using the mirror image of the usual lead placement for V_3 to V_4. Jugular vein distention indicates that the right side of the heart is not moving the blood forward normally as it returns from the body via the vena cava. Hypotension and clear lung fields are common findings. Nitroglycerin, morphine, and diuretics are contraindicated because they decrease preload and severe hypotension may ensue. If a patient with inferior lead changes develops hypotension after nitroglycerin therapy, right ventricular infarction should be suspected. Treat this hypotension with 500 ml boluses of normal saline IV up to 1 to 2 liters. If fluid loading does not reverse the hypotension, vasopressors, vasodilators, and intraaortic balloon pump therapy may be necessary.

21. **What are noncardiac causes of chest pain?**

Noncardiac chest pain can be caused by problems with the gastrointestinal (GI), vascular, respiratory, and musculoskeletal systems or trauma. Some of these situations are also life threatening. *When in doubt, treat the pain as cardiac pain or another life-threatening etiology until proven otherwise.*

Noncardiac causes of chest pain

Vascular
Aortic dissection
Aneurysm

GI
Esophageal spasms
Indigestion, acid reflux
Peptic ulcer
Hiatal hernia
Gallbladder disease

Musculoskeletal
Costochondritis
Muscle strain

Respiratory
Pulmonary embolus
Bronchitis
Pleuritis

Trauma
Aortic rupture
Chest wall contusion
Splenic injury
Rib fractures

Key Points

- Patients suffering from MI may present with atypical symptoms and no chest pain, especially the elderly, women, and patients with diabetes. When in doubt, assume cardiac origin until proven otherwise.
- Diagnosis and treatment for suspected MI must be fast to decrease the chance of permanent heart damage and death. The 12-lead ECG should be shown to an experienced emergency physician within 10 minutes of patient arrival.
- Patients with suspicious chest pain should receive morphine, oxygen, nitroglycerin, and chewable aspirin.
- Patients diagnosed with MI will also probably receive beta blockers, heparin or low–molecular-weight heparin, and a glycoprotein IIb/IIIa platelet inhibitor (abciximab or eptifibatide). If PCI is not available, fibrinolytics will be given (alteplase [TPA], tenecteplase [TNKase], reteplase).
- Right ventricle infarction should be suspected in any patient with inferior MI, especially in the presence of clear lungs and hypotension. Nitroglycerin and morphine may cause dangerous hypotension in these patients.

Internet Resources

American Heart Association Journal, *Circulation:*
www.circ.ahajournals.org

Cochrane Collaboration:
www.cochrane.org

eMedicine, Emergency medicine, Cardiovascular articles:
www.emedicine.com/emerg/CARDIOVASCULAR.htm

Wikipedia, Chest Pain:
http://en.wikipedia.org/wiki/Chest_pain

Bibliography

American Heart Association in collaboration with the International Liaison Committee on Resuscitation: Part 5: Acute Coronary Syndromes (pp III-55 - III-72) In 2005 International Consensus on Cardiopulmonary Resuscitation (CPR) and Emergency Cardiovascular Care (ECC) Science with Treatment Recommendations, *Circulation* 112(suppl I) 2005. Available at www.circ.ahajournals.org/cgi/reprint/112/22_suppl/III-55.

American Heart Association in collaboration with the International Liaison Committee on Resuscitation: Part 8: Stabilization of the Patient with Acute Coronary Syndromes (pp 89-110) In 2005 American Heart Association Guidelines for Cardiopulmonary Resuscitation and Emergency Cardiovascular Care, *Circulation* 112, 2005. Available at www.circ.ahajournals.org/cgi/reprint/112/24_suppl/IV-89.

Antman EM et al: ACC/AHA guidelines for the management of ST-elevation myocardial infarction: Executive summary, *Circulation* 110:1-49, 2004.

Pearson TA et al: Markers of inflammation and cardiovascular disease: Application to clinical and public health practice, *Circulation* 107:499-511, 2003.

Rexhous S: Chest pain. In Oman K, Koziol-McLain J, Scheetz L, editors: *Emergency nursing secrets*, Philadelphia, 2001, Hanley & Belfus.

Respiratory Distress

Ivy F. Shaffer

1. What are the main events that lead to respiratory distress?

Any condition that interferes with airway, ventilation, or respiration—including upper and lower airway respiratory conditions, as well as nonrespiratory conditions.

Upper airway distress includes the following pathological entities that impede the glottic opening and the supraglottic structures, such as the larynx, tongue, tonsils, uvula, and/or face:

- Laryngospasm
- Epiglottitis
- Foreign body obstruction
- Vocal cord dysfunction
- Croup
- Thermal/chemical injuries
- Postoperative ear, nose, or throat (ENT) hemorrhage
- Cancer of the throat or larynx
- Trauma to midfacial structures
- Trauma to larynx or trachea
- Angioneurotic edema
- Anaphylaxis with edema of tongue and upper airway structures
- Epistaxis
- Trismus of jaw
- Ludwig's angina
- Other deep neck infections that include cellulitis of the palate, tongue, and floor of the mouth

Lower airway distress involves pathology below the glottic opening, involving tracheal, bronchial, or alveolar structures or lung parenchyma, such as:

- Emphysema
- Bronchitis
- Pneumonia
- Asthma
- Tracheal displacement
- Pneumothorax
- Hemothorax
- Cancer of the lung, mediastinum, or esophagus
- Pulmonary edema
- Pleural effusions
- Noncardiogenic pulmonary edema

- Parenchymal lung injury from inhaled toxins (solvents, aerosols)
- Carbon monoxide poisoning
- Barotrauma
- Methemoglobinemia
- Pulmonary contusions

Respiratory complications can occur because of strangulation; hanging; near drowning; infections; interstitial lung diseases (sarcoidosis, asbestosis); stroke; severe mitral valve insufficiency; critical aortic valve stenosis; cystic fibrosis; alpha-1 antitrypsin deficiency; and fungal, viral, and bacterial lung infections. Severe metabolic imbalances and neuromuscular disorders such as amyotrophic lateral sclerosis, myasthenia gravis, Guillain-Barré syndrome, spinal cord injury, brain tumors, and head injury can also cause respiratory distress.

2. What are the subtle signs and symptoms of impending respiratory distress?

- Restlessness
- Agitation
- Confusion
- Inability to lie flat or slightly recumbent
- Progressive altered level of consciousness
- Increased respiratory rate and effort
- Cool, clammy skin
- Purulent cough and fever
- Frothy pink sputum
- Hemoptysis
- Pulse oximetry readings below 90%

3. What signs and symptoms indicate that respiratory management must be initiated?

- Persistent tachypnea with more than 30 breaths/min
- Difficulty speaking in short phrases
- Complaints of chest pain with ischemic electrocardiogram (ECG) changes
- Intercostal and suprasternal retractions
- Wheezing and stridor at rest
- Inability to speak, cough (choking victims), or swallow secretions
- Gasping or snoring respirations
- Pallor, cyanosis, and profuse diaphoresis
- Drooling in a patient with complaints of a "bad sore throat"
- Pulse oximetry readings below 90% despite titration of increased supplemental oxygen
- Arterial blood gases (ABGs) that indicate respiratory acidosis, hypoxemia, and hypercapnea
- Pulsus paradoxus greater than 25 mmHg during inspiration

4. What are the signs of impending respiratory arrest?

- Bradycardia
- Agonal or paradoxical respiratory efforts
- Hypercapnea
- Loss of consciousness

5. **What are the interventions for patients in respiratory distress?**

- Administer 100% oxygen via a nonrebreather mask.
- Clear the airway of secretions with a suction device.
- Elevate the head of the bed and remove constrictive clothing (and if possible any oral jewelry).
- If the patient is unconscious, place supine and position the head for optimal ventilation (head tilt–chin lift maneuver or jaw thrust if cervical spine injury may be present).
- If the patient becomes unable to maintain effective ventilation, intubate or support respirations using a bag valve mask device with a reservoir and 100% oxygen.
  - Squeeze the bag gently at a rate of 20 breaths/min, attempting to "breathe" with patient's own inspiratory efforts.
  - Ensure a good seal and observe for symmetrical rise of the chest wall.
  - Confirm intubation placement by presence of condensation in endotracheal tube (ETT), capnometry, improvement in pulse oximetry, absence of auscultated stomach contents over epigastrium, and presence of stomach contents in ETT.
  - Caution should be taken not to overinflate the lungs, especially in patients with high airway pressures or "stiff" lungs; forceful bagging can rupture lung bullae, leading to a pneumothorax.
  - Watch for abdominal distention and the possibility of emesis in the unprotected airway. As soon as possible place a gastric tube to avoid aspiration.
- Continue to monitor pulse oximetry, vital signs, and work of breathing.
- Treat underlying cause (e.g., diuretics for congestive heart failure [CHF], bronchodilators for reactive airway disease).
- Insert intravenous (IV) line as soon as possible, especially if a rapid sequence intubation protocol will be utilized or if the patient requires the aforementioned medications and IV sedation.
- Obtain a postintubation portable chest radiograph to ensure proper ETT placement, and rule out other pathology such as pneumothorax, pneumonia, CHF, or other potential reasons for respiratory decline.

6. **Why is pulse oximetry sometimes called the "fifth vital sign"?**

Many clinicians advocate assessment of oxygenation with pulse oximetry as another vital sign, especially during triage. The belief in the importance of routine assessment of oxygenation is supported by empirical evidence that pulse oximetry can detect early changes in respiratory function, often before the patient exhibits classic symptoms of distress. Because pulse oximetry is a quick, noninvasive assessment, it makes sense to incorporate its use into triage assessment, especially if the patient has a history of respiratory problems or a chief complaint related to the respiratory system.

7. **Is pulse oximetry reliable?**

Pulse oximetry is generally reliable (±4%) in patients whose levels of oxygen saturation in arterial blood (SaO_2) are above 80. For patients with lower saturation levels, pulse oximetry can produce falsely high readings. Patients who have a high baseline saturation can experience a significant change in the partial pressure of oxygen in arterial blood (Pa_{O_2}) with relatively little change in the oximetry reading. Look for a good pulse waveform in interpreting the pulse oximetry reading. Pulse oximetry is *not* reliable in carbon monoxide poisoning, methemoglobinemia, low flow states, and severe anemia (hemoglobin less than 5).

8. **What is the treatment of choice for acute respiratory failure?**

Intubation and mechanical ventilation have been the preferred treatment for years. Recently, however, noninvasive mask ventilation (e.g., bilevel positive airway pressure [BiPAP], continuous positive airway pressure [CPAP]) has been used successfully for patients with chronic obstructive pulmonary disease (COPD) and CHF. The advantage of noninvasive mask ventilation is avoidance of nosocomial pulmonary infection and barotrauma. In addition, ventilation-dependent respiratory failure and possibly a tracheotomy can be avoided. Other conventional therapies include oxygen, bronchodilators, steroids, diuretics, and antibiotics as indicated.

9. **What are the patient criteria for noninvasive mask ventilation?**

- Hemodynamic stability (no vasopressor agents needed)
- Alert and cooperative patient
- Ability of patient to protect airway
- Evidence of fatigue
- ABG data consistent with acute respiratory failure
  - Partial pressure of carbon dioxide in arterial blood (Pa_{CO_2}) greater than 50 mmHg with pH less than 7.30 (respiratory acidosis)
  - Pa_{O_2} less than 60 mmHg with fractional concentration of oxygen inspired gas (Fi_{O_2}) greater than 50%

  Patients predicted to do well with noninvasive mask ventilation are those whose ABGs are stable after a 30-minute trial run.

10. **Are there any new treatments for respiratory failure on the horizon?**

Yes. In circumstances in which noninvasive mask ventilation is not tolerated (combativeness, oxygen leak because of poorly fitting masks), new treatments on the horizon include the use of a mini-tracheotomy as a bridge between noninvasive and invasive mechanical ventilation. Although the efficacy and safety are still being researched, studies are promising for COPD exacerbations and respiratory failure. With transtracheal open ventilation (TOV), patients are able to speak (unlike with invasive intubations), there is minimal discomfort, breathing patterns normalize, and alveolar gas exchange improves.

11. **How does asthma affect the lungs?**

The large and small airways of the asthmatic are affected by acute bronchospasm, obstruction, inflammation, hyperresponsiveness, and hyperinflation (auto-positive end-expiratory pressure [auto-PEEP]). Asthma, a reactive airway disease, is often exacerbated by a trigger (e.g., allergen, infection, irritants, nonsteroidal antiinflammatory drugs [NSAIDs], beta blockers, sulfite agents, exercise, and psychological factors) that initiates hyperresponsiveness and cellular mediated inflammation in the bronchial tree. Disorders known to predispose a patient to asthma include esophageal reflux, sinusitis, aspiration, and chronic environmental and occupational exposures to irritants. Finally, swelling and spasm of the lower airways occur, and secretions produced from the inflammatory response collect, plugging the lower airways. The combined result is hyperinflation leading to decreased movement of air throughout the lung fields.

12. What is an asthma attack?

The patient complains of dyspnea, chest tightness, cough, sputum production, and wheezing, despite using rescue inhalers and prescribed nebulized treatments before arrival. The patient may use accessory muscles, speak in short broken sentences, and exhibit audible wheezing. Patients position themselves "straight" up in the chair or stretcher. The severity of the attack can be estimated initially by simple observation of the work of breathing, auscultated flow of air throughout the lung fields, a peak flow less than 200 L/min, and the inability of the patient to speak in complete sentences. A "quiet" chest during an exacerbation may be a foreboding sign, indicating that air movement is minimal. Patient fatigue, secondary to the enormous amount of energy expended in the work of breathing and the buildup of carbon dioxide, can lead to less air being moved to generate wheezing and thus a quiet chest.

13. How is an asthma attack treated?

Baseline peak flow should be measured and therapy initiated. Treatment of choice initially is the common beta-agonist albuterol, 2.5 to 5 mg by aerosolization. It has profound bronchodilation effects and can be repeated every 20 minutes, or delivered continuously in status asthmaticus.

The anticholinergics (e.g., iprotropium [Atrovent]) are potent antisecretory medications and can be used alone or in combination with albuterol. Current research has demonstrated these two drugs combined are more effective in improving pulmonary function and decreasing hospital admission rate. However, these drugs have side effects such as tremors and tachycardia, occasionally making them difficult for compromised cardiac patients to tolerate.

Levalbuterol (Xopenex) is a newer bronchodilator drug that contains the R isomer of racemic albuterol. Although early studies were promising, recent randomized controlled trials in children with asthma (Qureshi et al, 2005; Ralston et al, 2005) showed no difference in respiratory outcomes between racemic albuterol, levalbuterol, and iprotropium (with the exception that increase in heart rate was less with levalbuterol).

Other medications that may be given during the initial treatment of acute asthma are magnesium sulfate and leukotriene inhibitors (Accolate, Singulair), which augment bronchial smooth muscle relaxation and decrease the inflammatory response.

Oxygen is administered to maintain pulse oximetry at 90% or greater and PaO_2 at greater than 60 mmHg.

Corticosteroids, such as methylprednisolone 125 mg (Solu-Medrol), should also be initiated early in the treatment regimen, as research has demonstrated when corticosteroids are given within the first hour of admission there is a correlating reduction in hospital admissions because of recurrence.

The current trend is to administer nebulized medications continuously until the attack resolves. Remember to measure peak flow before and after treatment. It is not unusual to see a peak flow less than 200 L/min. As the restricted airways open, the patient should be able to generate higher peak flows throughout the course of treatment. Between treatments, position the patient comfortably, and administer oxygen via nasal cannula.

Most patients do well with a conventional treatment regimen; however, even the most astute clinician must be prepared for those patients who fail conventional treatment. Acetylcysteine may occasionally be used to break up mucus plugs, whereas other modalities such as nitric oxide or heliox (a mixture of oxygen and helium) assist by decreasing dyspnea and fatigue. In cases of extremis, in which an intubated patient's chest remains "tight" as evidenced by high peaked airway pressures on the ventilator, general anesthetic gas (e.g., halothane) may be used for further bronchodilatory effects.

14. How is treatment effectiveness determined?

Patients who demonstrate improvement after treatment say they feel less short of breath. Air flow throughout the lungs improves, wheezing decreases, peak flow improves, and there is decreased work of breathing.

15. What are the goals for the management of asthma?

Primary goals for asthmatics include self-awareness and preventing asthma exacerbations.
- Educate patients to recognize triggers (cigarette smoke is a major trigger), symptoms of early exacerbations, use of rescue inhalers, and when to seek clinic and emergency care.
- Teach proper use of medications, especially metered dose inhalers (MDIs). Instruct patients to take daily control medication (inhaled steroids) even when they feel well and are not wheezing. Spacer devices give the newly diagnosed asthmatic child, or adult with lack of manual dexterity, the ability to inhale MDI medications more easily and effectively.
- Teach monitoring of peak flow measurements (twice daily) so "baselines" are established and patients know to contact their healthcare provider when peak flow decreases greater than 20% from baseline.
- Encourage patients to maintain a healthy lifestyle, to avoid potential asthma triggers, and to get influenza and pneumococcal vaccines.
- Communicate with primary healthcare provider to evaluate the need for follow-up visits, testing (such as pulmonary function tests), and medication adjustments.
- Direct patients to resources and local support groups.

16. What is the pharmacological maintenance therapy for asthma?

Pharmacological management of asthma is generally with routine inhaled steroids, such as Beclovent, Vanceril, Pulmicort, AeroBid, and Flovent ("control" medicine) rather than bronchodilators ("rescue" medicine).

Prevention of bronchospasm through pharmaceutical control of inflammation is a key to preventing exacerbations. Mast cell stabilizers (Intal, Tilade) are a mainstay of chronic therapy and are administered via MDI to inhibit bronchospasm and inflammation resulting from antigen and environmental irritants. A new class of antiinflammatory drugs is gaining popularity. These pharmacological agents are called leukotriene receptor antagonists and work by promoting bronchodilation. Research by Perng et al (2004) demonstrates that the combination of low-dose corticosteroids with leukotriene-modifying agents is equally as effective as administration of high-dose inhaled steroid agents. Because of the success of newer medications, drugs such as the methylxanthines (theophylline) and terbutaline have fallen out of favor and are controversial because of toxicity and cardiovascular effects.

17. How does asthma differ from COPD?

Unlike asthma, the main cause of airway obstruction in patients with COPD is bronchoconstriction rather than inflammation. However, because COPD includes aspects of chronic bronchitis and emphysema, patients with chronic bronchitis often have some inflammation. Moreover, fibrotic constriction is present in COPD, contributing to air flow obstruction. Both asthma and COPD involve decreased air flow with resultant carbon dioxide retention and hypoxemia. In COPD, excessive mucus is produced and the airway is hyperresponsive. Long-term progression of COPD leads to a weakening of alveolar walls with subsequent entrapment of air within the alveoli.

18. What are the symptoms of a COPD exacerbation?

Increased dyspnea, sputum production, and sputum purulence.

19. Is the initial treatment for a COPD exacerbation similar to asthma?

Yes. Bronchodilators such as metaproterenol (Alupent), ipratropium (Atrovent), or albuterol (Proventil) are used, along with steroids and oxygen. Oxygen administration must be titrated according to carbon dioxide levels.

20. What kind of preventive information should be provided to patients with COPD?

Encourage patients to quit smoking. Smoking contributes 80% to 90% of the risk for the development of COPD. Continuation of smoking causes disease progression. Teach patients to recognize warning signs, such as an increased sputum production, change in sputum color or consistency, increased shortness of breath, fatigue, and elevated temperature. Patients should be advised to seek treatment at the initial appearance of these signs. Also instruct patients to get influenza and pneumococcal vaccines, exercise regularly, maintain optimal nutrition, and lose weight if obese.

21. What are the signs and symptoms of pulmonary embolism (PE)?

Pleuritic chest pain; hypoxia; shortness of breath at rest; wheezing without prior history; new onset right bundle branch block with tall P waves indicative of cor pulmonale; hemoptysis; tachycardia; an auscultated S_3 or S_4 gallop and pleural friction rub; episodic hypotension; history of syncope; and recent swollen, atraumatic calf pain. Other symptoms include back and shoulder pain, upper quadrant abdominal pain, mild low-grade fever, and basilar rales.

22. What are the risk factors for a pulmonary embolus?

- Smoking
- Sedentary lifestyle
- Obesity
- Dehydration
- Childbirth
- Birth control pills
- History of deep vein thrombosis (DVT)
- Polycythemia
- IV drug abuse
- Underlying malignancy
- Elderly
- Traveling long distance (truck drivers, long flights)
- History of recent minor or major surgical procedures
- Blunt trauma to lower extremities
- Fractures of long bones
- Indwelling catheters (peripherally inserted central catheter [PICC] lines, Swan-Ganz catheters)

23. How is PE differentiated from other causes of dyspnea or chest pain?

The presentation of dyspnea, syncope, and hemoptysis, alone or in combination with chest pain that worsens with respiration and new ECG changes (suggestive of right ventricular overload), are highly suspicious for PE. Pulmonary angiogram is the gold standard for diagnosis, but it is not available in all hospitals and is associated with risks. As an alternative, a ventilation-perfusion (VQ) scan suggestive of a moderate or high probability of PE, coupled with the clinical presentation, is usually sufficient confirmation to begin treatment. Approximately 86% of patients with a "high probability" VQ scan, 34% of patients with a "moderate probability" VQ scan, and 31% of patients with a "low probability" VQ scan have PE. In some centers spiral computed tomography (CT) scan of the chest has replaced the VQ scan. Although the D-dimer test is frequently used, it is often affected by other processes that can lead to a false positive. Therefore, the patient's risk factor profile, clinical status, and laboratory and radiographical findings should be concomitantly considered in differentiating a pulmonary embolic event. The role of Doppler ultrasonography is also being investigated.

24. If PE is suspected, what are the initial interventions?

Administer oxygen, monitor vital signs and pulse oximetry, place the patient on a cardiac monitor, establish venous access, and obtain baseline lab studies, including complete blood count (CBC), electrolyte panel, prothrombin time (PT), partial thromboplastin time (PTT), international normalized ratio (INR), D-dimer, and at least one set of cardiac enzymes to rule out a hypoxic cardiac event. A portable chest radiograph should also be done to rule out other pulmonary conditions and check for pulmonary congestion. If the patient is hypovolemic, cautious fluid resuscitation is indicated. Patients often have an impending sense of doom; be supportive and tell the patient what is being done.

Pharmacological intervention consists primarily of a bolus of IV heparin, followed by a continuous infusion of weight-based heparin to prevent further emboli and clotting. Thrombolytics, embolectomies, thoracotomy, and even cardiopulmonary bypass can be used when patients are in extremis if such resources are readily available and all other treatments fail. An inferior vena cava filter may be inserted for patients prone to DVT with pulmonary emboli.

25. What causes a pneumothorax?

Pneumothorax results from external trauma or barotraumas, or it can develop spontaneously. Air accumulates in the pleural space, resulting in collapse of the lung (or a portion thereof). Traumatic causes are addressed in Chapter 26. Barotrauma is often iatrogenic, seen in up to 15% of patients who are mechanically ventilated with PEEP. Spontaneous pneumothorax is classified as primary or secondary. Primary spontaneous pneumothorax is most common in tall, thin young people without lung disease, whereas secondary spontaneous pneumothorax is seen in elderly people with chronic lung disease.

26. How do patients with a spontaneous pneumothorax present?

Patients usually complain of chest pain, often localized on the side of the pneumothorax. The pain is often pleuritic in nature and described as "sharp." Varying degrees of dyspnea are usually present, depending upon the size of the pneumothorax. In some cases palpation of the chest wall will reveal subcutaneous emphysema and asymmetrical chest movement.

27. What are the priorities for a patient in whom spontaneous pneumothorax is suspected?

Administer oxygen, position the patient upright, obtain a chest radiograph, and prepare for evacuation of the pleural air. If the patient presents with left-sided chest pain, an ECG may be done to rule out transmural infarct.

Two methods are used to evacuate air: thoracic drainage with a chest tube and needle aspiration. Generally, needle aspiration is not performed if the pneumothorax is large. Patients who experience dyspnea are frightened and need support. Explain to the patient what is being done and offer reassurance. Small pneumothoracies (less than 10%) in patients who are otherwise healthy can be monitored without chest tube insertion. If the pneumothorax is traumatically induced, monitor the amount of blood collecting in the chest drainage unit.

28. What is epiglottitis?

Epiglottitis is an acute, life-threatening cellulitis involving the epiglottis and surrounding supraglottic tissues. It is most commonly caused by *Haemophilus influenzae* type b (Hib), *Streptococcus pneumoniae*, and/or group A streptococci. The epiglottis—which is normally a smooth, thin structure that covers the portal of the trachea—becomes enlarged and inflamed, appears beefy red, and can spontaneously occlude the trachea, resulting in complete airway obstruction.

29. What are the cardinal symptoms of epiglottitis?

Rapid onset of high fever, sore throat, muffled voice, and drooling are classic. Children may exhibit increased work of breathing, appear dyspneic, and have a slight stridor as the glottic opening is narrowed by periepiglottal inflammation.

An adult may appear anxious and slightly dyspneic with or without stridor. Children and adults will both position themselves with their neck slightly forward (tripod position) to obtain maximal air flow around the thickened epiglottis. Because children are frequently immunized against Hib, adults are becoming the more vulnerable population. However, despite immunizations in healthy, uncompromised children, some are still at risk because of an inability to launch an adequate immune response.

30. How is the diagnosis of epiglottitis made?

If there is a high index of suspicion for epiglottitis, *do not* attempt to visualize the pharyngeal structures on an adult or a child. Request an immediate radiograph of the neck to confirm the diagnosis, and have emergency medicine, anesthesia, and the OR on standby for emergent intubation and airway control.

31. What interventions can the nurse take?

From triage, epiglottitis must be suspected in presentations in which the patient complains of fever, sore throat, and difficulty swallowing; is constantly expectorating saliva; and appears distressed or anxious (despite normal pulse oximetry). In a child, allow the parents to hold and console the child and encourage speaking in a slow, calm manner to avoid upsetting the child and increasing the risk of respiratory distress and occlusion secondary to crying. Then, alert the charge nurse and immediately escort the patient to a resuscitation room.

Allow the adult and pediatric patient to sit up, apply oxygen, and have emergency airway equipment at the bedside with a bag valve mask. Do not agitate the child with attempts at IV line insertion or phlebotomy for lab specimens. It is not necessary to obtain ABGs for two reasons: Doing so will agitate both children and adults, potentially causing acute obstruction, and rising PCO_2 levels are not necessarily considered predictors of outcomes or impending obstruction. In fact, hypercapnea is a late indicator of impending respiratory decline.

The airway is optimally secured by fiberoptics in the OR. Priorities are to alert anesthesia and the OR team, constant surveillance of rate and quality of respirations, and administration of IV antibiotics if ordered for the adult patient.

32. What happens if the airway becomes obstructed?

If the airway becomes obstructed in either the adult or pediatric patient, immediately manage the airway with positive pressure ventilations using a bag valve mask device and 100% oxygen until intubation or a surgical airway can be accomplished. The edematous structures can be easily displaced with the force of positive pressure ventilation, thus buying time for definitive airway management. In cases in which intubation is unsuccessful, percutaneous cricothyroidotomy or needle cricothyroidotomy with high-frequency jet ventilation may be initiated to access the trachea.

33. What is the definitive treatment of epiglottitis?

Prophylactic intubation in a controlled setting, such as the OR, is recommended for children. Adults can be closely monitored without intubation; however, the severity of the symptomatology and the availability of clinicians skilled in managing an emergent surgical airway will ultimately assist the treating clinician in making the decision to secure the airway via intubation. IV fluid hydration and broad-spectrum antibiotics should be initiated as soon as possible.

34. **Respiratory illness is a common reason for emergency department (ED) visits. What is the emergency nurse's role?**

- "Cough with courtesy" should be encouraged by triage nurses, especially during flu season. The spread of respiratory-borne illnesses between patients and staff can potentially be prevented by simply requesting patients to cover their mouths when coughing or sneezing, supplying tissues and liquid hand sanitizer, or even requesting a patient to wear a mask for the protection of other waiting patients and staff.
- Routine triage questions for patients with respiratory symptoms should include recent travel (within 10 days) or contact with recent travelers outside the United States to areas where suspected severe respiratory distress syndrome (SRDS) or other potential flu outbreaks have been reported.
- In addition to protecting the public, it is important that ED staff first protect themselves. Wearing N95 respiratory masks, using universal precautions, and placing suspected contagious patients in negative air flow rooms should be the norm.
- Institutions with pneumonia protocols expedite patients with respiratory illnesses to the main department where they can be isolated. Such protocols allow the nurse to draw blood; order chest radiographs; initiate IV access; administer oxygen; and, after two sets of blood cultures have been drawn, consult the ED attending physician so that antibiotics are administered within 2 to 4 hours of admission to the department.
- Avoid being judgmental regarding tobacco use. Tobacco has profound addictive properties and most people are well aware of the dangers of smoking. They may need resources to assist with smoking cessation. Assess their level of knowledge about the effects of smoking on their health as well as others around them, and provide accessible, age-appropriate resources.
- Get involved in community outreach. Educate the public regarding when respiratory illness should initiate an ED visit. Useful information can be accessed through web sites such as the Centers for Disease Control and Prevention (CDC) or American Lung Association (ALA). Pamphlets that differentiate pneumonia from the flu can be ordered free from the ALA and made available to patients and visitors. During peak respiratory outbreaks, public education should be a collaborative effort by the community, hospital, ED, and CDC.

Key Points

- Respiratory illness presentations range from mild complaints of dyspnea to acute respiratory failure. Recognition and prompt treatment of exacerbations from asthma and COPD, suspected PE, and acute epiglottitis challenge the most seasoned clinician. The priority is always establishing and maintaining a patent airway while simultaneously ensuring adequate ventilation and perfusion.

- As unfamiliar respiratory illnesses such as severe acute respiratory syndrome (SARS), hantavirus, and the avian flu threaten to cause epidemic disease, ED staff will be on the front lines of recognizing, isolating, and treating these new medical enigmas before they spread into communities and hospitals. ED personnel must remain informed by public health workers, the CDC, the National Institutes of Health (NIH), and the World Health Organization (WHO) to be successful in fighting these emerging and potentially fatal illnesses.

- Asthma, COPD, and pneumonia are some of the more familiar respiratory illnesses seen in the ED setting. However, epiglottitis, a true life threat because of the sudden, unexpected airway obstruction, should always be suspected with symptoms of fever, drooling, muffled voice, and dyspnea. Although these symptoms often indicate a more common malady, peritonsillar abscess, the emergency nurse must always suspect epiglottitis until ruled out.

Internet Resources

American Academy of Allergy, Asthma, and Immunology:
www.aaaai.org

American Lung Association:
www.lungusa.org

Asthma Initiative of Michigan:
www.getasthmahelp.org

Centers for Disease Control and Prevention, Recent Outbreaks and Incidents:
www.bt.cdc.gov/recentincidents.asp

eMedicine, Emphysema:
www.emedicine.com/med/topic654.htm

eMedicine, Pulmonary Embolism:
www.emedicine.com/EMERG/topic490.htm

eMedicine, Pulmonology articles:
www.emedicine.com/med/PULMONOLOGY.htm

MedlinePlus, Asthma:
www.nlm.nih.gov/medlineplus/ency/article/000141.htm

Medline Plus, Lung Diseases Information:
www.nhlbi.nih.gov/medlineplus/lungdiseases.html

National Jewish Medical and Research Center
www.nationaljewish.org

Bibliography

Ames WA et al: Adult epiglottitis: An under-recognized, life-threatening condition, *Br J Anaesth* 85(5):795-797, 2000.

Andreoli TE et al: *Cecil essentials of medicine*, ed 6, Philadelphia, 2005, WB Saunders.

Brennan-Cook J, Scheetz L: Respiratory distress. In Oman K, Koziol-McLain J, Scheetz L: *Emergency nursing secrets*, Philadelphia, 2001, Hanley & Belfus.

Corbridge SJ: Severe exacerbations in asthma, *Crit Care Nurs Q* 27(3):207-228, 2004.

Farquharson C, Baugley K: Responding to the severe acute respiratory syndrome (SARS) outbreak: Lessons learned in a Toronto emergency department, *J Emerg Nurs* 29(3):222-228, 2003.

Higgins JC: The crashing asthmatic, *Am Fam Physician* 67(5):997-1004, 2003.

Jolliet P et al: Helium-oxygen versus air-oxygen noninvasive pressure support in decompensated chronic obstructive disease: A prospective, multicenter study, *Crit Care Med* 31(3):878-884, 2003.

Nickas BJ: A 60 year old man with stidor, drooling and " tripoding" following nasal polypectomy, *J Emerg Nurs* 31(3):234-235, 2005.

Lester JL, Lewis AM: A 59 year old man survives cardiac arrest from massive pulmonary emboli, *J Emerg Nurs* 29(4):310-313, 2003.

McFadden ER: Acute severe asthma, *Am J Respir Crit Care Med* 168:740-759, 2003.

McFadden ER: Asthma. In Kasper DL et al, editors: *Harrison's principles of internal medicine*, ed 16, New York, 2005, McGraw-Hill.

Perng DW et al: Leukotriene modifier vs inhaled corticosteroid in mild-to-moderate asthma, *Chest* 125(5):1693-1699, 2004.

Qureshi F et al: Clinical efficacy of racemic albuterol versus levalbuterol for the treatment of acute pediatric asthma, *Ann Emerg Med* 46(1):29-36, 2005.

Ralston ME et al: Comparison of levalbuterol and racemic albuterol combined with ipratropium bromide in acute pediatric asthma: a randomized controlled trial, *J Emerg Med* 29(1):29-35, 2005.

Sack JL, Brock CD: Identifying acute epiglottitis in adults: High degree of awareness, close monitoring are key, *Postgrad Med* 112(1):81-82, 85-86, 2002.

Tanner K et al: Haemophilus influenzae type b epiglottitis as a cause of acute upper airway obstruction in children, *BMJ* 325(7372):1099-1100, 2002.

Thys F: Transtracheal open ventilation and respiratory failure: The "missing link" between invasive and noninvasive approaches? *Crit Care Med* 33(5):1174-1175, 2005.

Truitt T, Witko J, Halpern M: Levalbuterol compared to racemic albuterol, efficacy and outcomes in patients hospitalized with COPD or asthma, *Chest* 123:128-135, 2003.

Abdominal Pain

Joyce A. Wright

1. **Is abdominal pain a common complaint of patients in the emergency department (ED)?**

   Yes. Pain, especially abdominal pain, is the chief complaint of many ED patients. A study released by the Centers for Disease Control and Prevention (CDC) on March 18, 2004, states there were 110.2 million ED visits in the United States; abdominal pain was the most common reason for seeking emergency treatment (6.5% of ED patients) (CDC, 2005).

2. **What are the different types of abdominal pain? How do they present?**

   The three types of abdominal pain are visceral, parietal, and referred. Visceral pain, sometimes referred to as primary pain, originates with an abdominal organ and is caused by the stretching of nerve fibers surrounding the organ. Parietal or somatic pain (secondary pain) results from a chemical or bacterial irritation of the surrounding structures and nerve fibers. Referred pain is caused by irritation of the shared dermatome of the affected organ. The following table depicts the types of pain, common presentations, and etiologies.

Abdominal pain

Type	Presentations	Etiologies
Visceral	Cramping, gaslike, colicky, ill-defined, intermittent pain that intensifies and then decreases	Appendicitis Cholecystitis Gastroenteritis
	Periumbilical location	Bowel obstruction
	Excruciatingly sharp, knifelike, twisting	Renal colic Pancreatitis
Parietal or Somatic	Rapid onset	Viral or bacterial peritonitis, late appendicitis, gastroenteritis
	Sharp, steady aching; severe in intensity	
	Localized to area of pathology	Sequela of laparoscopy because of retained carbon dioxide
	Knee-chest positioning	

Abdominal pain—cont'd

Type	Presentations	Etiologies
Referred	Distant from the site of pathology	Myocardial infarction (MI), angina (epigastric, jaw, neck, shoulder) Pancreatitis (left shoulder, back) Renal colic (thigh, genitalia) Abdominal aortic aneurysm (back) Female reproductive organs (inner thigh)

3. What are the common patterns of referred pain?

Pain can originate in the abdomen and manifest elsewhere. Likewise, pain can originate elsewhere and manifest as abdominal pain. Pain that manifests as abdominal pain but originates elsewhere may be caused by MI (especially in women), pneumonia (especially in children), or testicular problems. Pain that originates in the abdomen may be referred elsewhere. For example, gallbladder pain refers to the top of the right shoulder, stomach pain may refer to the spine between the shoulder blades, kidney pain may be felt in the groin area, pancreatic pain refers to the left shoulder and back, intestinal dysfunction may be felt in the middle or low back, splenic pain refers to the left shoulder, and an abdominal aortic aneurysm refers a tearing-type pain to the middle or lower back. Pain may radiate to either shoulder with ruptured ovarian cyst or ectopic pregnancy, dependent upon location.

4. Does the patient's body positioning give additional information about the etiology of the abdominal pain?

Yes. It is important to observe the patient when approaching the bedside because patients tend to assume the position that provides the most comfort. Flexion of the hips reduces movement of the psoas major muscle, reducing pain. Ask the patient whether shifting in bed, walking, or taking deep breaths relieves or intensifies the pain. Peritoneal pain, inflammatory in nature, intensifies with movement. Therefore, patients tend to lie quietly and avoid moving. Patients who have colicky pain (renal, biliary, bowel) are restless. If the patient appears comfortable, moving around at will, the problem probably is not severe.

5. What are the major life-threatening causes of abdominal pain? How do they present?

Recognition of life-threatening causes of abdominal pain is crucial. Acute, severe, worsening, or persistent abdominal pain suggests a surgical emergency. The conditions listed in the following table are the most common life-threatening conditions: abdominal aortic aneurysm, ruptured spleen, septic shock, ruptured ectopic pregnancy, MI, and bowel obstruction.

Life-threatening causes of abdominal pain

Causes	Presentations
Abdominal aortic aneurysm (dissecting or ruptured)	Severe, sudden, constant, uncontrollable middle-to-lower back pain, described as "tearing" or "ripping"
	Pain radiating to genitals, sacrum, flank
	Pulsatile abdominal mass with bruit is evident in 30% to 50% of cases
	Anxiety, agitation, syncope
	Rapid decompensation with fluctuating blood pressure (initially hypertensive, later dropping precipitously so that pressure is only palpable)
	Late classic sign is lower extremity ischemia with "purple toes" and mottling below the umbilicus
Ruptured spleen	Initial hypertension and tachycardia, followed by hypovolemic shock state and syncope
	Left shoulder pain (Kehr's sign), left upper quadrant abdominal pain
Septic shock (ruptured appendix or diverticulum, peptic ulcer, perforated or ischemic bowel, biliary sepsis, indwelling lines or urinary catheters)	"Warm, compensatory" or "cold, progressive, or refractory" shock
	Acute onset of abdominal pain of 6 hours to several days' duration, with acute tenderness and guarding
	Abdominal pain begins focally and later becomes diffuse
	Tachycardia, tachypnea, hypotension, diminished urine output, absent or diminished peristalsis
	Sensorium is listless or agitated, progressing to unresponsive
	Skin cool, clammy, with cyanosis progressing to mottled appearance
Ruptured ectopic pregnancy	History of late or missed periods, breast tenderness, abdominal tenderness
	Weight gain, nausea
	Rapid onset of lower quadrant abdominal pain, unilateral or bilateral
	Syncope
	Amenorrhea, may have some spotting
Myocardial infarction	Epigastric pain, nausea, diaphoresis, vomiting
	Cool, clammy, pale skin
	Vague symptoms of anxiety (e.g., "I just don't feel right," feeling of impending doom)
Bowel obstruction	Presentation differs for complete vs. partial obstruction
	Vomiting, cramping, distention, with inability to expel flatus
	Bowel sounds are high-pitched "tinkling" and /or a "rush" of air
	Radiographs show loops of dilated bowel with or without air-fluid levels
	Elderly have a higher incidence of infection and perforation
	Small bowel obstruction presents with rapid onset, frequent copious vomiting, colicky pain, and minimal abdominal distention; large bowel obstruction symptoms progress gradually with a cramping type of pain accompanied by constipation and abdominal distention

6. **Besides MI, what other non-abdominal conditions cause abdominal pain?**

Metabolic conditions (e.g., diabetic ketoacidosis [DKA]), systemic lupus erythematosus (SLE), porphyria, sickle cell disease, and insect envenomation present with abdominal pain. DKA-induced abdominal pain is usually accompanied by nausea and vomiting. SLE and porphyria present with abdominal pain and splenomegaly. Porphyria also presents with nausea and vomiting.

The most common insect envenomation is caused by spider bites (black widow or brown recluse). Other insects known for producing nausea include wasps, bees, ants, and ticks.

Sickle cell disease produces abdominal pain secondary to diminished blood supply to the gut.

Several neurological conditions, such as varicella zoster infection and degenerative disc disease, cause pain *around* the abdomen. Varicella zoster travels along nerve pathways; degenerative disc disease also impinges on nerve pathways, causing pain along the pathway. When the underlying pathology of each of these conditions is treated, the abdominal symptoms should resolve.

7. **What are the special etiological considerations for female patients with abdominal pain?**

Potential sources of abdominal pain in women include ectopic pregnancy, spontaneous or threatened abortion, ovarian cyst, and pelvic inflammatory disease (PID). In light of these etiological factors, the history should address the gynecological system and risk factors. Question the usage of birth control, sexual activity, and number of partners and obtain a pregnancy test (beta HCG). Of special note, one saturated tampon or pad is equal to approximately 30 ml of blood.

8. **What should be kept in mind about pediatric patients with abdominal pain?**

The most common causes of abdominal pain in children include gastroenteritis, appendicitis, and intussusception of the small bowel. However, always maintain a high index of suspicion for child neglect or abuse, including sexual abuse.

9. **What signs and symptoms often accompany abdominal pain?**

Accompanying signs and symptoms depend to some extent on the etiology of the pain. If the pain originates within the abdomen, patients often experience other gastrointestinal (GI) signs and symptoms, such as nausea, vomiting, diarrhea, constipation, and bloody or mucous stools. Intraabdominal irritation frequently causes vomiting. Vomiting, a classic sign of abdominal trouble, may occur as a result of intraabdominal irritation or bowel obstruction or in response to pain. An obstruction high in the intestine causes rapid onset of vomitus of bile or coffee-ground material, which may actually relieve pain. Coffee-ground vomitus occurs when hydrochloric acid mixes with blood in the gut. Intestinal obstruction below the pylorus is usually gradual in onset and may produce vomitus with feces or a strong fecal odor. Although vomiting frequently accompanies abdominal pain, it also presents in patients who have a central nervous system problem, such as increased intracranial pressure (ICP), causing irritation to the vomiting center in the brain.

Additional signs and symptoms that accompany abdominal pain may include fever, change in bowel or bladder habits, dehydration, abdominal distention, and vaginal discharge. These manifestations may signal intraabdominal or extraabdominal problems.

Pain that refers to the abdomen from an extraabdominal source is accompanied by additional signs and symptoms. For example, a patient experiencing epigastric pain of cardiac origin may present with other cardiac symptoms. A patient with pneumonia who experiences abdominal pain also presents with respiratory signs and symptoms.

10. What history should be obtained from a patient who presents with abdominal pain?

Use a systematic approach to pain assessment, such as the PQRSTT mnemonic:
Provokes: What provokes the pain? What position of comfort does the patient assume? How did the pain begin? What makes it better or worse?
Quality: Ask the patient to describe the character of the pain in his or her own words. Is the pain tight, crushing, tearing, pressing, or cramping?
Radiation: Where does the pain start? Does the pain spread anywhere? Ask the patient to point to where the pain is. Localized versus diffuse pain provides clues to the origin.
Severity: Ask the patient to rate the severity of the pain, using one of the pain scales, such as 0 to 10 or the Faces scale. Have there been any changes in severity?
Timing and Treatment: Does the pain come and go, or is it always present? Did you try anything to relieve the pain? Was it effective? When did the pain begin?
Additional focused history should include questions about diet, relationship of pain to eating, when last foods or fluids were taken, medications (prescription, over-the-counter, herbal, and recreational drug use), alcohol use, previous problems of a similar nature, allergies (including food), travel outside the United States, additional signs and symptoms, recent endoscopic procedures (endoscopy), and other recent surgeries and trauma (especially abdominal, chest, or flank). Female patients should be questioned about their menstrual cycle, including the date of the last menses, changes in menstrual patterns, use of contraceptives, possible pregnancy, vaginal bleeding, pain during intercourse, and risk factors for sexually transmitted diseases (STDs). If interviewing the patient privately, ask if she has been injured by an intimate partner or forced to have sex against her will.

11. What are the components of the abdominal assessment?

- **Visual inspection** must always precede palpation of the abdomen to avoid increasing intestinal activity with manual stimulation. Inspection identifies symmetry of the abdomen, visual peristaltic waves, and character of the skin. Observe for bruising, dilated veins, abdominal distention, rashes, change in the skin pigmentation, and scars. Observe closely for laparoscopic scars, especially around the umbilicus, because they are easy to miss. Having the patient cough may elicit bulges or pain.

- **Auscultation** with the bell of the stethoscope to hear low-pitched sounds, such as a bruit; note the frequency and character of the sounds. The diaphragm of the stethoscope is used to detect normal peristalsis. High-pitched, tingling sounds are auscultated proximal to a bowel obstruction, whereas low-pitched sounds or silence is auscultated distal to an obstruction. Other important findings on auscultation include absent or decreased sounds in the presence of a paralytic ileus and high-pitched sounds with diarrhea. Abdominal bruits, associated with dissecting aneurysms and renal artery stenosis, can be auscultated with the bell of the stethoscope.
- **Percussion** helps to identify the density of underlying structures, air, or fluid. Tympany is present over most of the abdomen because of the air throughout the stomach and intestinal tract. Percussion tones are dull over solid organs, tumors, or stool-filled intestines.
- **Palpation** is the last assessment technique and should begin at a nonpainful area and progress to the identified painful area last following the pattern of gentle, deep, then rebound palpation. Use firm downward pressure with the flat areas of the fingers. Instruct the patient to bend the knees to promote comfort and relax the abdominal musculature. Pay attention to the patient's facial expression, which provides an important diagnostic clue. Rebound tenderness is usually significant with peritoneal inflammation. If the patient exhibits symptoms of perforation (such as abdominal rigidity, involuntary guarding, or a boardlike abdomen), do not check for rebound tenderness or perform deep palpation.

12. What factors may complicate assessment of patients with abdominal pain?

- **Young age:** Patients may be poor historians and fearful of people wearing white lab coats. Use visual smiley faces to assess pain intensity, or use descriptors such as, "Is the pain sharp like a needle?" Young patients may also have difficulty relaxing to cooperate with abdominal palpation and may be ticklish. Distraction may help, as does palpating with the child's hand below yours.
- **Old age:** Elderly patients present with muted and delayed symptoms (e.g., atypical pain, which is usually milder and less specific; low or absent fever in the presence of infectious or inflammatory disease). Elderly patients also may be poor historians. A majority of elderly patients have a preexisting condition that complicates the presentation of their symptoms. They may have catastrophic illnesses rarely seen in young patients, including mesenteric ischemia, leaking or ruptured abdominal aortic aneurysm, and MI.
- **Obesity:** Assessment of abdominal pain can be especially challenging in obese or pregnant patients. A large abdomen and layers of fat can displace or hide abdominal organs, making assessment more difficult.
- **Compromised immune systems:** These patients often do not mount a telltale response to infectious or inflammatory disease. Patients with HIV may also have enterocolitis with profuse diarrhea and dehydration, perforation of the large bowel caused by cytomegalovirus (CMV), obstruction caused by Kaposi's sarcoma, or severe pancreatitis caused by certain retroviral drugs.

13. Patients who present with severe abdominal pain often undergo ultrasound and may have a surgical or gynecological consult. Providing early pain relief is important, but not all physicians agree. How should the nurse handle this dilemma?

Considerable evidence indicates that all pain is undermedicated, a recent survey of emergency physicians indicate that 80% of United States ED medicine respondants withheld opiod analgesia pending surgical assessment (Wolf et al, 2000). Sometimes clinicians are hesitant to administer analgesia for fear of masking diagnostic clues, such as a change in the pattern or severity of pain. To get at the root of the problem, ask these questions:

- Who is reluctant to cooperate with pain management in the ED? Attending physicians? Residents? A specific physician service?
- Is the resistance from just *one* person or *many*?
- Why does the reluctance exist? Ask the question in a nonthreatening way. Many myths exist about analgesic administration. A good body of literature supports the quest for better pain management.
- What strategies, if any, have been tried in the past to overcome resistance?

A suggestion is to lead the effort in the hospital or ED to develop multidisciplinary pain management protocols. Follow these steps:

- Provide documentation of the need or problem.
- Conduct a literature review and/or survey of other EDs to identify solutions and practices elsewhere.
- Solicit physician input to develop the guidelines. Refer to the Agency for Healthcare Research and Quality (AHRQ—formerly the Agency for Health Care Policy and Research [AHCPR]) pain management guidelines. Often the barrier to pain management is not attributable to the physician, but to nurses or even the patient.
- Document the effectiveness of the guidelines (consider piloting them first).
- Make revisions to the guidelines as needed.

14. What drugs provide effective pain relief for patients with abdominal pain?

The etiology of the pain guides the choice of analgesics. Renal colic responds well to ketorolac, whereas gallbladder pain responds better to opiods (e.g., fentanyl, hydromorphone, morphine). One advantage of ketorolac is that, as a non-steroidal antiinflammatory drug (NSAID), it can be given to patients before surgery to facilitate pain relief without causing sedation (which interferes with obtaining informed consent) or masking localizing symptoms. Ketorolac is contraindicated for long-term therapy and for patients with renal disease or coagulopathies. The safety and efficacy of ketorolac and morphine have not been established for pediatric patients. Intravenous (IV) administration of morphine and ketorolac provides more effective pain relief than oral or intramuscular (IM) administration.

15. What are the anticipated nursing measures for the patient with abdominal pain?

- Focus the exam not only on the abdomen but also on the full body to document posturing.

- Have a higher index of suspicion for the elderly, who frequently present with nonspecific findings and may necessitate an electrocardiogram (ECG), or any patients that present with nonspecific epigastric pain.
- Blood tests to consider for the patient with abdominal pain include complete blood count (CBC) with differential, electrolytes, blood urea nitrogen (BUN), creatinine, glucose, amylase, lipase, prothrombin time (PT), and partial thromboplastin time (PTT).
- With the hypovolemic patient, make sure to start IV access with two large-bore cannulas, normal saline, or Ringer's solution for fluid resuscitation.
- Type and cross match for two to four units of blood if the patient is hypovolemic, and perform orthostatic vital signs if not contraindicated.
- Radiographs, which are frequently utilized for abdominal pain, include the abdominal ultrasound, spiral computed tomography (CT) scan, chest and abdominal x-ray, and IV pyelogram.
- Obtain a beta HCG level for women of childbearing age.
- Insert a gastric tube in the unconscious patient.

Key Points

- There are three types of abdominal pain. Visceral pain usually presents as cramping and is poorly defined because of the stretching of nerve fibers. Parietal pain has a rapid onset and is sharp because of chemical or bacterial irritation. Referred pain is distant from the pathology; common sites of referred pain are the shoulders and back.

- Pain is the most important presenting symptom. Three common drugs used to relieve abdominal pain include fentanyl, morphine, and ketorolac. Timely pain management promotes patient comfort and therefore aids in establishing a diagnosis.

- The primary goal for the diagnosis of abdominal pain is to accurately determine, through a thorough work-up, the identity of abdominal pain and treat the cause. A differential diagnosis needs to be made because many causes of abdominal pain do not require surgery.

Internet Resources

Nursewise, Abdominal Assessment:
www.nursewise.com/courses/abdassess_hour.htm

Nursing Continuing Education, Abdominal Pain and Abdominal Emergency:
www.nursingceu.com/courses/1/index_nceu.html

RNWeb, Triaging Lower Abdominal Pain:
www.rnweb.com/rnweb/article/articleDetail.jsp?id=118602

Bibliography

American College of Emergency Physicians: Clinical policy for the initial approach to patients presenting with a chief complaint of nontraumatic acute abdominal pain, *Ann Emerg Med* 23:906-922, 1999.

Bliss DZ, Sawchuk L: Nursing management of lower GI problems. In Lewis SM, Heitkemper MM, Dirksen SR, editors: *Medical surgical nursing assessment and management of clinical problems,* St Louis, 2004, Mosby.

Bohrn M, Siewart B: Acute abdominal pain: What not to miss, *Patient Care* 38:31-39, 2004.

Bryan DE: *Abdominal pain in elderly persons,* eMedicine, 2005. Available at www.emedicine.com/emerg/topic931.htm. (accessed March 23, 2005).

Center for Disease Control: National Center for Health Statistics, *CDC releases latest data on emergency department visits, March 18, 2004.* Atlanta, Ga., 2004. Available at www.cdc.gov/nchs/pressroom/04facts/emergencydept.htm. (accessed March 23, 2005).

Cheung W, Heeney L, Pound JL: An advance triage system, *Accid Emerg Nurs* 10:10-16, 2002.

Cook K: Evaluating acute abdominal pain in adults, *JAAPA* March 2005. Available at www.jaapa.com/issues/j20050301/articles/belly0305.htm.

Gallagher J et al: Clinical policy: Critical issues for the initial evaluation and management of patient presenting with a chief complaint of non-traumatic acute abdominal pain, *Ann Emerg Med* 36:4, 406-413, 2000.

Heiser R: Abdominal conditions. In Kidd PS, Sturt PA, Fultz J, editors: *Mosby's emergency nursing reference,* ed 2, Philadelphia, 2000, Mosby.

Karch AM: Alphabetical listing of drugs by generic name. In *Lippincott's nursing drug guide,* New York, 2004, Lippincott Williams & Wilkins.

Newberry L: Gastrointestinal emergencies. In *Sheehy's emergency nursing principles and practice,* ed 5, St Louis, 2003, Mosby.

O'Connor RE: *Abdominal aneurysm,* eMedicine, 2004. Available at www.emedicine.com/emerg/topic27.htm.

Thomas SH et al: Effects of morphine analgesia on diagnostic accuracy in emergency department patients with abdominal pain: A prospective, randomized trial, *J Am Coll Surg* 196:18-31, 2003.

Trautman D: Pain management. In *Sheehy's emergency nursing principles and practice,* ed 5, St Louis, 2003, Mosby.

Wolfe JM et al: Analgesia administration to patients with acute abdomens: A survey of emergency physicians, *Am J Emerg Med* 18:250, 2000.

Environmental Emergencies

Kathleen Flarity

RABIES

1. **How is rabies contracted?**

   Rabies, caused by an RNA virus, is usually transmitted by the bite of an infected animal. However, some reported cases are thought to be contracted by contact with infected saliva of bats and other animals. Transmission in such cases is through the mucous membranes (eyes, nose, mouth) or open wounds.

2. **Who are the carriers?**

   The most common carriers in the United States are coyotes, skunks, foxes, raccoons, bats, jackals, wolves, groundhogs, ferrets, dogs, cats, and other carnivores. Rabies is rarely carried by rodents or hares. If previously bitten by a rabid animal, livestock such as cattle, horses, sheep, or goats can transmit rabies. In other countries dogs are the most common carriers.

3. **Where is rabies most common?**

   In the United States rabies is reported most commonly in Northern California, Connecticut, Florida, Iowa, Maine, Georgia, Maryland, Massachusetts, New York, New Jersey, Pennsylvania, North and South Carolina, Virginia, and Texas. The majority (99%) of human deaths are in areas where canine rabies (unvaccinated dogs) is endemic such as Asia, Africa, and Latin America.

4. **What are the symptoms of rabies?**

   During the prodromal phase (2 to 10 days), symptoms include pain and paresthesia at the wound site, malaise, fatigue, anxiety, agitation, irritability, insomnia, depression, fever, headache, nausea and vomiting, slurred speech, sore throat, abdominal pain, anorexia, productive cough, inability to swallow, and visual hallucinations. During the acute neurological period, encephalitic symptoms include lethargy, increasing agitation, hyperactivity, seizures, disorientation, hallucinations, bizarre behavior, fever, headache, pharyngeal spasm, hydrophobia, aerophobia, hypertension, hyperthermia, hypersalivation, laryngeal/diaphragm spasms, and death (may occur abruptly or be preceded by paralysis and coma); paralytic symptoms include diffuse weakness, lethargy, incoordination, ascending paralysis (including respiratory and pharyngeal musculature), minimal alteration in consciousness, coma, and death.

5. How is rabies diagnosed?

A presumptive diagnosis is made from the exposure history and the presence of neurological signs. Definitive diagnosis is made by isolating the virus before or after death from saliva, neurological tissue, cerebrospinal fluid, urine sediment, or other body tissues of either the host or victim. No currently available premortem diagnostic testing can be considered absolutely reliable. The absolute definitive diagnostic test remains the presence of fluorescent viral antigen particles within neurons of biopsied brain tissue.

6. What is the postexposure treatment regimen?

Postexposure prophylaxis consists of three primary elements: wound care, infiltration of rabies immune globulin, and vaccine administration. Modern rabies vaccines are very efficacious and will prevent rabies if they are administered promptly and correctly after a rabies exposure. There are several postexposure regimens available. The standard five-dose schedule is given as one intramuscular (IM) dose of cell culture vaccine on days 0, 3, 7, 14, and 28. Also in the United States one dose of human rabies immunoglobulin (HRIG) 20 International Units per kg is given only for transdermal wounds at the time of the incident or within 7 days after the first dose of the vaccine. The protocol is as follows:

UNVACCINATED PATIENT

- Clean wound immediately with soap and water. Irrigate with several hundred ml of normal saline, using a 12-ml syringe and 18-gauge needle. Some facilities repeatedly irrigate with a virucidal agent, such as povidone-iodine solution.
- Debride devitalized and crushed tissue. Do not suture wounds.
- Administer HRIG 20 International Units per kg, by infiltrating as much of this dose as possible into and around the wound; administer the remainder in divided IM doses at distant sites. If the calculated dose of HRIG is insufficient to infiltrate all wounds, sterile saline may be used to dilute it twofold to threefold to permit thorough infiltration.
- Administer rabies vaccine. Administer antibiotics and tetanus vaccine as indicated.

PREVIOUSLY VACCINATED PATIENT

- Clean wound immediately with soap and water. Irrigate with several hundred ml of normal saline, using a 12-ml syringe and 18-gauge needle. Some facilities repeatedly irrigate with a virucidal agent, such as povidone-iodine solution.
- Debride devitalized and crushed tissue. Do not suture wounds.
- *Do not* administer HRIG.
- Obtain a rabies titer.
- Administer rabies vaccine. Administer tetanus vaccine and antibiotics as indicated.

7. How is rabies vaccine administered?

Several types of rabies vaccines are available in the United States, including human diploid cell vaccine (Imovax), rabies vaccine adsorbed (RVA), and purified chick embryo cell (PCEC) vaccine (RabAvert).

The rabies vaccine is administered intramuscularly in the deltoid in adults. Only children may receive the vaccine in the anterolateral aspect of the thigh. In adults, less than deep IM administration in the deltoid may result in ineffective dosing.

For postexposure prophylaxis in patients who have never received the rabies vaccine, administer 1 ml intramuscularly on the first day, then one dose on days 3, 7, 14, and 28 for a total of five doses. HRIG 20 ml/kg should also be administered.

For postexposure prophylaxis in patients who have received the rabies vaccine previously, administer 1 ml intramuscularly on the first day, then one dose on day 3 for a total of two doses.

8. What are the adverse effects of HRIG and rabies vaccine?

Adverse effects from HRIG include soreness at the injection site and mild fever. Adverse effects from rabies vaccine include soreness, redness, swelling, itching at the injection site, nausea, headache, muscle aches, or even abdominal pain. Moderate reactions (which are rare) include hives, joint pain, and illness resembling Guillain-Barré syndrome with complete recovery.

9. Is there a cure for rabies once contracted?

No. HRIG, antiviral drugs, and immunomodulators do not change the clinical course when given during the presence of clinical disease. Supportive measures, such as airway maintenance and cardiovascular support, are keystones of care; however, they usually do not prevent death.

TETANUS

10. What is tetanus?

Tetanus is a toxin-induced process, neither infective nor inflammatory, caused by *Clostridium tetani*, a gram-positive anaerobic spore-forming rod.

11. What are the sources of tetanus?

C. tetani is found almost everywhere. It enters the body through puncture wounds; crush injuries; burns; wounds heavily contaminated with feces, soil, or debris; dental infections; elective surgery; ischemic peripheral ulcers; embedded penetrating objects; injections; and contaminated instruments used for illegal abortions. The spores gain entry and can remain dormant for months to years. Spores convert to a vegetative state in conditions of decreased oxygen tension, which cause an anaerobic environment. The vegetative form produces the neurotoxin tetanospasm, causing central nervous system dysfunction.

12. What is the incubation period for tetanus?

The average incubation period is 7 days, but it ranges from 1 to 54 days.

13. What is the clinical presentation of tetanus?

Localized tetanus presents with spasms of focal muscles and may remain localized for weeks and slowly resolve. Generalized tetanus presents with tachycardia, trismus, hyperactivity, profuse sweating, dysphagia, arrhythmias, labile hypertension, opisthotonos, laryngeal spasms, hyperthermia, and boardlike abdominal rigidity.

14. What are trismus and opisthotonos?

Trismus is spasm of the masticator muscle in the jaw. Opisthotonos is an abnormal posturing characterized by rigidity and severe arching of the back, with the head thrown backwards. It is seen with tetanus and strychnine poisoning.

15. How is tetanus diagnosed?

There are no tests to measure tetanus toxin in body fluids. Diagnosis is based on the clinical picture and the exclusion of differential diagnoses, such as bacterial meningitis, epilepsy, strychnine poisoning (often found in heroin users), phenothiazine reaction, subluxation of the temporomandibular joint, increased intracranial pressure (ICP) with decerebrate posturing, narcotic withdrawal, intracranial bleeds, and hypocalcemia. Culture of the wound may be negative even if tetanus is present.

16. What treatments are available for tetanus?

- Control and reverse the tetany with antitoxin (tetanus immune globulin)
- Diazepam for muscle spasms
- Remove and destroy the toxin through surgical exploration and debridement
- Antibiotics, including penicillin, clindamycin, erythromycin, or metronidazole
- Cardiovascular and respiratory support
- Control of arrhythmias
- Reduction in sympathetic nervous system stimulation (decreasing external light and sound sources; promoting a calm, quiet environment)

17. What treatments are indicated for tetanus exposure?

The administration of human hyperimmune antitetanus globulin of at least 500 units (with doses ranging from 3000 to 6000 units) and administration of an antibiotic effective against *C. tetani* for 10 days (penicillin, erythromycin, or metronidazole). In addition, provide wound care, including washing, irrigation, and debridement as appropriate.

18. Can tetanus be prevented?

Yes. The Centers for Disease Control and Prevention (CDC) recommends mandatory primary immunization and booster immunization, regardless of age. The CDC guidelines for administration of passive or active immunization are presented in the following table.

Tetanus prophylaxis in routine wound management

History of tetanus toxoid	Clean, minor wounds		All other wounds*	
	Td†	*TIG*	*Td†*	*TIG*
Less than 3 doses	Yes	No	Yes	Yes
More than 3 doses‡	No§	No	No¶	No

Modified from www.cdc.gov/nip/recs/adult-schedule.htm.

Td, tetanus-diphtheria toxoid; *TIG*, tetanus immunoglobulin.

*Such as, but not limited to, wounds contaminated with dirt, feces, soil, and saliva; puncture wounds; avulsions; and wounds resulting from missiles, crushing, burns, and frostbite.

†For children younger than 7 years old, diphtheria-tetanus-pertussis vaccine (DTaP) is preferred to tetanus toxoid alone. If pertussis vaccine is contraindicated, give Td vaccine. For persons 7 years of age or older, Td is preferred to tetanus toxoid alone.

‡If only three doses of fluid toxoid have been received, a fourth dose, preferably an adsorbed toxoid, should be given.

§Yes, if more than 10 years since last dose.

¶Yes, if more than 5 years since last dose. (More frequent boosters are not needed and can accentuate side effects.)

BITES, STINGS, AND FLYING THINGS

19. Are tick-borne illnesses common?

Currently 10 diseases are commonly included in the differential diagnoses of tick-borne illness. The following table outlines these diseases.

Tick-borne diseases

Disease	Organism	Agent
Lyme disease	*Borrelia burgdorferi*	Spirochete
Rocky Mountain spotted fever	*Rickettsia rickettsii*	Rickettsia
Colorado tick fever	Orbivirus	RNA virus
Q fever	*Coxiella burnetii*	Rickettsia
Ehrlichiosis	*Ehrlichia canis*	Rickettsia
Encephalitis	Arbovirus	Virus
Relapsing fever	*Borrelia parkeri,* *Borrelia hermsii,* *Borrelia turicatae*	Spirochete
Tick paralysis	None	Toxins
Babesiosis	*Babesia microti*	Protozoan
Tularemia	*Francisella tularensis*	Bacteria

20. How do Lyme disease and Rocky Mountain spotted fever differ in presentation, diagnosis, and treatment?

The following table outlines these differences. Lyme disease is the most frequently reported vector-borne disease in the United States.

Comparison of lyme disease and rocky mountain spotted fever

	Lyme disease	Rocky mountain spotted fever
Presentation	**Stage 1** (1-4 weeks post–tick bite): bull's-eye rash on the thigh, groin, or axilla in 10% to 20% of cases; migratory secondary annular lesions; malaise; fatigue; tender regional lymphadenopathy; migratory musculoskeletal problems; meningeal or cerebral changes; arthritis. **Stage 2** (4-10 weeks post–tick bite; latent period): neurological changes; sleep disturbances; memory losses. **Stage 3** (weeks to years post–tick bite): recurrent asymmetrical episodes of joint swelling or pain; can be localized or migratory.	High fever, chills, headache, nausea, vomiting, abdominal pain, rash, myalgia, conjunctivitis, peripheral edema, seizures, lethargy, confusion, cardiac involvement, interstitial pneumonitis (cough, chest pain, shortness of breath).
Diagnosis	ELISA or IFA; if inconclusive, do Western blot, 2-tier method.	History of rash, fever, tick bite; Weil-Felix test and complement fixation tests.
Treatment	Doxycycline, amoxicillin, cefuroxime axetil, erythromycin, ceftriaxone, penicillin G, azithromycin. Patients presenting with clinical symptoms and living in an endemic area should be treated with antibiotics without laboratory confirmation.	Tetracycline, chloramphenicol, doxycycline, fluoroquinolone. Supportive care is imperative.

ELISA, enzyme-linked immunosorbent assay; *IFA*, immunofluorescence assay.

21. What does the Rocky Mountain spotted fever rash look like?

The rash originates as pink macules, 2 to 5 mm in circumference, which blanch with pressure. It begins on the palms, hands, soles, feet, and ankles, moving up the body to the face. After 2 to 3 days, the rash becomes stationary, darker red, and papular and evolves into petechiae.

22. How should a tick be removed?

The tick should be grasped as close as possible to the skin with curved forceps, tweezers, or fingers protected with gloves or tissues. Use a steady pulling motion, and avoid squeezing or crushing the tick's body. The bite site should be cleansed and disinfected.

23. What discharge instructions should patients be given about preventing tick-borne diseases?

People should wear light-colored clothing with long pants and long sleeves to cover exposed skin, use tick repellents, inspect all body parts carefully and regularly (at least twice daily), remove ticks immediately, keep lawns mowed, cut back dense shrubs or brush, and avoid tall grass and wooded areas.

24. What reactions can occur from Hymenoptera stings (yellow jackets, hornets, bees, wasps)? How do they present? How are they managed?

Hymenoptera stings

Reaction	Presentation	Management
Normal (inflammatory, local)	Pain, itching, redness, slight swelling (5 cm); symptoms disappear in 1-2 hours.	Gently scrape stinger away, apply ice, elevate, administer over-the-counter antihistamine.
Extended (large, local)	Pain, itching, redness, swelling (greater than 5-15 cm) in area contiguous to sting; peaks in 24-48 hours and disappears after 7-10 days.	As for normal reaction, plus administer histamine blocker and oral corticosteroid.
Toxic (results from repeated stings)	Pain, itching, redness, swelling, hypotension.	Antihistamines, corticosteroids, epinephrine, calcium gluconate, systemic support.
Anaphylactic	Severe swelling, hives, throat tightness, laryngeal edema, coughing, weakness, dizziness, wheezing, dyspnea, dysphagia, cardiovascular changes, hypotension, shock, loss of consciousness, nausea, vomiting, diarrhea, abdominal cramps.	Supportive care, epinephrine, antihistamines, corticosteroids. Patients on beta-adrenergic blockers may be refractory to epinephrine; glucagon bolus or isoproterenol infusion may be indicated.
Delayed	Occurs 6 hours to 2 weeks after the sting. Urticaria, generalized rash, joint swelling, arthralgias, pharyngeal swelling, serum sickness.	Management varies with the severity of symptoms and presence of glomerulonephritis, carditis, and/or septic meningitis.

25. How should a stinger be removed?

Use a gentle, side-to-side scraping motion using a credit card or similar tool. Never squeeze or use tweezers; such techniques may cause contraction of the venom sac and release more contents into the puncture site.

26. What is the medical treatment for bites/stings?

Remove any stinger; apply ice; administer ibuprofen or acetaminophen for pain; wash the site with soap and water; administer tetanus booster and oral antihistamines as indicated.

27. What should patients be told about preventive measures if they have a history of an allergic reaction to a Hymenoptera sting?

Patients with a history of allergic reaction should carry an emergency kit that includes injectable epinephrine and an oral antihistamine. Two commonly available epinephrine kits include Ana-Kit (Hollister-Stier) and Epipen/Epipen Jr. (Center Laboratories). Make sure the patient can use the prescribed epinephrine delivery device prior to discharge. EpiPen trainers are available from Center Laboratories and distributors of American Heart Association (AHA) educational materials. The patient should prepare the epinephrine device immediately if stung, call 911, and take the oral antihistamine. The patient should self-inject with the epinephrine if he or she experiences difficulty breathing, lightheadedness, or dizziness. These patients should also be referred to an allergist for potential desensitization therapy and be instructed in avoidance of stings. Use of medical alert or medical identification tags is also recommended. Teach the patient strategies to help avoid future stings, including:
- Do not wear perfumes or scented products when outside; stay away from flowers
- Avoid eating outside; keep drinks covered
- Keep garbage containers covered; stay away from rotting fruit or food
- Do not walk barefoot outside
- Keep windows closed or screened

28. Which presents a greater hazard: brown recluse or black widow spiders?

The brown recluse spider is a greater health hazard because of its gentle, innocent appearance; indoor habitats; and larger numbers in endemic areas. However, the black widow spider bite is more toxic.

29. What are the differences between the brown recluse spider, black widow spider, and scorpion in regard to appearance, habitat, wound, and treatment?

Comparison of brown recluse spiders, black widow spiders, and scorpions

	Brown recluse spider	Black widow spider	Scorpion
Appearance	2-5 cm; cephalothorax and abdomen vary from dark brown to tan color; characteristic violin-shaped dark brown spot on its abdomen; three sets of eyes.	2.5 cm; glossy black; female carries bright red or orange marking that may be hourglass shaped or appear as two spots.	5-20 cm; three-segment body with whiplike telson; tail contains two venom glands connected to tip of stinger.
Habitat	Hot, dry, little-used environments (vacant garages, sheds, buildings, basements, rock piles, closets, and woodpiles). Nocturnal creatures; most active from April to October. Can live 6 months without food.	Prefer hot, dry climates. Under stones, logs, bark piles, clumps of vegetation, grain fields, vineyards, stables, outhouses, and unoccupied buildings.	Prefer warmer climates. Nocturnal, with tendency to burrow, hiding under rocks and debris.
Wound	The bite is often painless. Both localized and systemic symptoms 1-4 hours after bite. Cutaneous sharp, stinging pain; intense local ache; pruritus; edema; mottled purple center with irregular margins and larger erythematous halo. Blister/bleb may appear; eschar evolves over 72 hrs to reveal an ulcer of variable depth and size that may extend to the muscle; slow healing. Fever, scarlatiniform rash, leukocytosis, chills, arthralgias, nausea and vomiting, malaise.	Initial bite causes little or no pain. Skin lesions are rare; small red papule without pain or swelling. Painful skeletal muscle spasms, cramps develop 1 hr after envenomation, causing truncal and abdominal rigidity. Autonomic disturbances, hypertension, diaphoresis, burning paresthesia, thready pulse, slurred speech, headache, dizziness, dysphagia, nausea and vomiting, facial edema, ptosis, increased	North American species: local pain, swelling, occasional fever; occasionally a small puncture site with margin of erythema can be identified. Sympathetic, parasympathetic, and neurological symptoms may also be seen. Initial hypertension and tachycardia occurs in close to half the patients with even mild envenomations. Envenomations are categorized by

Continued

Comparison of brown recluse spiders, black widow spiders, and scorpions—cont'd

	Brown recluse spider	Black widow spider	Scorpion
Wound—cont'd	Hemolytic anemia, hemoglobinuria, thrombocytopenia, and disseminated intravascular coagulation (DIC) can occur.	salivary flow, mild fever, seizures, hyperactive deep tendon reflexes, increased spinal pressure, oliguria.	severity from grade 1 to 5.
Treatment	Wound cleansing, continuous ice/cool compresses, immobilization and elevation of site for 2-3 days. Antibiotics if signs/symptoms of infection. Leukocyte inhibitor (dapsone). Travase ointment for debridement. Some evidence that systemic steroids may be helpful if started within 24 hrs of bite.	Wound cleansing, ice/cool compresses, sedation, nitroprusside, nifedipine, labetalol, hydralazine, or diazoxide for hypertension reduction and cardiovascular and respiratory efforts. Calcium gluconate for abdominal cramping; diazepam for sedation and/or muscle spasms. Equine-derived *Latrodectus mactans* antivenom for severe reactions.	Wound cleansing, cool compresses, analgesics. Prazosine or captopril for hypertension. Controversial use of scorpion sting antivenin (only available in Arizona, where it is used for severe grade 3-5 envenomations). Sedatives, hypnotics.
Admission and observation	Observed in emergency department (ED) for minimum of 6 hrs.	Observe in ED for minimum of 8-10 hrs after treatment to monitor for relapse or reoccurrence of symptoms. Admission for children, elderly, hypertensive, or pregnant patients.	May require admission for children. Scorpion bite is considered a likely etiology of pediatric coma of unknown cause in infested areas.

30. Are tarantulas dangerous?

Bites from the 30 species of tarantulas that live in the United States are relatively innocuous and result in only low-grade histamine reaction. If handled, tarantulas release tiny hairs from their abdomen, causing a local urticarial reaction. Bites from tarantulas found in the Panama Canal area may cause paresthesia and localized pain. South American tarantulas are more toxic and an antivenin is available.

31. **What is the treatment for tarantula bites and injuries?**

Treatment for tarantula bites should be supportive (e.g., antihistamines, oral analgesics). The hairs, which may be barbed, can be removed with a piece of tape.

32. **How do fire ants inflict injuries?**

Fire ants both bite and sting. They anchor themselves with their strong mandibles to leverage the thrust of the stinger. Their venom has both hemolytic and necrotic effects. Fire ants tend to swarm and sting in unison, resulting in multiple stings. Reactions tend to be local, systemic, or anaphylactic (rare).

33. **What is the treatment for fire ant stings?**

Treatment involves local wound care, cold compresses, antihistamines, and topical steroids for mild cases. Severe reactions should be treated with intravenous (IV) fluid, epinephrine, antihistamines, and corticosteroids, as well as advanced cardiac life-support measures as indicated.

34. **What are kissing bugs and bed bugs?**

The kissing bug (*Triatoma* species) is found mostly in the southern United States. It feeds at night on the blood of vertebrates, including humans. These insects have a long proboscis through which they suck their victim's blood without causing pain. Bed bugs are also painless nocturnal bloodsuckers. They are not vectors for disease, but their bites may cause an allergic reaction or trigger asthma.

SNAKEBITES

35. **What are the poisonous snakes in the United States?**

The Crotalidae family (pit vipers) includes rattlesnakes, cottonmouths or water moccasins, and copperheads. Although there are approximately 40 to 50 species of venomous elapids (cobra family) in North and South America, the only elapids native to the United States are coral snakes (the eastern coral snake and the Texas coral snake). Coral snakes are shy creatures, and bites are uncommon. Most people bitten by coral snakes are intentionally handling the snakes.

36. **What are the effects of crotalid venom (pit vipers)?**

After envenomation, substantial local and systemic effects may develop within minutes to hours. The venom is neurotoxic, cytotoxic, cardiotoxic, and hemolytic. Its purpose is to immobilize, kill, and digest prey.

37. **How is coral snake envenomation different from pit viper envenomation?**

The coral snake venom apparatus is comprised of a pair of small, fixed, hollow fangs through which the snake injects venom via a chewing motion. Unlike pit vipers, which strike quickly, coral snakes must hang on for a brief period to achieve significant envenomation in humans. Coral snake venom is the most potent of any of the poisonous snakes in the United States.

38. What are the effects of elapid (coral snake) venom?

Onset of symptoms may be delayed as long as 10 to 12 hours but then be rapidly progressive. Coral snake venoms tend to have significant neurotoxicity (altered mental status, ptosis, generalized weakness, and muscle fasciculations). Other symptoms include pharyngeal spasm, hypersalivation, trismus, respiratory distress, cyanosis, hypotension, tachycardia, and cardiovascular collapse. Coral snake venom has little enzymatic activity or necrotic potential compared with most pit vipers. Coral snake venom is some of the most potent, yet the venom yield per snake is less than most of the vipers. Because of the relatively ineffective venom delivery system, up to 60% of people bitten by North American coral snakes may not be envenomed. Very few deaths related to coral snakebites have been reported in the United States since antivenom has been available. Patients who survive the bite may require respiratory support for up to a week and may suffer persistent weakness for weeks to months.

39. What determines the severity of a snakebite?

- The size, age, and health of the victim
- Level of exertion after the bite
- Amount of venom delivered
- Age, size, species of snake, and condition of its fangs
- Location, depth, and number of bites
- Length of time of snake attachment
- Presence of bacteria in snake's mouth or on victim's skin
- First aid measures
- Time to treatment

40. How is envenomation graded?

Envenomations are classified according to a five-level system that correlates to the amount of antivenin needed.

Crotalid envenomation classifications		
Grade	Degree of envenomation	Physical findings
0	None	Fang marks; no local or systemic reactions, or minimal local edema or pain.
1	Minimal	Fang marks; moderate local pain; edema 2.5-15 cm; ecchymosis/reddish discoloration; delayed findings; vesicles; hemorrhagic blebs; petechiae; necrosis. No systemic manifestations.

PT, prothrombin time; *APTT*, activated partial thromboplastin time; *CPK*, creatine phosphokinase.

Crotalid envenomation classifications—cont'd

Grade	Degree of envenomation	Physical findings
2	Moderate	Fang marks; more severe pain over larger area; edema 25-40 cm spreads toward the trunk; petechiae and ecchymosis in the edematous area; redness; nausea; vomiting; paresthesia; diaphoresis; orthostatic changes; serosanguinous ooze; hypotension; hematemesis; melena; hemoptysis; epistaxis; hemoconcentration; mild prolonged bleeding and clotting times; decreased red blood cells; thrombocytopenia; hematuria; proteinuria.
3	Severe	Fang marks; edema 40-50 cm; subcutaneous ecchymosis; diffuse pain; generalized ecchymosis and petechiae; fever; hypotension; tachycardia; hyperpnea; visual disturbances; convulsions; shock; marked coagulopathy; hypofibrinogenemia; prolonged PT/APTT times; increased fibrin split products; increased CPK; hematuria; proteinuria.
4	Very severe	Early manifestation of systemic systems with extremely rapid progression.

41. What treatments/interventions are recommended for crotalid snake envenomation?

Prehospital:
- Calm the victim; physical exertion or excitement will speed the spread of venom.
- If possible, retrieve the dead snake (decapitated heads can envenomate for as long as 60 minutes). Retrieval of the snake is a low priority, because treatment will ultimately be based on the patient's clinical presentation.
- Immobilize the bitten extremity. Note that tourniquets should not be used because they interfere with estimation of severity of envenomation.
- Transport the victim to the nearest medical facility.

In hospital: Determine the severity of envenomation and need for antivenin. Antivenin is most therapeutic when given within 4 hours of the bite and has limited value after 12 hours.
- Grade 0: no antivenin; local wound care; tetanus immunization as indicated; observe in ED at least 4 hours.
- Grade 1: 2 to 5 vials (20 to 50 ml) of antivenin; antihistamines.
- Grade 2: 6 to 10 vials (60 to 100 ml) of antivenin.
- Grade 3: 10 to 15 vials (100 to 150 ml) of antivenin.
- Grade 4: more than 15 vials (more than 150 ml) of antivenin.

Supportive care is given as indicated to maintain circulatory, respiratory, central nervous system, and hematological function. Secondary wound infection is prevented by administration of a broad-spectrum antibiotic, such as cephalosporin or dicloxacillin. The extremity should be kept slightly dependent until after the antivenin is given and then elevated. Surgical debridement of hemorrhagic blebs, vesicles, and superficial necrotic tissue can begin after day 3 to 5 and before day 7. Skin grafting is a consideration. Fasciotomy may be needed to prevent compartment syndrome.

42. **What treatments/interventions are recommended for elapid snake envenomation?**

Prehospital: As stated in question 41 for crotalid snakebites, plus:
- Some advocate the use of the Australian pressure-immobilization technique for field management.
- Start IV therapy.

In hospital: Aggressively manage any signs of impending respiratory failure with endotracheal intubation. Place on monitor and pulse oximeter, and monitor vital signs closely. Do not use grading scales for elapid bites. Administer appropriate antivenom. Because of the potential delay in onset of symptoms, admit all coral snakebites.

MARINE LIFE

43. **What is seabather's eruption, and how is it treated?**

Seabather's eruption, also known as sea lice, is a self-limited dermatitis found in swimmers and divers. It is caused by jellyfish larvae trapped as water flows through bathing suits. The larvae discharge nemotocysts when disturbed, causing a stinging sensation to the patient. Patients present with an intensely pruritic, maculopapular, and vesicular rash in the swimsuit area.

The cutaneous eruptions typically clear completely in 2 weeks with or without treatment. Localized symptoms can be treated with topical corticosteroids and oral antihistamines.

44. **What hazards are found among marine animals?**

Hazards from marine animals include bites, puncture wounds, and envenomation. Marine animals that bite include sharks, eels, barracudas, sea lions, killer whales, needlefish, giant clams, and giant squid. Wounds vary from punctures to large, avulsion-type wounds. Marine animals that envenomate include jellyfish, Portuguese man-of-war, anemones, hydrozoa fire coral, sea wasps, and box jellyfish. Contact with these animals results in burning, itching, pain, linear erythema, and dermatitis. Spiny creatures such as stingrays, scorpionfish (stonefish), sea urchins, pencil urchins, and catfish cause puncture wounds, lacerations, and envenomation. These wounds produce burning pain with an erythemic to dusky appearance and severe swelling. Wounds from spiny animals have a high incidence of ulceration, necrosis, and secondary infection. The venom can produce paresthesia, muscle weakness, hypotension, tachycardia, seizures, and cardiopulmonary arrest.

45. What are some toxic marine life, and how is their envenomation treated?

Comparison of toxic marine life

	Invertebrates	Vertebrates	Spiny creatures
Appearance	Coelenterates include Portuguese man-of-war, feather hydroids, fire corals, jellyfish, sea nettles, sea anemones, and corals. Characterized by stinging organoids.	Stingrays; the stingray is armed with one to four barbed venomous spines on a whiplike tail. The spines on the tail have a sharp tip with serrated edges that can cause a jagged laceration in addition to the puncture wound.	Scorpaenidae family includes scorpionfish, stonefish, lionfish, and zebrafish. They are all very well camouflaged; envenomations usually occur when creatures are inadvertently stepped on. Venom is injected as the spine punctures the skin. The spine may also break off into the skin.
Presentation	Clinical features of coelenterate envenomations range from mild dermatitis to rapid cardiovascular collapse. Can include stinging sensation, paresthesias, pruritus, local edema, blistering, and wheal formation. The man-of-war sting produces intense pain, radiating proximal with linear, edematous, erythematous eruptions on the skin. Systemic reactions can include nausea, vomiting, headache, myalgias, respiratory distress, hypotension, anaphylaxis, and cardiovascular collapse.	Stingray envenomations include an intense, localized pain that radiates centrally. Local edema and bleeding may also occur. The pain intensifies and peaks in 30-60 minutes. The wound may progress to deep tissue involvement and frank necrosis. Systemic effects may include muscle cramping, nausea, vomiting, weakness, headache, diaphoresis, dizziness, and in rare cases seizures, cardiovascular collapse, and death.	Clinical presentations vary from mild with the lionfish to life threatening with the stonefish. Intense pain may occur at the sting site, with radiation centrally that may intensify for several hours. Wound may appear ecchymotic, cyanotic, erythematous, and edematous. Local tissue necrosis may occur. Systemic symptoms may include nausea, vomiting, abdominal pain, headache, myalgias, weakness, hypotension, syncope, seizures, cardio-vascular collapse, and death.

Continued

Comparison of toxic marine life—cont'd

	Invertebrates	Vertebrates	Spiny creatures
Treatment	Includes advanced life-support measures, symptomatic care, analgesics. Rinse immediately with seawater, vinegar, or isopropyl alcohol (avoid vinegar with man-of-war). Remove tentacles with gloved hand or hemostats. For sea nettles or lion's mane stings, a baking powder slurry applied to the area may be helpful. Meat tenderizer may be used for the pruritic dermatitis caused by larval forms of certain coelenterates. Topical anesthetics, antihistamines, and corticosteroids may be helpful. Tetanus and analgesics as indicated. No prophylactic antibiotics.	Includes advanced life-support measures. Immerse wound in hot water for 60 minutes for pain relief and to deactivate the venom, which is heat labile. Wound debridement, analgesics, and tetanus as indicated. Prophylactic antibiotics are often given, along with diligent wound care and close follow-up.	Includes advanced life-support measures. Immediately immerse the affected part in hot water (110° to 115° F) for 60-90 minutes for pain relief and to deactivate the venom, which is heat labile. Remove any retained spines. Tetanus and analgesics as indicated. There are antivenins available from Australia's Commonwealth Serum Laboratories for serious stonefish and box jellyfish envenomations.

HEAT- AND COLD-RELATED EMERGENCIES

46. How is core body temperature regulated?

The anterior hypothalamus plays a key role in regulating core temperature of the brain, heart, lungs, liver, and kidneys. Skin components, subcutaneous fat, and skeletal muscles regulate the body's surface temperature.

Heat is produced through the body's metabolic processes; muscle activity; shivering; and effects of thyroxine, epinephrine, and norepinephrine.

Heat is lost through the following mechanisms:

- Radiation: Infrared energy radiated directly into the environment.
- Conduction: Transference of heat to another object by direct contact.
- Convection: Air movement surrounding the skin surface carries heat away.
- Evaporation: Insensible water vapor loss removes heat via perspiration and respiration.

47. What is hypothermia?

Hypothermia exists when the body's core temperature drops below 95° F (35° C).

48. What causes hypothermia, and who is at risk?

Causes of hypothermia include exposure to excessive cold or wind, immersion in water, wearing wet clothing, inability to produce heat, increased heat loss, and impaired thermoregulatory ability.

Those at high risk for hypothermia include the very young; elderly; socio-economically deprived people; homeless people; outdoor recreation employees; substance abusers; alcoholics; and people with chronic cardiovascular, endocrine, or musculoskeletal disorders.

49. What physiological changes occur in hypothermia?

Physiological changes with hypothermia

System	Change
Cardiac	Initially, increased heart rate and decreased cardiac output, followed by decreased heart rate and cardiac output with prolonged QT interval and J or Osborne wave (which is a positive deflection on the terminal 0.04 seconds of the QRS complex) that develops as core temperature drops below 92° to 90° F or 33.3° to 32.2° C and is fully prominent at 84° F or 28.8° C. Ventricular fibrillation can occur with stimulation and a further decline in core temperature to 82° F or 27.7° C. Asystole presents by 75° F or 23.8° C.
Neurological	Subtle decrease in logical thinking, mood swings, relative amnesia (95° F or 35° C); dilated pupils and progressive coma (88° to 80° F or 31.1° to 26.6° C); progressive and severe paralysis (87° to 85° F or 30.5° to 29.4° C); flat electroencephalogram (EEG) (68° F or 20° C).
Acid-base	Respiratory alkalosis in initial compensatory hyperventilation stages, progressing to respiratory acidosis with decreasing respiratory rate and shallower efforts, then to metabolic acidosis as a shift to anaerobic metabolism occurs.
Fluid and electrolytes	Cold diuresis, fluid shift from intracellular to extracellular space.
Hematological	Dehydration effect increases hematocrit and viscosity of blood.
Immunological	Decreased resistance to bacterial and viral pathogens.
Metabolic	Basal metabolic rate increases initially and rapidly declines; insulin release decreases; hypoglycemia results from fluid shifts and increased urine output.

50. What is the treatment for hypothermia?

Treatment for hypothermia focuses on returning the core body temperature to normal and providing supportive care. The methods of rewarming depend on the severity of hypothermia.

51. What rewarming methods are currently recommended?

Prehospital: Removal of wet clothing and application of heated inhalations and warmed blankets helps to prevent additional heat loss.
In hospital: Three methods for rewarming are used.
- Mild hypothermia (90° to 95° F or 32.2° to 35° C) can be treated with passive rewarming such as warm blankets, forced warm-air blankets, and warmed environment.
- Moderate hypothermia (82.5° to 90° F or 28° to 32.2° C) requires active core rewarming with warm IV fluids, warmed oxygen, and warmed peritoneal lavage.
- Severe hypothermia (less than 82.5° or less than 28° C) requires active core internal rewarming such as warmed IV solutions, warmed peritoneal lavage, and warmed thoracotomy/mediastinal lavage. Consider cardiopulmonary bypass or continuous arteriovenous rewarming (CAVR) with a Level 1 fluid warmer if available.

52. Which arrhythmias might be observed during hypothermia and rewarming?

Atrial fibrillation is a common arrhythmia after exposure to cold weather. Premature ventricular contractions and ventricular fibrillation are frequent rewarming arrhythmias. Treatment consists of following advanced cardiac life-support protocols.

53. What causes afterdrop of the core temperature?

Afterdrop, the decline of core temperature during rewarming, is caused by the continued return of cold peripheral blood to the core.

54. What is the best way to tell if rewarming is effective?

Core temperature is a key indicator; temperature measurement should be continuous during rewarming efforts. A return to normal level of consciousness and normal urine output are better indicators of effective rewarming than pupillary response, heart rate, or blood pressure.

55. How is the core temperature measured?

Rectal, esophageal, tympanic, and urinary bladder devices are available. The rectal temperature may be affected by the presence of cold stool, and esophageal temperature may be affected by heated inhalations or warmed gastric lavage.

56. What is frostbite?

Frostbite is a local tissue-freezing injury. Ice crystals form during metabolic standstill, initially extracellularly, because of intracellular to interstitial fluid shifts. Ninety percent of frostbite cases involve the hands and feet, followed by ears, nose, cheeks, and penis.

57. What types of frostbite occur?

Superficial frostbite involves the skin and subcutaneous fat and presents with numbness and clumsiness of the affected part. A throbbing pain develops with rewarming. The affected area feels soft on palpation and during rewarming flushes and turns red or deep purple.

Deep frostbite involves the deeper structures and produces no pain or sensation. The affected area feels quite hard on palpation and may appear white or waxy. The skin appears dehydrated and becomes purple, blue, or blackish on rewarming. Blisters generally form in 24 to 48 hours; blisters and color changes indicate reperfusion.

58. How is rewarming for frostbite performed, and what further treatment is needed?

Because most tissue damage occurs during the thaw-and-refreeze cycle, rewarming is begun when the body part can be warmed and not reexposed to cold. Rewarming occurs in a warm (100.8° to 106° F or 38.2° to 41.1° C), agitated water bath. Elevate the affected area to limit edema. Rewarming activity continues until the body part appears pink or reddened. Debride nonhemorrhagic blisters, because they contain high levels of inflammatory mediators. Rinse with sterile water (90° to 95° F or 32.2° to 35° C). Pat dry, and apply a nonconstrictive protective bulky barrier dressing. Administer tetanus prophylaxis as indicated. Ibuprofen has been advocated for systemic and topical thromboxane inhibition.

59. What is chilblains?

Chilblains, also known as perniosis, is an inflammatory skin lesion that occurs in nonfreezing climates, usually as a result of repeated exposure to cold (30° to 60° F) and typically affecting the hands and feet. The vasoconstriction-vasodilation cycle leads to vasospasms, intense pain, and itching. The affected parts redden and are slightly edematous; nodules and ulcerations may develop.

60. What is immersion foot (trench foot)?

Immersion foot is also a nonfreezing injury of prolonged exposure to wet cold (32° to 60° F or 0° to 15.5° C) either through actual immersion or wearing tight or wet socks and ill-fitting boots. Patients who wear waterproof footwear for an extended period are also at risk because of moisture from sweat. The affected parts appear cold, swollen, and dusky red or cyanotic in color. The complication is liquification gangrene rather than frostbite.

61. What techniques are used for rewarming in patients with chilblains and immersion foot?

Soft, gentle handling of affected tissue, and rewarming in water 104° to 108° F (0° to 42.2° C). Stop ingestion of nicotine and caffeine. Administer drugs with antiplatelet activity and hydrotherapy two to three times daily.

62. What are the common heat syndromes?

- Anhidrotic heat exhaustion
- Heat cramps

- Heat edema
- Heat exhaustion
- Heat stroke
- Heat syncope
- Heat tetany
- Prickly heat

63. How do the heat emergencies compare with respect to presentation and treatment?

Heat emergencies and treatment

Type	Presentation	Treatment
Anhidrotic heat exhaustion	Syncope, lightheadedness, shortness of breath, tremors, relative or complete lack of normal sweating on trunk or limbs, and excessive sweating on face and forehead.	Desquamation agent (salicylic acid 1%) and antibacterial agents (chlorhexidine solution or lotion); in diffuse inflammation states, antibiotics (erythromycin, dicloxacillin, and cloxacillin) are added.
Heat cramps	Brief, intermittent severe muscular cramps in muscles fatigued by heavy work, excessive fatigue, decreased coordination, nausea, vomiting, headache, and dizziness.	Place patient in cool environment and massage affected muscles; patient should rest until symptoms subside. Administer salt solution— 0.9% normal saline, 1000 ml IV, over 1-3 hrs or 23.5% normal saline in 10-ml to 20-ml increments IV; or 0.1% saline solution orally. Monitor electrolytes and magnesium levels, with replacement as needed.
Heat edema	Hydrostatic pressure changes, vasodilation of cutaneous vessels, and orthostatic blood pooling.	Elevate the extremities, use thigh-high support hose, and decrease exposure to heat.
Heat exhaustion	Dehydration, malaise, weakness, flulike symptoms, thirst, tachycardia, frontal headache, and muscle cramps.	Fluid and electrolyte replacement based on serum electrolytes and calculation of body water deficit. Spontaneous cooling to 102° F (39° C). Acetaminophen or ibuprofen may be used.
Heat stroke	Hot, dry skin; altered level of consciousness; psychotic behavior; delirium; coma; seizures; and severe muscle cramps. Temperature ranges from 106° to 116° F. This is a neurological emergency.	Aggressive cooling to 102° F (39° C) within 1 hour. Mannitol may be considered to decrease ICP. Initiate respiratory and cardiovascular support early.

Heat emergencies and treatment—cont'd

Type	Presentation	Treatment
Heat syncope	Decreased venous return, decreased cardiac output, and decreased cerebral perfusion.	Place patient in supine position and remove from heat source.
Heat tetany	Severe intermittent tonic spasms, hyperventilation, and distal extremity paresthesias.	Massage affected muscles.
Prickly heat	Superficial glistening vesicles on red base; intense itching and absence of sweat on unclothed body parts; blocked sweat pores and tissue maceration.	Restrict exercise, keep patient in cool environment, and increase oral fluid intake.

64. **What are the three types of heat exhaustion?**

- **Water depletion:** caused by inadequate fluid intake; leads to progressive dehydration and hypernatremia; if untreated, progresses to heat stroke.
- **Salt depletion:** caused by adequate fluid intake and inadequate sodium/salt intake; leads to hyponatremia and hypochloremia; body core temperature is nearer to normal in this type.
- **Mixed salt and water depletion:** caused by loss of both salt and water, usually in hot environment with exertion; leads to dehydration and heat stroke.

65. **How is body water deficit replaced?**

The number of liters to be infused is determined from a calculation of total body water, desired sodium content, and measured sodium content. Normal saline should be infused until the patient is hemodynamically stable; then free water is administered over 48 hours.

66. **What additional treatments are indicated?**

- Place the patient in a cool environment.
- Use cooling methods to obtain a core temperature of 102° F (39° C).
- Correct dehydration to normalize serum osmolarity at the rate of 2 mOsm/hr (faster correction may result in cerebral edema and seizures).

67. **How is cooling achieved?**

The safest method is evaporative cooling by spraying or sponging the patient with lukewarm water in an environment of air movement (large circulating fans). Placing padded ice packs along lateral aspects of the trunk and groin is also helpful. Methods to be used with caution include ice water immersion, gastric lavage, peritoneal lavage, rectal lavage, cardiopulmonary bypass, or hemodialysis. Caution also is urged with the use of ice packs, which significantly increase shivering and heat production and may cause local tissue damage, including frostbite.

68. What are the three types of heat stroke?

- **Classic:** occurs over several days when the environmental temperature is high, often with elevated humidity. Also called the endemic form, it often affects elderly, infirm, homeless, or sedentary people.
- **Exertional:** occurs with strenuous exercise, generating 800 kcal/hr. It also can occur in the presence of moderate temperatures and humidity and affects healthy people.
- **Drug-induced (malignant hyperthermia):** precipitated by drugs that increase muscular hyperactivity, inducing hypermetabolism; associated with impaired thermoregulation, cardiovascular compensation, and heat dissipation.

69. What happens with heat stroke?

All three types may progress to a shock state, permanent neurological deficits, and cardiac compromise with hematological insult (e.g., disseminated intravascular coagulation). Other sequelae include hepatic impairment, renal impairment, respiratory alkalosis, lactic acidosis, and bone marrow damage. Rhabdomyolysis and myoglobinuria lead to acute oliguric renal failure.

70. What interventions are recommended?

Aggressive cooling is the cornerstone of therapy and is initiated early to prevent high mortality rates. The goal is to cool to 102° F (39.0° C) within 1 hour. Discontinue the cooling at 102° F (39.0° C) to avoid iatrogenic hypothermia. Mannitol may be considered to reduce intracerebral swelling. Respiratory and cardiovascular support are initiated early in the treatment plan.

WATER-RELATED EMERGENCIES

71. What is the difference between drowning, near-drowning, and secondary near-drowning?

Drowning is the death of a victim from suffocation by asphyxiating immersion or submersion in any fluid or liquid media when the cause of death cannot be attributed to other lethal disorders. Near-drowning occurs when the victim recovers spontaneously or is successfully resuscitated, at least temporarily. Secondary near-drowning is the delayed onset of respiratory insufficiency resulting from submersion.

72. What is immersion syndrome?

Immersion syndrome occurs immediately on contact with cold water. Sudden death occurs from cold-induced ventricular arrhythmia or asystole. This rapid-onset problem rarely results in rescue and resuscitation; most victims drown. The cause is a reflex mechanism (diving reflex) that occurs when cold-water immersion of the face causes apnea, bradycardia, and intense peripheral vasoconstriction.

73. What is a shallow-water blackout?

Shallow-water blackout is hyperventilation-induced hypocapnea. Swimmers dangerously use this to remain under water for a longer time. This syndrome suppresses the two dominant respiratory drives, causing hypoxia and unconsciousness, which leads to drowning. Victims are found dead with no evidence of a struggle.

74. What is breath-hold diving?

Divers withhold breathing on ascension, causing a decrease in the partial pressure of oxygen. This action results in hypoxia and, ultimately, loss of consciousness. More skilled divers rather than neophytes are noted for this behavior.

75. What is the difference between dry drowning and wet drowning?

Dry drowning occurs in the absence of aspiration. Prolonged respiratory obstruction is secondary to laryngospasm. As the level of consciousness decreases, glottic closure occurs, causing asphyxia.

Wet drowning involves aspiration of fluid. It is precipitated by laryngospasm, which causes loss of consciousness, followed by glottic relaxation that results in aspiration and suffocation. Wet drowning often occurs with much struggling; the victim blows off air, which enhances aspiration of water.

76. What is the pathophysiology of drowning?

The underlying pathophysiology of all events is hypoxia, hypercapnia, and acidosis (metabolic and respiratory).

77. How does the awake victim present?

The victim can appear asymptomatic or present with the following symptoms:
- Dyspnea
- Cyanosis
- Cough
- Pink frothy expectorant
- Wheezes, rales, rhonchi
- Apnea
- Laryngospasm
- Substernal burning or pleuritic pain
- Arrhythmia
- Hypovolemic or hypervolemic states
- Hypothermia
- Restlessness, irritability
- Flaccidity
- Confusion
- Seizures
- Decorticate posturing or hyporeflexia
- Vomiting
- Abdominal distention
- Azotemia, proteinuria, and oliguria
- Disseminated intravascular coagulation

78. What treatments are indicated?

Supportive care for the neurological, cardiac, and respiratory systems is indicated. Mechanical ventilation assisted by continuous positive airway pressure (CPAP) and positive end-expiratory pressure (PEEP) is the mainstay of treatment. Bronchodilators, osmotic and loop diuretics, and muscle relaxants also are used, along with barbiturate coma.

79. What are the pressure-related diving syndromes?

- **Mask and ear canal squeeze:** In scuba diving, negative pressure in the mask can cause capillary rupture, skin ecchymosis, and conjunctival hemorrhage. Entrapped air in the external auditory canal from a tight-fitting diving hood causes painful ear squeeze on descent. The same problem can occur when earplugs are used in the presence of cerumen or bony growths. The result is pain, bleeding, hemorrhagic blebs, or tympanic membrane rupture.
- **Barotitis (ear squeeze):** A vacuum develops in the middle ear during descent, causing pain and a sensation of fullness. Fluid shifts can cause serous otitis.
- **Barosinusitis (sinus squeeze):** During descent a vacuum develops, causing pain and bleeding. When this syndrome occurs during ascent or decompression, it is known as reverse sinus squeeze.
- **Barodontalgia (dental barotrauma):** Air is trapped under a faulty filling as a result of pressure changes on descent. Abscesses and dental infections also can cause this syndrome.
- **Pulmonary overcompression syndrome:** Forcible breath-holding or a closed glottis leads to bronchospasm. Air is forced across the pulmonary capillary membrane and enters either pulmonary capillaries or pulmonary interstitial spaces.

80. What is arterial gas embolism (AGE)?

AGE bubbles originate not from supersaturation of gases in the blood and tissue but from rupture of the alveoli caused by the barotrauma of ascent. The bubbles enter the pulmonary vein and are carried to the heart and systemic circulation. The classic presentation is a sudden onset of unconsciousness within minutes of reaching the surface after a dive. Symptoms occur immediately and the effects are devastating:

- Cardiac flow: arrhythmias
- Cerebral flow: focal or general seizures, unconsciousness, altered mental status, diverse neurological signs and symptoms depending on the location of emboli

Treatment includes advanced life-support measures, recompression, and hyperbaric oxygen as quickly as possible.

81. What is nitrogen narcosis?

Nitrogen narcosis is an increase in the partial pressure of nitrogen that occurs when the diver breathes dissolved nitrogen under pressure. As partial pressure of nitrogen increases, more nitrogen is dissolved in the blood, impairing the conduction of nerve impulses. Nitrogen narcosis can occur when the diver dives too deep or stays down too long. Some divers appear to be more susceptible than others. Symptoms mimic alcohol intoxication and include euphoria and deterioration in judgment, logic, and reasoning, progressing to drowsiness, unconsciousness, weakness, and death from drowning. Treatment is ascent to shallower depth. Gas mixtures other than compressed air may be used to prevent this.

82. **What is decompression sickness?**

Decompression sickness results from the expansion and release of dissolved nitrogen in the tissues as atmospheric pressure rapidly decreases (e.g., during rapid ascent from a deep dive). These bubbles may disrupt cellular function or cause obstruction. The nitrogen bubbles can be interstitial, intralymphatic, or intravascular. Symptoms can evolve over minutes or up to 12 hours; they rarely appear after 12 hours.

83. **What signs and symptoms can be observed in decompression sickness?**

Decompression sickness

Type of decompression	Signs and symptoms
Cutaneous	Itching (may be intense) without visible source, local or generalized mottling, hyperemia, ischemic marbled skin.
Limb ("the bends")	Severe tendonitis, joint pain, and joint tenderness may or may not be present; single or multiple joints may be involved; paresthesia over joints and grating sensation with joint movement are common, but lymphedema is rare.
Neurological: brain	Headache, dysphagia, visual field deficit, confusion, island like spotty motor and/or blind gap in visual field, sensory deficit, mental dullness, disorientation.
Neurological: spinal cord	Back pain, abdominal pain, extremity weakness, hypo- or hyperparesthesia, paresia, anal sphincter weakness, heaviness, paresthesia, ataxia, vertigo, urinary bladder distention.
Pulmonary	Dyspnea, substernal tachypnea, pain with increased tachycardia or deep inspiration, cyanosis, nonproductive cough.
Vasomotor	Weakness, sweating, hypotension, unconsciousness, tachycardia, pallor and/or mottling, hemoconcentration, decreased urine output, profound general heaviness or fatigue.

84. **How is decompression sickness treated?**

The only effective treatment for decompression sickness is recompression in a chamber with hyperbaric oxygen therapy administered according to standardized protocols published by the United States Navy. The Navy dive treatment tables are very effective, especially when recompression is initiated early. The treatment selected is based on the severity of the patient's condition. The number of treatments is determined by physical examination and identifiable improvements from the baseline condition.

85. **How does recompression work?**

Recompression works in two ways: by promoting inert gas elimination and by decreasing the size of the gas bubbles in the body. Recompression also provides oxygen to damaged tissue, treats platelet and clotting damage, and assists excretion of metabolites.

86. Where can information about decompression emergencies and recompression centers be obtained?

Duke University's Divers Alert Network (DAN) is available 24 hours per day at 919-684-8111. Education and resource materials are available from DAN at 919-684-2948 (http://anesthesia.duhs.duke.edu/divisions/dan.html or www.diversalertnetwork.org/about).

The Undersea and Hyperbaric Medical Society (UHMS), which publishes a directory listing of all approved chambers in the United States and resources for international referral, can be contacted at 301-942-2980 or 410-257-6606 (www.uhms.org).

HIGH-ALTITUDE EMERGENCIES

87. What are high-altitude syndromes?

High-altitude syndromes are caused by hypobaric hypoxia. The exact causative mechanisms are not clear. There is a delay from the onset of hypoxia to the onset of altitude illness. High-altitude syndromes develop with travel to altitudes above 8000 feet (greater than 560 mmHg). Altitude is further defined as moderate (8000 to 12,000 feet) or extreme (above 19,000 feet).

88. What is high-altitude illness?

High-altitude illness refers to a spectrum of conditions that occur at altitudes of 8000 feet or higher, including acute mountain sickness (AMS), high altitude pulmonary edema (HAPE), and high altitude cerebral edema (HACE). High-altitude illness is a collection of symptoms caused by rapid ascent of an unacclimatized person to 8000 feet or higher from altitudes below 5000 feet. For the partially acclimatized, AMS may result from an abrupt ascent to a higher altitude, overexertion, and/or use of respiratory depressants. AMS is a result of hypoxia or insufficient oxygen to the tissue. Because of decreased partial pressure of oxygen at altitude, there is less oxygen available to the tissue because of incomplete hemoglobin loading. For example, if at sea level an individual's oxygen saturation is 97% and the person travels quickly to 18,000 feet, the saturation falls to 71%. If strenuous exercise is added, the saturation is correspondingly lower.

89. What symptoms present in AMS?

In most cases, AMS symptoms begin about 12 to 24 hours after reaching altitude. AMS is defined as a syndrome that occurs after altitude gain and presents with a headache and at least one of the following symptoms:
- Gastrointestinal symptoms (anorexia, nausea, vomiting)
- Fatigue or weakness
- Dizziness or lightheadedness
- Difficulty sleeping (fragmented sleep)
- Other symptoms, including irritability, chills, malaise, lassitude, dyspnea on exertion, tachycardia, dry cough, postural hypotension, fluid retention, and absence of normal urination

Ataxia is the clinical indicator used to denote progression from mild to severe AMS. Altered level of consciousness follows, with progression of confusion, disorientation, and impaired judgment. Coma may evolve within 24 hours after the development of ataxia.

90. How is AMS treated?

Treatment of mild AMS begins with halting the ascent to allow acclimatization; improvement of symptoms should occur within 12 hours to 4 days. Descent to a lower altitude reverses AMS and is critical in cases of severe AMS. Acetazolamide, dexamethasone, aspirin, and prochlorperazine can mediate symptoms.

91. What is HAPE?

HAPE is a life-threatening condition occurring at altitudes above 8000 feet. It usually occurs within the first 4 days of ascent. Early symptoms include dry cough, dyspnea at rest, substernal pain, headache, anorexia, and lassitude. Later symptoms include tachypnea, wheezing, orthopnea, hemoptysis, tachycardia, pulmonary rales and rhonchi, pink frothy sputum, mental changes, and ataxia. HAPE is believed to be a form of neurogenical pulmonary edema, which is a high-protein permeability edema.

92. How is HAPE treated?

Descent is the key to effective treatment. Bed rest and administration of supplemental oxygen are central to the treatment plan. If the condition progresses to adult respiratory distress syndrome, intubation and mechanical ventilation are indicated. Portable hyperbaric chambers (also called "gamow bags" after Dr. Igor Gamow) may be useful for patients who are unable to descend.

93. What is HACE?

HACE is clinical progression of the neurological and cerebral signs of AMS.

94. What additional symptoms are seen in HACE?

Ataxia, severe lassitude, changes in mental status, drowsiness, obtundation, stupor, and coma. Also evident are hallucinations, cranial nerve palsy, hemiparesis, seizures, hemiplegia, and various focal neurological signs, including cortical blindness, aphasia, and an islandlike blind spot in the visual field. The progression from AMS to HACE occurs over 12 hours to 4 days. Stroke may result from polycythemia, dehydration, increased ICP, cerebrovascular spasm, or other problems.

95. What is the treatment for HACE?

Immediate descent. Evaluation for evidence of a stroke should ensue. Steroids and oxygen are frequently administered until HACE improves.

96. What causes high-altitude pharyngitis and bronchitis?

An increase in ventilatory rate, mouth breathing, and movement of dryer and colder air causes dehydration, irritation, and pain similar to pharyngitis.

Key Points

- Postexposure rabies vaccines are very efficacious and will prevent rabies if they are administered promptly and correctly after a rabies exposure.
- For a patient who has completed the tetanus series, a tetanus booster should be given if it has been more than 10 years for clean wounds and more than 5 years for dirty wounds. TIG is also administered for high-risk wounds or to patients without adequate baseline immunizations.
- Treatment of Lyme disease with standard antibiotics is very effective at preventing long-term sequelae.
- All bites and stings have the potential to cause allergic and anaphylactic reactions.
- There is antivenin available for serious snakebites, as well as stonefish and scorpion (only in Arizona) envenomation.
- Because most tissue damage occurs during the thaw-and-refreeze cycle, rewarming of frostbite is begun when the body part can be warmed and not reexposed to cold.
- The treatment of hypothermia focuses on returning the core body temperature to normal and providing supportive care. The methods of rewarming depend on the severity of hypothermia.
- The initial treatment for AMS, HAPE, and HACE is immediate descent of at least 2000 to 3000 feet.

Internet Resources

Centers for Disease Control and Prevention, *Rabies Vaccine* (pdf document, Adobe Acrobat Reader software required):
www.cdc.gov/nip/publications/vis/vis-rabies.pdf

Centers for Disease Control and Prevention, Rabies:
www.cdc.gov/ncidod/dvrd/rabies

Divers Alert Network, On-Site Neurological Examination:
www.diversalertnetwork.org/medical/neuroexam.asp

eMedicine, Bites, Insects:
www.emedicine.com/emerg/topic62.htm

eMedicine: Heat Exhaustion and Heatstroke:
www.emedicine.com/emerg/topic236.htm

National Outdoor Leadership School, Wilderness Medicine Institute:
www.nols.edu/wmi

World Health Organization, *WHO Recommendations on Rabies Post-Exposure Treatment and the Correct Technique of Intradermal Immunization against Rabies* (pdf document, Adobe Acrobat Reader software required):
http://whqlibdoc.who.int/hq/1996/WHO_EMC_ZOO_96.6.pdf

Bibliography

American Academy of Pediatrics, Committee on Infectious Diseases: Prevention of Lyme disease, *Pediatrics* 105:142-147, 2000.

Auerbach PS: *Wilderness medicine*, ed 4, St Louis, 2001, Mosby.

Briggs DJ: Rabies vaccination: Protecting vulnerable travelers, *Infect Med* 19(12):561-565, 2002.

Centers for Disease Control and Prevention: Compendium of animal rabies prevention and control, *MMWR* 49(RR08):19-30, 2000.

Centers for Disease Control and Prevention: Human rabies prevention—United States: 1999 recommendations of the Advisory Committee on Immunization Practices (ACIP), *MMWR* 48(RR-1):1-21, 1999.

Centers for Disease Control and Prevention: Hypothermia-related deaths: United States, 2003, *MMWR* 53(8):172-173, 2004.

Centers for Disease Control and Prevention: Recommendations for the use of Lyme disease vaccine: Recommendations of the Advisory Committee on Immunization Practices (ACIP), *MMWR* 51:29-31, 2002.

Fenner PJ: Dangers in the ocean: The traveler and marine envenomation. I: Jellyfish, *J Travel Med* 5:135-141, 1998.

Fenner PJ: Dangers in the ocean: The traveler and marine envenomation. II: Marine vertebrates, *J Travel Med* 5:213-216, 1998.

Garcia R: Preventing human rabies before and after exposure, *Nurse Pract* 24:91-92, 95-97, 101, 1999.

Greenberg MI et al: *Greenberg's text—Atlas of emergency medicine*, Philadelphia, 2005, Lippincott.

Harris MD et al: High altitude medicine, *Am Fam Physician* 57:1907-1917, 1998.

Hayney MS, Grunske MM, and Boh LE: Lyme disease prevention and vaccine prophylaxis, *Ann Pharmacother* 33:723-729, 1999.

Kanzenbach TL, Dexter WW: Cold injuries: Protecting your patients from the dangers of hypothermia and frostbite, *Postgrad Med* 105:72-77, 1999.

Krebs JW, Rupprecht CE, Childs JE: Rabies surveillance in the United States during 1999, *J Am Vet Med Assoc* 217(12):1799-1811, 2000.

Lewis LM, Levine MD, Dribben WH: Bites and stings. In Dale DC, Federman DD, editors: *Interdisciplinary medicine II*, WebMD, Scientific American Medicine, 2002.

Markovchick V, Pons PT, editors: *Emergency medicine secrets*, ed 2, Philadelphia, 1999, Hanley & Belfus.

Norris R: *Snake envenomations, coral*, eMedicine, 2005. Available at www.emedicine.com/emerg/topic542.htm.

O'Reilly M: Environmental emergencies. In Oman K, Koziol-McLain J, Scheetz L: *Emergency nursing secrets*, Philadelphia, 2001, Hanley & Belfus.

Pray WS: Preventing acute mountain sickness, *US Pharmacist* 26(3), 2001.

Spira A: Diving and marine medicine review. Part II: Diving physics and physiology, *J Travel Med* 6:180-198, 1999.

Vetrano SJ, Lebowitz JB, Marcus S: Lionfish envenomation, *J Emerg Med* 23:379-382, 2002.

Ingestions and Poisonings

Cheryl Montanio

1. **What is the initial emergency department (ED) management of the comatose patient suspected of having taken an overdose?**

The approach is similar to that for any patient who presents to the ED with altered mental status:
- Assess the ABCs (airway, breathing, circulation).
- Place the patient on 100% oxygen with a cardiac monitor.
- Establish intravenous (IV) access.
- Obtain a full set of vital signs, including core temperature and pulse oximetry reading.
- Administer 2 mg naloxone, a competitive antagonist of opiates at the opiate receptor. Opiates frequently are abused, and they are a common means of attempted suicide. Naloxone can induce opiate withdrawal.
- Administer dextrose or perform a rapid glucose determination. Hypoglycemia is a common cause of altered mental status that is easily treated with dextrose. Adults should be given 50% dextrose (50 ml) and children 0.5 to 1 gm/kg of D10 to D25 (2 to 4 ml/kg). Common medications (including insulin and oral hypoglycemics) as well as many medical conditions can cause hypoglycemia. Because dextrose may worsen hyperglycemic states and cerebral ischemia, a rapid glucose determination, if possible, is advised before administering dextrose blindly.
- Administer thiamine (100 mg IV in adults) concomitantly with glucose to adult patients who are suspected of being alcoholics or malnourished to prevent worsening of Wernicke-Korsakoff syndrome. Wernicke-Korsakoff syndrome is caused by vitamin B_1 (thiamine) deficiency and presents with ocular motor abnormalities, ataxia, and confusion.
- Serum levels of acetaminophen, salicylate, and ethanol; serum electrolytes (including blood urea nitrogen [BUN] and creatinine); and an electrocardiogram (ECG) should be obtained for most comatose patients suspected of having taken an overdose.

2. **What dose of naloxone should be administered to adults and children who present with respiratory arrest or apnea after a suspected opiate exposure?**

All patients, adults and children alike, who present with respiratory arrest or apnea should be given 2 mg of naloxone. Some patients may require larger doses, but the initial dose of 2 mg is the same for children and adults. Administration of naloxone to opiate-addicted patients can precipitate opiate withdrawal. A smaller initial dose of naloxone may be considered for patients who do not present with respiratory arrest or apnea and are suspected to be addicted to opiates. Narcotic drugs such as meperidine, propoxyphene, diphenoxylate, and methadone may be relatively naloxone resistant and require large doses of naloxone, up to 10 mg. Generally, failure to achieve a positive clinical response after 10 mg of naloxone signifies that further doses are not indicated and the patient's clinical presentation is probably not related to opioid toxicity.

3. Is opiate withdrawal a concern before administering naloxone?

No. Although opiate withdrawal can be life threatening for neonates, it is not life threatening for children and adults. Opiate withdrawal does not cause seizures, except in neonates born to opiate-addicted mothers. Although patients experiencing opiate withdrawal are uncomfortable, they should not have an altered mental status. Opiate withdrawal causes yawning, sneezing, mydriasis (dilated pupils), nausea, vomiting, abdominal cramping, diarrhea, piloerection (goose bumps), and agitation. Physical exam findings that are useful for detecting opiate withdrawal include dilated pupils, increased bowel sounds, and piloerection.

4. What specific information should be gathered in taking the history of a patient who presents to the ED after a suspected ingestion?

- Determine the reason for the ingestion (unintentional versus intentional). Ask a straightforward question, such as, "Why did you take 20 aspirin? Were you trying to hurt yourself?"
- Attempt to identify and record all substances involved, including coingestants. However, always suspect that additional substances may be involved.
- Attempt to locate all containers and pill bottles. Send family, friends, EMS personnel, or co-workers to retrieve the containers or pill bottles.
- Quantify the magnitude of the exposure. Perform pill counts and measure liquids. Determine the amounts missing.
- Determine where the ingestion occurred and any other potential toxins to which the patient may have had access.
- Record a history of past ingestions and the substances involved.
- Determine the time of the ingestion.
- Determine what, if any, treatment has been provided in the prehospital phase.
- Consult the regional Poison Control Center at 800-222-1222 for information about management of the patient.
- Ask whether anyone else may have taken the ingestion along with the patient, especially in cases involving children.

5. Should all patients with an ingestion undergo gastrointestinal (GI) decontamination?

The decision to decontaminate a patient's GI tract is complex and must be individualized. Factors that should be considered include the substances involved, the degree of toxicity of the ingested substances, the amount ingested, the time after ingestion, and the patient's clinical status. Patients ingesting nontoxic substances or nontoxic doses of toxins often do not require GI decontamination. Some examples include unintentional pediatric ingestions of topical corticosteroids, a small number of ibuprofen tablets, oral contraceptives (without iron), throat lozenges (without local anesthetic), diaper rash creams and ointments, pen ink, and chalk. Although these are minimally toxic substances, each patient's situation and circumstances must be evaluated separately for appropriate care.

6. What methods are used to decontaminate a patient's GI tract?
  - Administration of syrup of ipecac (see question 8 for contraindications)
  - Administration of activated charcoal
  - Orogastric lavage
  - Whole bowel irrigation

7. How do the different methods of GI decontamination prevent absorption?

Syrup of ipecac contains two plant alkaloids, cephaline and emetine, derived from the ipecacuanha plant, which induce vomiting by stimulating peripheral sensory receptors in the GI tract and the central chemoreceptor trigger zone in the brain. Syrup of ipecac is useful only for removing toxins from the stomach—not from the remaining GI tract.

Activated charcoal binds most drugs and chemicals well and prevents their absorption across the GI wall into the systemic circulation. Toxins bound to charcoal pass through the GI tract and are excreted in the stool. Activated charcoal can bind toxins in the stomach and throughout the GI tract.

Orogastric lavage is performed by inserting a tube down the esophagus and into the patient's stomach. Water or saline is inserted through the tube and subsequently removed, with the goal of removing toxins from the stomach. Pediatric tube sizes range from 24 to 32 French and adult tube sizes range from 36 to 42 French. Orogastric lavage is useful only for removing toxins from the stomach. The small size of the pediatric orogastric tube relative to the size of most pills limits the usefulness of lavage in most children and argues against its use. Severe aspiration pneumonia and permanent lung damage have resulted from orogastric lavage in children.

Whole bowel irrigation decreases GI transit time. A nonabsorbable solution containing polyethylene glycol is administered by mouth and passes through the GI tract. By decreasing GI transit time toxins have less time to be absorbed and are excreted in the stool. Administering multiple doses of cathartics is not recommended and should not be confused with whole bowel irrigation. Cathartics can cause fluid and electrolyte abnormalities not associated with polyethylene glycol administration.

8. What are the indications for the different methods of GI decontamination?

Syrup of ipecac is rarely indicated for administration in the ED setting. In the past, Poison Control Centers occasionally recommended home administration of syrup of ipecac for some accidental pediatric ingestions; however, this practice is no longer supported nor advised. It is extremely rare for an emergency nurse to administer syrup of ipecac today.

Activated charcoal is indicated for most patients that present to the ED within a few hours of a potentially toxic ingestion. Activated charcoal is not recommended for isolated ingestions of metals (lithium, iron), alcohols (ethanol, methanol, and ethylene glycol), and caustics. Because aspiration of activated charcoal can cause pneumonitis, caution should be taken to make sure that the airway is adequately protected. Activated charcoal often causes vomiting.

Orogastric lavage is indicated for patients who present to the ED with an ingestion that is believed to be potentially life threatening and at a time when it is believed that the substance may still be present in the stomach. Because of the risk of aspiration, orogastric lavage should not be performed unless a patient's airway is adequately protected. Orogastric lavage can cause esophageal injury.

Whole bowel irrigation is indicated for patients with large ingestions of substances poorly bound to activated charcoal (lithium, iron), for patients with GI stores of wrapped illicit drugs (body packers and body stuffers), and for patients with large ingestions of enteric-coated or sustained-release preparations (sustained-release beta blockers and calcium channel blockers, enteric-coated aspirin).

9. Is there any benefit in administering more than one dose of activated charcoal?

Activated charcoal is commonly dosed at 1 to 2 gm/kg. It makes sense that the dose of activated charcoal should depend on the amount of toxin ingested and how well the poison is bound to activated charcoal. Generally a 10:1 ratio of activated charcoal to the substance ingested is recommended, but practically this ratio is difficult if not impossible to achieve clinically. One or two repeat doses of activated charcoal may be of benefit after large ingestions of potentially life-threatening substances that are well bound to activated charcoal (salicylate, theophylline) or when sustained-release or enteric-coated preparations are involved. If a repeat dose is to be given, administer half the original dose between 4 and 6 hours after the first dose. Remember, activated charcoal aspiration can produce severe and permanent lung damage.

10. What is the toxicological differential diagnosis of a patient who presents with an increased anion gap metabolic acidosis (AGMA)?

CATMUDPILES is a helpful mnemonic for remembering the toxicological causes of an increased AGMA:

C	Cyanide, carbon monoxide
A	Alcoholic ketoacidosis
T	Toluene
M	Methanol
U	Uremia (elevated BUN)
D	Diabetic ketoacidosis, alcoholic ketoacidosis, starvation ketoacidosis
P	Phenformin or metformin, paraldehyde
I	Isoniazid, iron
L	Lactate (carbon monoxide, cyanide)
E	Ethylene glycol
S	Salicylate

A normal anion gap is 12 ± 4 mEq/L and is calculated as follows:

Serum sodium (mEq/L) − (serum chloride [mEq/L] +

serum bicarbonate [mEq/L])

11. **Does any grouping of toxins guide the emergency care of patients with an ingestion?**

Yes. The emergency nurse should determine whether the patient's presentation is consistent with an anticholinergic, cholinergic, opioid, or serotonin syndrome.

12. **What signs and symptoms are associated with anticholinergic toxicity?**

Anticholinergic toxicity is caused by blockade of acetylcholine receptors, which results in decreased stimulation. Signs and symptoms include:
- Sinus tachycardia
- Increased temperature ("hot as hell")
- Dilated pupils ("blind as a bat")
- Red flushed skin ("red as a beet")
- Dry mucous membranes and skin ("dry as a bone")
- Hallucinations and agitation ("mad as a hatter")
- Urinary retention
- Decreased GI motility with decreased bowel sounds
- Seizures ("seizing like a squirrel")

   Different patients with anticholinergic toxicity exhibit differing degrees of these symptoms. Patients with a constellation of these symptoms are said to have the anticholinergic toxidrome.

13. **What are some common causes of anticholinergic toxicity?**

- Antihistamines (diphenhydramine [Benadryl], meclizine [Antivert], cyproheptadine [Periactin])
- Phenothiazines (chlorpromazine [Thorazine])
- Cyclic antidepressants (amitriptyline [Elavil])
- Antispasmodics (dicyclomine [Bentyl], scopolamine, hyoscine, oxybutynin)
- Mucous membrane–drying agents (glycopyrrolate)
- Agents used to dilate the eyes (cyclopentolate [Cyclogyl], homatropine, tropicamide [Mydriacyl])
- Bronchodilators (ipratropium [Atrovent])
- Skeletal muscle relaxants (cyclobenzaprine [Flexeril])
- Antivirals (amantidine [Symmetrel])
- Anti-Parkinson agents (benztropine [Cogentin])
- Numerous plants and mushroom species

14. **What antidote can be used to diagnose anticholinergic toxicity?**

Physostigmine reverses anticholinergic effects. It inhibits the metabolism of acetylcholine by acetylcholinesterase, thereby increasing the amount of acetylcholine at the receptor. Physostigmine may be helpful in diagnosing anticholinergic toxicity. However, it should not be used to treat the patient because of the risk of cholinergic symptoms, including bradycardia, seizures, and asystole. Patients with confirmed anticholinergic toxicity should be sedated with benzodiazepines.

15. What signs and symptoms are associated with cholinergic toxicity?

Cholinergic toxicity is caused by an abundance of acetylcholine at muscarinic and nicotinic acetylcholine receptors, resulting in increased stimulation. Acetylcholine is abundant at these receptors because acetylcholinesterase, the enzyme that breaks down acetylcholine, is inhibited.

SLUDGE is a useful mnemonic for remembering signs and symptoms of acetylcholine excess at the muscarinic receptor. Other muscarinic effects include miosis (small pupils), bradycardia, and bronchoconstriction.

S	Salivation
L	Lacrimation
U	Urination
D	Diarrhea/diaphoresis
G	Increased **GI** motility
E	Emesis (vomiting), pulmonary edema

Another useful mnemonic to remember the cholinergic syndrome is DUMBBBELS:

D	Defecation
U	Urination
M	Miosis
B	Bronchorrhea
B	Bradycardia
B	Bronchospasm
E	Emesis
L	Lacrimation
S	Salivation

The signs and symptoms of acetylcholine excess at the nicotinic receptor are fasciculations and muscle weakness. Patients with a constellation of the above symptoms are said to have the cholinergic toxidrome.

16. What are the common causes of cholinergic toxicity?

- Organophosphate insecticides (malathion, parathion, diazinon)
- Carbamate insecticides (aldicarb, carbaryl)
- Carbamate drugs (physostigmine, neostigmine, edrophonium chloride [Tensilon])
- Chemical warfare agents (sarin, soman, VX)

17. What antidotes are used to treat cholinergic toxicity?

The two antidotes used for cholinergic toxicity and cholinergic toxidrome are atropine and pralidoxime (2-PAM). Cholinergic toxicity is caused by an abundance of acetylcholine at the muscarinic and nicotinic receptor sites. Atropine competes with acetylcholine at the receptor sites. Atropine doses are titrated to clear the patient's secretions, specifically pulmonary edema. The atropine endpoint is dry lungs. Pralidoxime reactivates acetylcholinesterase. By pulling the poison from acetylcholinesterase, pralidoxime allows it to metabolize acetylcholine. Reactivation of the acetylcholinesterase decreases the abundance of acetylcholine at both muscarinic and nicotinic receptors.

18. **What signs and symptoms are associated with the opioid syndrome?**

Opioid drugs bind to opiate receptors with various affinities in the brain. The classic opioid syndrome triad includes coma, miosis (pinpoint pupils), and depressed respirations (slow, shallow breathing). Blood pressure and pulse are usually decreased. The skin is dry, and bowel sounds are decreased. Patients may be hypothermic. Common opiates that may cause this toxidrome are morphine, heroin, meperidine, hydromorphone, codeine, oxycodone, hydrocodone, and propoxyphene.

19. **What antidote is used to treat opiate toxicity?**

Naloxone (Narcan) is a specific opiate antagonist. See question 2.

20. **What signs and symptoms are associated with serotonin syndrome?**

Serotonin is a neurotransmitter involved in many central and peripheral nervous system functions. Serotonin syndrome is divided into three categories:
- Altered mental status, including confusion, agitation, seizures, and coma.
- Muscular abnormalities, including shivering, tremor, myoclonus, and rigidity, especially of the lower extremities.
- Autonomic instability, including hyperthermia, hyper- or hypotension, salivation, and diarrhea.

21. **What are some common causes of serotonin syndrome?**

Serotonin syndrome is believed to be caused by use of certain drugs, which decrease serotonin metabolism, increase serotonin release, or inhibit serotonin reuptake. Some drugs causing serotonin syndrome are:
- Monoamine oxidase inhibitors (MAOIs) (phenelzine [Nardil])
- Amphetamines
- Cocaine
- Selective serotonin reuptake inhibitors (SSRIs) (fluoxetine [Prozac], paroxetine [Paxil], sertraline [Zoloft])
- Tricyclic antidepressants (amitriptyline [Elavil], doxepin [Sinequan], imipramine [Tofranil])
- Dextromethorphan
- Meperidine (Demerol)
- Codeine
- Fentanyl

22. **What antidote is used to treat serotonin syndrome?**

There is no specific antidote used to treat serotonin syndrome. Aggressive use of benzodiazepines is important to decrease muscular rigidity, and external cooling may be needed to treat hyperthermia. Serotonin syndrome usually resolves with supportive care. Creatinine kinase (CK) may be markedly elevated so it is a good idea to monitor CK enzyme concentrations.

23. What other antidotes/chelators may be useful during management of toxin toxicity?

Management of toxin toxicity

Toxin	Antidote	Nursing implications
Acetaminophen	N-acetylcysteine (NAC, Mucomyst, Acetadote)	Acetaminophen is metabolized by the liver to a toxic intermediate that binds to cells and causes liver damage. NAC prevents the toxic intermediate from binding to liver cells and increases the body's ability to detoxify the toxic intermediate.
Benzodiazepines	Flumazenil (Romazicon)	Flumazenil is a competitive antagonist at the benzodiazepine receptor site. It may precipitate benzodiazepine withdrawal and seizures in patients addicted to benzodiazepines and should be used with caution in this patient population. It should be avoided in patients with tricyclic antidepressant overdose because of seizure risk.
Calcium channel blockers and beta-adrenergic blockers	Glucagon, calcium	Patients with hypotension and bradycardia that are refractory to standard therapy can be treated with glucagon. Glucagon increases both cardiac contractility and cardiac rate. Calcium is also useful for calcium channel blocker toxicity.
Carbon monoxide	Oxygen	Carbon monoxide decreases oxygen delivery to the tissues. 100% oxygen and hyperbaric oxygen can decrease the half-life of carbon monoxide in the body.
Cyanide	Amyl nitrite pearls, sodium nitrite solution, sodium thiosulfate solution	The cyanide antidote kit has three parts. Amyl nitrite pearls and sodium nitrite cause methemoglobinemia, which pulls cyanide from the cytochrome oxidase and allows aerobic respiration to continue. Sodium thiosulfate increases the body's normal detoxification process for cyanide. Methylene blue (not included in the antidote kit) is then used to manage the methemoglobinemia.
Digoxin	Digibind (Digoxin Immune Fab [Ovine]), DigiFab (Digoxin Immune Fab [Ovine])	Digoxin Immune Fab is an antibody that binds digoxin. The digoxin-antibody complex is excreted via the kidneys.
Hydrofluoric acid	Calcium	The fluoride ion binds calcium and can cause life-threatening hypocalcemia. Topical calcium preparations are useful for topical burns, and systemic calcium is useful for systemic hypocalcemia.

Continued

Management of toxin toxicity—cont'd

Toxin	Antidote	Nursing implications
Iron	Deferoxamine mesylate (Desferal) for injection USP	Deferoxamine is a chelator that binds iron, and the deferoxamine-iron complex is excreted via the kidneys.
Isoniazid	Pyridoxine (vitamin B_6)	Isoniazid can cause seizures. Pyridoxine (vitamin B_6) is used to treat isoniazid-induced seizures.
Lead	DMSA (succimer [Chemet]), BAL, IV calcium disodium EDTA	Asymptomatic patients with elevated lead levels are commonly treated with the oral chelator DMSA. Symptomatic patients with lead toxicity may be treated with intramuscular (IM) BAL and IV calcium disodium EDTA.
Methanol and ethylene glycol	Fomepizole (Antizol) or ethanol	Both methanol and ethylene glycol are metabolized to toxic intermediates by alcohol dehydrogenase. Methanol can cause blindness, and ethylene glycol can cause renal failure. Either fomepizole or ethanol can be used to prevent alcohol dehydrogenase from metabolizing the parent compounds to the toxic intermediates.
Warfarin	Vitamin K_1	Warfarin impairs the body's ability to synthesize the vitamin K–dependent coagulation factors. Patients with bleeding from overanticoagulation may be treated with both plasma and vitamin K_1.

DMSA, dimercaptosuccinic acid; BAL, British antilewisite; EDTA, ethylene diamine tetraacetic acid.

24. A patient's ECG reveals a widened QRS duration of longer than 0.1 seconds, a prominent R wave in aV_r, and a QTc duration of longer than 0.45 seconds. What drugs may account for the ECG abnormalities?

These findings are suggestive of a drug with type 1 arrhythmic sodium channel-blocking effects. Drugs that should be considered include tricyclic antidepressants, certain antihistamines (diphenhydramine), procainamide, quinidine, and disopyramide.

25. Why is sodium bicarbonate used to treat both tricyclic antidepressant toxicity and salicylate (aspirin) toxicity?

Sodium bicarbonate is used to treat both tricyclic antidepressant toxicity and salicylate toxicity, but its mechanism of action is different for each poison. For salicylate toxicity, an IV infusion of sodium bicarbonate is used to alkalinize the urine. Sodium bicarbonate is excreted by the kidneys into the urine. Increasing the urine pH increases the excretion of salicylate, trapping the salicylate ion in the urine. For tricyclic antidepressant toxicity, IV boluses of sodium bicarbonate are used to reverse arrhythmias by reversing sodium channel blockade. Unlike in treatment of salicylates, administration of sodium bicarbonate does not increase excretion of tricyclic antidepressants.

26. What agents may result in toxicity in a small child after ingestion of only one pill or sip?

- Tricyclic antidepressants (cause arrhythmias, hypotension, and seizures)
- Antiarrhythmics (cause arrhythmias, hypotension, and seizures)
- Beta blockers and calcium channel blockers (cause bradycardia and hypotension)
- Opiates (cause central nervous system depression and respiratory depression)
- Lomotil (diphenoxylate + atropine; antidiarrheal that causes central nervous system depression and respiratory depression)
- Methanol (component of windshield washer fluid that causes acidosis and blindness)
- Ethylene glycol (component of antifreeze that causes acidosis and renal failure)
- Ethanol (causes central nervous system depression, hypoglycemia, and respiratory depression)
- Caustics (acids and bases)
- MAOIs (antidepressants that cause seizures and hyperthermia)
- Cyanide (causes cardiovascular instability, metabolic acidosis, and seizures)
- Benzocaine (topical anesthetic that causes seizures and methemoglobinemia)
- Brodifacoum (long-acting anticoagulant rodenticide that causes bleeding)
- Camphor (topical liniment that causes seizures)
- Imidazoline products (tetrahydrozoline, Visine and oxymetazoline [Afrin] eye drops and nasal sprays, which cause central nervous system depression, bradycardia, and hypotension)
- Selenious acid (component of gun-bluing solutions that causes caustic injury)
- Methylsalicylate (highly concentrated salicylate solution that causes salicylate toxicity)
- Hydrocarbons (aspiration causes hydrocarbon pneumonitis)
- Chloroquine, hydroxychloroquine, and quinine (cause arrhythmias and seizures)
- Hydrofluoric acid (component of rust removers or glass etchers that causes hypocalcemia)
- Theophylline (causes tachycardia and seizures)

27. What vital sign changes are associated with ingestions?

- Bradycardia (buspirone, clonidine, digoxin, propranolol, verapamil)
- Hypertension (disulfiram-ethanol interaction, phencyclidine, phenylpropanolamine, theophylline)
- Hypotension (barbiturates, carbamazepine, tetrahydrozoline, verapamil, captopril)
- Hyperthermia (amphetamines, atropine, cocaine, MAOIs, phencyclidine)
- Hypothermia (chloral hydrate, ethanol, narcotics, nutmeg, phenothiazines [haloperidol])
- Respiratory depression (codeine, diazepam, ethanol, meprobamate, morphine)
- Tachycardia (albuterol, levothyroxine, oleander, pseudoephedrine, tricyclic antidepressants)
- Tachypnea (benzocaine, caffeine, hydrogen sulfide gas, salicylates, strychnine)

28. Are urine toxicology screens clinically useful during the management of patients with suspected overdose?

Urine toxicology screens rarely change the management of a patient who presents to the ED with a suspected overdose. They are expensive and time consuming. Because there is no "standard" urine toxicology screen, different healthcare facilities screen for different drugs. Many urine screens test only for drugs of abuse, whereas others are more comprehensive. Even "comprehensive" urine toxicology screens, however, fail to detect many toxins. Reliance on the results of urine toxicology screens has led to morbidity and mortality from both overtreatment and undertreatment. Urine toxicology screens are *not* recommended as part of the management of most patients who present to the ED with a suspected overdose.

29. Why are serum acetaminophen and aspirin levels recommended during the management of suicidal patients who present to the ED with a history of an overdose of unknown medications?

Hundreds of different over-the-counter and prescription medications contain acetaminophen and/or aspirin. Acetaminophen is a common medication ingested by suicidal patients. Each year it is one of the leading causes of poisoning-related deaths in the United States. Within the first 24 hours after acetaminophen ingestion, no signs or symptoms reliably predict which patients will develop hepatic damage. Within the first 24 hours, even patients with normal liver function tests and coagulation studies can develop hepatotoxicity. The serum acetaminophen level is the best way to predict which patients are at risk for acetaminophen toxicity and to determine which patients require treatment with the antidote, N-acetylcysteine. The most reliable way to exclude potential acetaminophen toxicity is to check the serum acetaminophen level. Because aspirin and acetaminophen are often confused by patients and salicylate poisoning poses a serious threat, it is a good idea to always get a salicylate blood level as well.

30. For what toxins are serum levels clinically useful during the management of suspected overdose?

Serum levels may be useful in managing cases of suspected overdose from methanol, ethylene glycol, lithium, salicylate (aspirin), theophylline, digoxin, ethanol, carbon monoxide, acetaminophen, and antiseizure medications such as phenytoin (Dilantin), carbamazepine (Tegretol), valproic acid (Depakote), and phenobarbital.

31. What are the most common ingestions?

According to Watson et al (2004), the top 10 drug and nondrug substances for which patients were treated in a healthcare facility are:
Drugs
- Analgesics: acetaminophen, nonsteroidal antiinflammatory drugs (NSAIDs), salicylates, narcotics
- Anticonvulsants: carbamazepine, phenytoin, valproic acid
- Antidepressants: cyclic antidepressants, lithium, MAOIs, SSRIs, trazodone

- Antihistamines: H2 receptor antagonists, diphenhydramine
- Cardiovascular drugs: angiotensin-converting enzyme (ACE) inhibitors, antiarrhythmics, beta blockers, calcium antagonists
- Cold and cough preparations
- Hormones: thyroid, oral contraceptives, corticosteroids
- Muscle relaxants: carisoprodol, cyclobenzaprine, methocarbamol
- Sedatives, hypnotic drugs: barbiturates, benzodiazepines, over-the-counter sleep aids
- Stimulants and street drugs: amphetamines, cocaine, heroin, lysergic acid diethylamide (LSD), diet aids

Nondrugs

- Alcohols: ethanol, isopropyl, methanol, beverage ethanol
- Chemicals: acetone, acids/alkalis, formaldehyde, phenol, glycols, ketones, methylene chloride
- Cleaning substances: detergents, bleaches, disinfectants, rust removers, laundry products, drain and oven cleaners
- Cosmetics, personal care products: dental, hair, nail, and eye products; bath oils, creams, and lotions; makeup
- Food products, food poisonings
- Foreign bodies: coins, toys, glass, ornaments, thermometers, glow products
- Fumes, gases, vapors: carbon monoxide, methane, chlorine, propane
- Hydrocarbons: benzene, diesel fuel, gasoline, kerosene, turpentine
- Insecticides, pesticides

32. **Should a Poison Control Center be consulted for all cases of suspected poisoning?**

Poison Control Centers typically are consulted by ED staff when assistance is needed in managing a patient with an exposure to an unusual toxin, when patients develop severe toxicity, when antidotes and chelators are used, or when patients have an unusual presentation of a common toxin. ED staff may forgo consulting the Poison Control Center for cases that they are comfortable managing or when patients have only minimal symptoms. The regional Poison Control Center phone number is 800-222-1222.

Although the focus of most interactions between ED staff and a Poison Control Center revolves around individual patient management, Poison Control Centers serve an important public health function. A nurse can assist the public health function of the local Poison Control Center by reporting all cases of suspected poisoning. Data collected by Poison Control Centers are used by regional and national public health officials, including the Food and Drug Administration (FDA), Environmental Protection Agency (EPA), and Centers for Disease Control and Prevention (CDC). Poison Control Centers have been instrumental in improving product safety, detecting incidents of poison-related product tampering, identifying epidemics of contaminated food products, and identifying new patterns of drug and chemical toxicity.

Key Points

- All patients who present with respiratory arrest or apnea should be given 2 mg of naloxone. Some patients may require larger doses, but the initial dose of 2 mg is the same for children and adults.

- The decision to decontaminate a patient's GI tract is complex and must be determined on a case-by-case basis. Several factors, including the patient's status, amount and substance involved, and time since ingestion are considered when developing a treatment plan.

- Urine toxicology screens may fail to detect many toxins; thus the term "negative drug screen" could be misleading. Urine toxicology screens rarely change the management and are not recommended in the management of a patient who presents to the ED with a suspected overdose.

- Routine use of syrup of ipecac as an emetic is no longer recommended or advised in either the home setting or the ED. There is no evidence that use of ipecac syrup improves patient outcome, and it may delay administration of charcoal, antidotes, and other drugs.

- Acetaminophen and aspirin are commonly ingested by suicidal patients. Although aspirin poisoned patients may develop acidosis, which offers a diagnostic clue, an aspirin level is still recommended. Patients with acetaminophen ingestions often take more than 24 hours to show signs or symptoms that predict hepatotoxicity. The most reliable way to exclude potential acetaminophen toxicity is to check the serum acetaminophen level.

 Internet References

American Academy of Clinical Toxicology, Position Statements:
www.clintox.org/Pos_Statements/Intro.html

American Association of Poison Control Centers:
www.aapcc.org

American College of Medical Toxicology:
www.acmt.net

Centers for Disease Control and Prevention, National Center for Injury Prevention and Control, Poisonings: Fact Sheet:
www.cdc.gov/ncipc/factsheets/poisoning.htm

European Association of Poison Centres and Clinical Toxicologists:
www.eapcct.org

Internet Journal of Medical Toxicology:
www.ijmt.net

Poison Prevention:
www.poisonprevention.org

Bibliography

American Academy of Clinical Toxicology, European Association of Poisons Centres and Clinical Toxicologists: Position paper: Gastric lavage, *J Toxicol Clin Toxicol* 42:933-943, 2004.

American Academy of Clinical Toxicology, European Association of Poisons Centres and Clinical Toxicologists: Position paper: Whole bowel irrigation, *J Toxicol Clin Toxicol* 42:843-854, 2004.

Bartlett D: The coma cocktail: Indications, contraindications, adverse effects, proper dose, and proper route, *J Emerg Nurs* 30:572-574, 2004.

Belson MG et al: The utility of toxicologic analysis in children with suspected ingestions, *Pediatr Emerg Care* 15:383-387, 1999.

Bledsoe BE: No more coma cocktails. Using science to dispel myths & improve patient care, *JEMS* 27:54-60, 2002.

Chyka PA et al; American Academy of Clinical Toxicology; European Association of Poisons Centres and Clinical Toxicologists: Position paper: Single-dose activated charcoal, *Clin Toxicol (Phila)* 43:61-84, 2005.

Committee on Poison Prevention and Control; Board on Health Promotion and Disease Prevention; Institute of Medicine of the National Academies: *Forging a poison prevention and control system,* Washington, DC, 2004, The National Academies Press.

Emery D et al: Highly toxic ingestions for toddlers: When a pill can kill, *Pediatr Emerg Med Rep* 3:111-122, 1998.

Goldfrank LR: Principles of managing the poisoned or overdosed patient: An overview. In Goldfrank LR et al, editors: *Goldfrank's toxicologic emergencies,* ed 7, New York, 2002, McGraw-Hill.

Keim ME, Pesik N, Twum-Danso NA: Lack of hospital preparedness for chemical terrorism in a major US city: 1996-2000, *Prehospital Disaster Med* 18:193-199, 2003.

Keyes DC, Dart RC: Initial management of the poisoned patient. In Dart RC, editor: *Medical toxicology,* ed 3, Philadelphia, 2004, Lippincott Williams & Wilkins.

Manoguerra AS, Cobaugh DJ: Guidelines for the management of poisoning consensus panel. Guideline on the use of ipecac syrup in the out-of-hospital management of ingested poisons, *Clin Toxicol (Phila)* 43:1-10, 2005.

Mokhlesi B et al: Adult toxicology in critical care: Part I: General approach to the intoxicated patient, *Chest* 123:577-592, 2003.

Mokhlesi B et al: Adult toxicology in critical care: Part II: Specific poisonings, *Chest* 123:577-592, 2003.

Watson WA et al: 2003 annual report of the American Association of Poison Control Centers toxic exposure surveillance system, *Am J Emerg Med* 22:377-392, 2004.

Yip L: Salicylates. In Dart RC, editor: *Medical toxicology,* ed 3, Philadelphia, 2004, Lippincott Williams & Wilkins.

Psychiatric Emergencies

Bari K. Platter and Anne M. Felton

1. What constitutes a psychiatric emergency?

The American Psychiatric Association (APA) defines psychiatric emergency as an acute disturbance in mood, thought, behavior, or social relationship that requires immediate intervention and treatment. The patient is unable to cope with the current situation and has not been able to mobilize sufficient resources to provide support. Changes in mental status, severe impairment in general functioning, and determination of grave disability all constitute a psychiatric emergency.

2. Why are psychiatric emergencies so prevalent in the emergency department (ED)?

For many patients, the ED is often the entry point into the mental health system. Nationally, access to mental health services has been a growing problem. Community mental health centers have become more restrictive regarding their ability to provide care for their chronically mentally ill patients. This restriction in care has forced patients to access EDs for their mental healthcare. According to the Centers for Disease Control and Prevention (CDC; www.cdc.gov/nchs/data/hus/hus04.pdf), over the past decade psychiatric hospitals have decreased inpatient census by 31%, thus significantly increasing the length of time psychiatric patients must remain in the ED before placement.

3. What are the most common psychiatric emergencies?

Common psychiatric emergencies include suicidal ideation and attempts, acute psychosis, substance abuse, significant behavioral disturbance, and other acute mental status changes. Although there are often precipitating factors, a psychiatric emergency may occur at any time.

4. What other psychiatric presentations are likely to be seen in the ED?

In addition to the previously mentioned psychiatric emergencies, common psychiatric presentations can include or be associated with the following:
- Depression
- Mania
- Anxiety/panic attack
- Grief
- Domestic violence
- Sexual assault

- Homelessness
- Eating disorders
- Victims of disaster

It is important to be aware of common psychiatric presentations. A patient may present to the ED with a sense of urgency, having one or more of these complaints. Without proper identification and intervention, an urgent presentation may quickly escalate into a psychiatric emergency.

5. What is the difference between an urgent psychiatric presentation and a psychiatric emergency?

The possible outcome of a patient's presentation to the ED is what differentiates an urgent presentation from a psychiatric emergency.

Psychiatric emergency versus urgent psychiatric presentation

Case Example A: Psychiatric Emergency

A 22-year-old man is brought to the ED by ambulance following a 911 call by family after discovering the patient with a suicide note and loaded handgun. The family is distraught and tells you that the patient has become more withdrawn lately and has been talking to himself at times. This patient is clearly presenting with a psychiatric emergency. The patient requires immediate intervention secondary to imminent risk to self. His presentation indicates possible alteration in both mood and thought.

Case Example B: Urgent Psychiatric Presentation

A 58-year-old woman presents to the ED with her 35-year-old daughter. The woman is complaining of depression and later tells you that she has been feeling very lonely, hopeless, and anxious about having to go to work in the mornings. You learn that her husband of 26 years died several years ago. The patient denies being suicidal, yet admits to daily thoughts of wanting to see her husband again. This is an urgent presentation that requires intervention. The patient is not imminently dangerous to herself, but without intervention, the situation could easily escalate.

The goals of ED care in these two cases are very different. The first case would require psychiatric hospitalization, whereas the patient in the second case demonstrates the cognitive ability and problem-solving skills to mobilize her resources and to be discharged with plans to establish appropriate outpatient care and treatment.

6. What information is important to know about ED patients with psychiatric emergencies?

Patients who are experiencing psychiatric emergencies often lack the resources and insight to address their current stressors. Internal resources, such as cognitive and intellectual ability, organizational skills, interpersonal skills, and problem-solving skills, can be impaired secondary to increased levels of stress and symptoms related to psychiatric illness. External resources, such as friends, family, and other caregivers, may not be available to assist the patient in coping with the current stressors. Many chronically mentally ill patients have "burned their bridges" with friends and family and cannot count on them during an emergency.

Patients often present with irritability, hostility, and provocative behavior. This behavior is directly related to both the level of stress and the presence of severe psychiatric symptoms.

7. **Which patients require hospitalization?**

Assessment for hospitalization includes consideration of several factors. The most important determinant for hospitalization is the patient's ability to maintain safety in the community. This includes assessment of the dangerousness to self and/or others and of grave disability (inability to attend to one's daily needs).

The assessment to determine if the patient requires hospitalization includes the following:
- History of present complaint with complete psychiatric history
- Formal mental status exam
- Assessment of medical co-morbidity, including acute and chronic medical conditions
- Evaluation of the patient's internal and external resources

This information, along with expert consultation, is summarized to formulate a complete picture of the need for hospitalization.

8. **How prevalent are suicides and suicide attempts in the United States?**

Suicidal behavior is evident in at least 30% of patients presenting in emergency psychiatric services. Fourteen percent of the American population report having suicidal ideation at least once in their lives. Four percent of Americans have had a plan to commit suicide, and 4.6% have made an attempt. Suicide is the eighth leading cause of death in the United States. Every year, more than 30,000 people take their own lives. Every day, approximately 86 people commit suicide and over 1000 people make a suicide attempt.

9. **What are the common demographical risk factors for suicide?**

- **Race.** Caucasians complete suicide twice as frequently as African Americans and Hispanics. The suicide rate of Native Americans is 1.7 times higher than Caucasians.
- **Age.** Caucasians age 75 to 84 complete suicide twice as often as those age 15 to 24. With African Americans, men age 25 to 34 are most likely to kill themselves.
- **Gender.** Women make 60% to 70% of suicide *attempts*, but men are more likely to *complete* suicide.
- **Marital status.** Married people are least likely to attempt or complete suicide. Single people are more likely to complete suicide, and divorced or widowed people have the highest rate of completed suicides.

10. **What are other important risk factors for suicide?**

- *History of previous suicidal ideation and suicide attempts.* Patients who have had a history of previous suicidal ideation and attempt are at higher risk for completing suicide.
- *Sexual orientation.* Homosexual or bisexual adolescents are at particularly high risk for suicide attempt and completed suicide.
- *History of violence.* If the patient has a history of violent behavior, the risk for suicide is increased. Violent behavior within 1 year of an ED presentation is a significant predictor of suicide.

- *Medical illness.* Patients with chronic medical illness and/or chronic pain are at an increased risk for suicide attempts and completed suicide. There is not a clear relationship between terminal illness and suicide; less than 1% of cancer patients commit suicide, and of those, 30% are considered to be terminal.
- *Anxiety.* Anxiety and anxiety-related symptoms (insomnia, decreased concentration, and panic attacks) are strong predictors of suicide.
- *Hopelessness and life satisfaction.* Men who are dissatisfied with their lives are more than 25 times as likely to complete suicide as men who are satisfied with their lives.
- *Intoxication.* Patients with alcoholism are likely to verbalize feelings of hopelessness and are generally more challenging to treat in the ED setting. They are also more likely to commit suicide late in the course of their illness.

11. **What is the best way to intervene with a suicidal patient?**

Safety is the most important consideration when working with a suicidal patient. Suicidal patients should never be left alone during an ED visit. If a family member is unable to stay with the patient, the nurse will need to delegate the responsibility to another available staff person. Ensure that any dangerous items are removed from the patient and placed in a safe location. It is generally advisable to have the patient change into a hospital gown upon admission to the ED. This allows the nurse to be sure that all potentially dangerous items such as pills or razors are removed. The patient is also less likely to elope when wearing a hospital gown.

Many suicidal patients feel uncomfortable with the perceived intrusive treatment in the ED. It is helpful to approach them in a calm, hopeful, and reassuring manner. Provide empathy, assuring the patient that measures taken in the ED provide them with the best possible care. It is sometimes helpful to let patients know that changing into a gown and having someone watch them and accompanying them to the bathroom are hospital policies that are required to be followed for all patients with possible threats of suicide. Patients often feel targeted when placed on suicide precautions. Explaining hospital policy decreases the likelihood of the patient acting out.

Suicide contracts or "No Harm Contracts" should not be used in the ED. The basis of a suicide contract is that the patient agrees not to harm himself based upon his relationship with the healthcare provider. This is an impractical arrangement in the ED, given that the patient has known the provider for a very brief period of time.

12. **What is the best way to assess for suicidality (or suicide intent)?**

All patients with a psychiatric presentation should have an assessment to determine their level of suicide risk. The following questions will help the emergency nurse assess suicide risk:
- What were the patient's previous suicide attempts and their level of lethality? Did the patient require medical admission?
- How withdrawn or hopeless does the patient appear?
- Is the patient isolated in his or her social environment?
- Does the patient have a current plan for suicide with the means to complete this plan?

A simple risk assessment will help ensure that all patients with psychiatric complaints receive the appropriate level of care.

13. How does one evaluate the acutely psychotic patient?

The patient experiencing acute psychosis, or altered mental status, is generally a poor historian. The patient is usually brought to the ED by a friend, family member, or support system. In these cases, it is essential to utilize these third parties to gather as much clear and concise history as possible. The third party should be encouraged to give information about the patient's behavior for the past several weeks. Careful observation of the patient's presentation, including appearance, willingness to make eye contact, activity level, and unusual behavior and movements, should be considered and carefully documented. It is also important to obtain a medication history, including the medications the patient is currently prescribed and those the patient may have abused. This history, combined with laboratory findings and medical examination, will help differentiate a medical emergency such as delirium from a functional organic state.

14. What is the difference between functional psychosis and organic psychosis?

Psychosis implies an impaired sense of reality. The signs of loss of reality include deterioration in the patient's thought content, perceptions, and communication skills. Functional psychoses, also referred to as primary psychoses, are disorders resulting completely from psychiatric illness, such as schizophrenia. Although once common, organic psychosis is no longer a term favored by most clinicians. Instead, the terms secondary psychosis, delirium, acute confusion, or altered mental status are preferred. It is important to know that these terms are often used interchangeably. Organicity is generally considered more of a descriptive term relating symptoms to a condition, rather than an adequate term for the specific disease process. In these cases, the psychotic symptomatology is different in character from that of a primary psychosis, and it results from an underlying medical or neurological disease process.

Symptoms associated with primary and secondary psychosis

Primary Psychosis
Fixed and complex delusional system
Auditory hallucinations
No alteration in alertness
Age onset in early 20s

Secondary Psychosis
Illusions
Visual hallucinations
Alteration in consciousness
Abrupt onset
Age onset after age 40

15. Why is it important to treat acute psychosis promptly?

Acute psychosis is a syndrome found in a number of psychiatric and medical conditions. It is distressing to the patient and family, friends, or support system.
   Symptoms of acute psychosis include:
- Hallucinations/perceptual disturbances
- Delusions
- Behavioral disturbances, including aggression and irritability
- Anxiety
   Patients experiencing these symptoms can quickly escalate and become difficult to manage in the ED setting. Prompt care ensures safety and provides for the relief of painful symptoms.

16. What is the goal of treatment for patients with acute psychosis?

There are two immediate and crucial objectives when treating acute psychosis in the ED. These goals are the reduction of distressing symptoms and the determination of etiology so that appropriate care and treatment are initiated. Agitation and violence are complications to be aware of with acute psychosis and altered mental status. Sedation may be therapeutic but should be used with caution because it may further impair cognition in patients predisposed to delirium and dementia.

17. What is the best way to intervene with a psychotic patient?

- Use clear, direct statements when talking with the patient.
- Make sure that your body language is congruent with what you are saying.
- Accept and validate feelings and expressions of emotion.
- Move the patient to a quiet area of the ED to decrease external stimulation.
- Reassure the patient that he or she will be safe in this environment; instruct him or her about how to contact you for assistance if necessary.
- Consider increased monitoring of the patient, using audio-visual monitoring if available.
- Offer food and fluids that are wrapped or in closed containers.
- Reorient the patient as needed.

18. What is delirium? Why is it a medical emergency?

Delirium is an acute state of altered mental status characterized by rapid onset, altered consciousness, disorientation, and a fluctuating course. Delirium is "organic," the result of an acute medical condition. It is an emergency condition that is often misdiagnosed and referred for psychiatric treatment based on the presenting "psychotic" symptoms. The following are clues that the patient is suffering from delirium rather than psychosis as a result of psychiatric illness:
- The patient's confusion and disorientation tends to change throughout the day, with periods of lucidity.
- The patient may experience *illusions*, which are misperceptions of reality, rather than *hallucinations*, which are typically not reality based.
- The patient is more likely to exhibit extreme emotional lability.
- The patient may have agitation lapsing to somnolence.
- The patient demonstrates disorganized speech or difficulty with word finding.

Compared with other patient groups, patients with delirium have very poor outcomes. Delirium is generally considered to be a reversible condition; however, recent studies have shown delirium to have a more persistent state, especially when mismanaged. With timely discovery of the primary etiology there is the best chance of complete reversal. The longer a patient suffers with delirium, the greater the likelihood of negative consequences and continued permanent mental status changes. Do not make the mistake of assuming that every patient presenting to the ED with "psychotic" symptoms, especially older adults, has a psychiatric illness.

19. What are common precipitants to delirium?

These common conditions can be linked to delirium:
- Infection
- Metabolic imbalance
- Fluid or electrolyte imbalance
- Hypoxia
- Cerebrovascular event
- Seizures
- Hypoglycemia

Medications, toxins, impaired nutritional status, and use of illicit substances have also been found to be precipitants to delirium.

20. How should a delirious patient be interviewed?

The evaluation of a patient with delirium is much the same as that of any patient experiencing altered mental status or acute psychosis. If a patient is suspected to be suffering from delirium, it is crucial to assist the patient to remain calm and comfortable while attempting to uncover the root cause for the delirium. Reassure and reorient the patient as needed while using brief questions to assess the level of consciousness, orientation, and memory. Attempt to obtain accurate information about the patient's baseline mental status and functioning. It is more important for the patient to remain calm than to provide answers to the questions. The patient's behavior may escalate if confronted with the fact that his or her mental status is unstable. Instead, utilize family and outside caregivers as much as possible to provide a history.

21. How is delirium managed?

Identification of the underlying medical condition is critical. Monitor vital signs and anticipate the following laboratory tests:
- Urinalysis
- Complete blood count (CBC) with differential
- Toxicology screens
- Electrocardiogram (ECG)
- Thyroid function tests
- Chest films
- Computed tomography (CT) scan of the head

The combination of subclinical findings, such as mild dehydration, minor urinary tract infection (UTI), and decreased sleep, can easily cause delirium in compromised patient groups. Common groups include the elderly, patients with dementia, and those with chronic mental illness. This is an area in which the nurse may take a more active role in decreasing the risk of morbidity and mortality in these patients; 15% to 30% of older adults diagnosed with delirium die.

Maintain a safe environment by recognizing the following:

- *The patient with delirium should never be left alone.* Families are important members of the healthcare team and can play a vital role in ensuring the patient's well-being. Although the role of the family is often under utilized, do not overlook the family's need for reassurance and education.
- *Agitation is commonly seen in patients with delirium.* The use of benzodiazepines for sedation and physical restraint has been shown to further impair cognitive status and increase risk for negative outcomes. They should be used as a last resort when reassurance, reorientation, and other comfort measures have failed.

22. What is the difference between delirium and dementia?

Dementia is similar to delirium in that it affects mental functioning, primarily that of memory and other cognitive abilities. Dementia is gradual and relatively stable over the course of several months compared with delirium, which is an acute change in mental status. Although many of the presenting symptoms of delirium and dementia may be consistent with one another, patients with delirium usually have impaired levels of consciousness or alertness. Although a patient with dementia may experience "sun-downing," or increased confusion in the early evening, this is a predictable and stable pattern. With delirium, the patient's impairment is not predictable or stable and has developed over a short period of time. Patients with dementia are at increased risk for delirium. It is therefore important for the nurse to note chronic cognitive deficits and acute mental status changes.

23. How are acute psychosis and delirium pharmacologically managed in the ED?

When medicating a patient suffering with acute psychosis, there are several factors to consider:

- Is the psychosis primary or secondary?
- What is the patient's known history with emergency medications?
- Will the patient be able to tolerate taking medications orally?
- What are the target symptoms?

Agitation is often the target symptom requiring the use of medications in the ED. Based on the patient's underlying complaint and presentation, pharmacological management of agitation differs from patient to patient.

When a patient presents with psychotic agitation and has a history of primary psychiatric illness, first offer oral medications that have been therapeutic in the past. Benzodiazepines, such as lorazepam, remain the first-line medication of choice for acute agitation when intramuscular (IM) medication is needed and delirium is not suspected. Haloperidol and lorazepam are commonly used in combination in the ED. Psychiatric experts currently suggest that neuroleptic medications have a more therapeutic effect and decreased side effects when administered either orally or intravenously after administration of benzodiazepines.

Current literature regarding pharmacological management of delirium varies widely. Experts agree that the following approaches can be helpful:

- Avoid use of benzodiazepines.
- Avoid use of anticholingeric medications.
- Treat specific symptoms as they arise.
- Consider use of sedating oral medications, such as risperidone or olanzapine.

24. What is lethal catatonia?

Lethal catatonia is a rare and serious syndrome seen primarily in patients with schizophrenia. Signs and symptoms include rigidity of the musculature and stupor alternating with periods of hyperactivity. As this syndrome progresses, symptoms can include mutism, refusal of food and fluids, fever, hypotension, diaphoresis, convulsions, delirium, coma, and even death.

25. What is neuroleptic malignant syndrome (NMS)?

NMS is a rare but life-threatening reaction to neuroleptic medications. Both high- and low- potency, as well as traditional and new-generation neuroleptics have been implicated in the development of NMS. However, haloperidol and fluphenazine HCL (both high-potency traditional neuroleptics) are the agents most frequently associated with NMS. Other drugs commonly used in the ED, such as proclorperazine and promethazine, may precipitate the syndrome as well. The occurrence of NMS is not highly correlated with dosage and is considered idiosyncratic rather than a toxic reaction to these medications. The onset of symptoms can develop within hours of initiation of medication therapy; however, the average onset is 4 to 5 days after beginning therapy. Of patients who develop NMS, 90% do so within 10 days. Initial symptoms include:

- Rapid onset of severe muscular rigidity (lead pipe) with akinesia
- Hyperthermia
- Elevated creatine phosphokinase (CPK)
- Change in mental status, including level of consciousness
- Tachycardia
- Increase in diastolic blood pressure
- Diaphoresis
- Tachypnea
- Drooling
- Tremor
- Incontinence

After an episode of NMS, the patient must be told that he or she is at risk for recurrence if rechallenged with any neuroleptic medication.

26. How is NMS treated?

Early recognition of NMS is critical. Neuroleptic medications should be discontinued immediately when NMS is first suspected. Initial treatment interventions include restoring electrolyte disturbances with adequate fluid intake and providing supportive measures to lower body temperature. The patient should be monitored closely for signs of possible respiratory failure as a result of muscle rigidity and an inability to swallow.

Severe cases of NMS may require pharmacological intervention. Bromocriptine, amantadine, and dantrolene are commonly used to decrease muscle rigidity and restore normal body temperature. Benzodiazepines are often used to control agitation.

27. What psychiatric emergencies are caused by drug toxicity and/or drug withdrawal?

Drug toxicity and drug withdrawal states are commonly seen as psychiatric emergencies and often are a source of confusion in evaluating patients. Nearly all drugs can cause alterations of mood, thoughts, and behavior when taken in excess or when taken by individuals predisposed to idiosyncratic responses because of concurrent illness, psychological makeup, or ingestion of other drugs. Psychiatric symptoms are, in some instances, the first and only symptoms of potentially lethal toxicity.

28. What drugs cause psychiatric symptoms at toxic levels?

Many common medications can become toxic and produce psychiatric symptoms even when taken as ordered. Examples include:
- **Digitalis** toxicity is relatively common. Symptoms include incoherent thinking, hallucinations, delusional thoughts, irritability, distractibility, labile mood, illusions, and disorientation. Symptoms present in a differential include anorexia, nausea, blurred vision, and chromatopsia (appearance of yellow-green tint to objects).
- **Steroids** (e.g., prednisone) may cause mania, depression, psychosis, delirium, and dementia.
- **Levodopa and amantadine (Symmetrel)**, used in the treatment of Parkinson's disease, have been associated with psychiatric symptoms. Levodopa toxicity can cause mania, depression, delirium, and psychosis. Delirium has been associated with amantadine use.

29. What factors can be used to predict violent behavior?

Violence is an unpredictable act; even after thorough assessment and intervention, patients may exhibit dangerous violent behavior in the ED. With careful observation, planning, and intervention, nurses can decrease the likelihood of patients acting out in a violent manner.

Perception, judgment, mood, inhibition, and cognition are all involved in planning and executing a violent act. Any or all of these functions can be impaired or intensified by psychiatric symptoms. Patients have been found to be more likely to act upon violent ideation when the following is present:
- Alcohol and/or substance impairment
- Psychosis
- Mania
- Dementia

- Temporal lobe epilepsy (TLE)
- Head trauma
  The nurse should be aware of behaviors that are often present before a violent act:
- Agitation
- Pacing
- Inability to follow direction
- Pressured speech
- Threats of violence
- Menacing and threatening stance

30. **What steps should be taken when it is suspected that a patient has the potential for violence?**

Successfully managing psychiatric patients who present to the ED with agitation and aggression can be quite challenging. A violence risk assessment should be completed with every psychiatric patient in the ED. The following data is collected and considered in a violence risk assessment:

- *Relevant demographical data:* Patients with the highest potential for violence include men, youth age 15 to 24, and those with lower socioeconomic status.
- *Current functional symptoms* versus organic symptoms.
- *Historical findings:* Patients with a history of violent behavior and/or severe and persistent mental illness are more likely to become violent. Antisocial personality disorder and substance abuse are also strong predictors of violent behavior.
- *Environmental factors:* Patients who live in poverty-stricken neighborhoods are more likely to exhibit violent behavior. Mentally ill patients are more likely to become violent toward people with whom they are familiar.

Findings from this assessment guide the clinician in decision making regarding management in the ED and appropriate disposition. Violence develops along a behavioral continuum. In the first level, the patient exhibits signs of anxiety. The most effective approach is to provide support and empathy. Avoid either being judgmental and/or dismissing the patient as a complainer. Listen to the patient's concerns and move the patient to a quieter area of the ED. If the patient's behavior continues to escalate, the next step is to provide a directive approach. This includes explaining behavioral expectations and setting limits on inappropriate behavior. Limits must be clear, simple, and enforceable. If these measures are not success-ful, the staff must intervene to create a safe environment. Interventions include providing a "show of force" (a group of staff approach the patient together to give a message about behavior expectations) and involvement of security officers to give additional verbal direction to the patient. Mechanical restraint should be used only as a last resort when the patient is imminently dangerous to self or others and is unable to maintain physical control.

31. **What do nurses need to know about mechanical restraint use?**

Lower-level interventions should always be attempted to prevent restraint use and to respect patient rights. When all options fail, restraints may need to be applied to keep the patient and staff safe. EDs must follow state and federal regulations regarding the use of restraint. It is important to remember that regulations vary from state to state. Verbal and/or written restraint education should be provided to the patient and family as appropriate. The family should be notified of the restraint as soon as possible. Federal regulations require obtaining an order to apply a restraint. For a nurse to be able to apply restraints, the nurse's employee record must reflect that he or she has demonstrated competency to do so. Remember the following guidelines:

- Do not apply restraints alone. Have at least one other person to ensure patient and staff safety.
- The restraint must be fixed to the immovable frame of the bed.
- If using a nonlocking restraint, use a slip knot for immediate and quick release.
- Ensure the restraint is not applied too tightly by inserting one to two fingers between the restraint and patient's skin.
- Check body alignment after applying the restraint and adjust as needed.
- Perform and document one-to-one or intermittent observations as required by the institutional policy and state or federal regulations.
- Assess range of motion at least every 2 hours. Follow state regulations if required more frequently.
- When applying two-point restraints, use only opposite limbs so the patient cannot flip out of the stretcher.
- Offer frequent toileting, food, and fluids, at least every 2 hours.
- When providing in-person observation, sit within an arm's length of the patient. Do not read, watch TV, or verbally interact with others while providing one-on-one observation.

32. **What should the nurse know about psychiatric emergencies with children and adolescents?**

Psychiatric emergencies with children and adolescents are most often disturbances in behavior, thought, or mood defined by the parents, primary caregivers, or the community as requiring immediate intervention and treatment. Children and adolescents lack insight, judgment, and cognitive process necessary to mobilize adequate problem-solving skills. It is most often a behavior or traumatic event that brings a child or adolescent to the ED for evaluation.

33. **What is the best way to manage the child or adolescent with a psychiatric emergency?**

Violent behavior is the most common predictor for psychiatric-related ED visits in children and adolescents. In many of these cases, the parents, school, foster home, or community placement has not been able to appropriately manage the patient's behavior, and the ED becomes the reasonable safe haven. Approximately 4 million (1 in 10) children have functional impairment as a result of psychiatric illness, yet only 20% will receive appropriate treatment.

Safety is the primary goal in the ED. Most children are able to calm themselves and do not require emergency sedation or physical restraints. The nurse should assess whether the presence of the family and/or caregivers is beneficial to the patient. If behavior escalates when the family and/or caregivers are present, the nurse should consider separating the patient from the family. The patient should never be left alone in the ED; the nurse should designate a staff person to remain with the patient.

Because children and adolescents lack the internal resources found in adults, disposition should focus on the ability of the child's support system to provide a safe environment after the patient has been discharged from the ED. Suicidal ideation and violent behavior are often not thoroughly assessed in the ED; it is crucial for the nurse to ensure that the patient has been connected with follow-up care before discharge if the patient is not admitted to the hospital.

 Key Points

- Psychiatric emergencies can occur at any time and are increasingly prevalent in EDs.
- Suicide contracts should not be used in the ED setting.
- Do not assume that symptoms of psychosis are related to a psychiatric illness; instead assess for the presence of delirium before referring the patient for psychiatric consultation.
- Dementia is gradual and relatively stable over the course of several months compared with delirium, which is an acute change in mental status.
- Less restrictive interventions should always be attempted to prevent restraint use and to respect patient rights. When all options fail, restraints may need to be applied to keep the patient and staff safe.
- When working with children and adolescents, the nurse should assess whether the presence of the family and/or caregivers is beneficial to the patient. If behavior escalates when the family and/or caregivers are present, the nurse should consider separating the patient from the family.
- Any drug can be taken as a lethal overdose. Don't assume that high-risk drugs are the only drugs used in purposeful or accidental overdoses.

 Internet References

Centers for Disease Control and Prevention, *Health, United States, 2004: With Chartbook on Trends in the Health of Americans* (pdf document, Adobe Acrobat Reader software required): www.cdc.gov/nchs/data/hus/hus04.pdf

National Alliance on Mental Illness:
www.nami.org

National Institute of Mental Health:
www.nimh.nih.gov

United States Department of Health and Human Services, Substance Abuse & Mental Health Services Administration:
www.samhsa.gov

Bibliography

Allen MH, editor: *Emergency psychiatry: Review of psychiatry,* vol 21, Washington, DC, 2002, American Psychiatric Publishing.

Allen MH et al: Treatment of behavioral emergencies: A summary of the expert consensus guidelines, *J Psychiatr Pract* 9:16, 2003.

Anderson DA, Filley CM: Behavioral presentations of medical and neurologic disorders. In Jacobson AM, editor: *Psychiatric secrets,* ed 2, Philadelphia, 2001, Hanley & Belfus.

Antai-Otong D: Managing geriatric psychiatric emergencies: Delirium and dementia, *Nurs Clin North Am* 38:123, 2003.

Centers for Disease Control and Prevention, *Health, United States, 2004: With Chartbook on Trends in the Health of Americans* (pdf document, Adobe Acrobat Reader software required):

Citrome L: Atypical antipsychotics for acute agitation, *Postgrad Med* 122:85, 2002.

Dulcan MK, Martini DR, Lake M: Special clinical circumstances. In Hales RE, editor: *Child and adolescent psychiatry,* ed 3, Washington, DC, 2003, American Psychiatric Publishing.

Edelsohn G et al: Predictors of urgency in a pediatric psychiatric emergency service, *J Am Acad Child Adolesc Psychiatry* 42:1197, 2003.

Ewing JD, Rund DA, Votolato NA: Evaluating the reconstitution of intramuscular ziprasidone (Geodon) into solution, *Ann Emerg Med* 43:419, 2004.

Jensen LA: Managing acute psychotic disorder in an emergency department, *Nurs Clin North Am* 38:45, 2003.

Kimball R, Baldwin N: Psychiatric emergencies. In Oman K, Koziol-McLain J, Scheetz L, editors: *Emergency nursing secrets,* Philadelphia, 2001, Hanley & Belfus.

Kobayashi JS: Delirium. In Jacobson AM, editor: *Psychiatric secrets,* ed 2, Philadelphia, 2001, Hanley & Belfus.

Menninger JA: Involuntary treatment: Hospitalization and medications. In Jacobson AM, editor: *Psychiatric secrets,* ed 2, Philadelphia, 2001, Hanley & Belfus.

Richardson R: Dementia. In Jacobson AM, editor: *Psychiatric secrets,* ed 2, Philadelphia, 2001, Hanley & Belfus.

Chapter 20

Endocrine Emergencies

Ivy F. Shaffer

1. What is an endocrine emergency?

Endocrine emergencies arise as a result of either overproduction or underproduction of hormones responsible for the humoral homeostasis within the body. Additionally, concurrent disease, endocrine tumors, and pathological responses to hormones may also contribute to endocrine dysfunction.

The endocrine system consists of specific glands that respond to a complex feedback system mediated by the central nervous system, precursors to hormones, the target organ, and/or circadian rhythm. Additional factors such as stress, depression, blood pressure, levels of circulating glucose, calcium, and other chemicals are also responsible for synthesis, release, or inhibition of hormones.

The endocrine system plays a key role in physiological homeostasis. Symptomatology can be subtle to severe; therefore, focusing on the patient's history and reason for seeking care will lead to successful recognition and treatment of these medical emergencies.

2. What are frequent causes of diabetic ketoacidosis (DKA)?

DKA can be a result of new onset diabetes (especially in infants and children younger than 5 years of age), uncontrolled diabetes mellitus, refractory vomiting, diarrhea, complications from pregnancy, infections in any person with known diabetic disease, inadvertent omission of insulin, acute myocardial infraction (MI) or cerebrovascular accident (CVA), alcohol, sepsis, pancreatitis, prescribed medications (steroids, thiazides, Dilantin, Dobutamine, calcium channel blockers), anorexia, or trauma.

3. How does DKA become a life-threatening emergency?

Without circulating insulin required for cellular metabolism of glucose, the body and vital organs cannot use glucose for energy. Blood glucose levels begin to rise, causing an increase in serum osmolarity. This hyperosmolar state leads to profound diuresis. As diuresis progresses, hypovolemic shock will ensue if not treated. Simultaneous breakdown and oxidation of fatty acids produce ketones, the adjunct energy source that ultimately leads to metabolic acidosis, hypokalemia, and hyperketonemia.

Potassium, usually an intracellular ion, shifts out of the cell, replacing hydrogen to initially compensate for the metabolic acidosis. Therefore initial laboratory tests will reveal a potassium level greater than 5.5 mEq/L. However, it is imperative to remember that as acidosis is corrected, potassium will shift back into the cell, producing hypokalemia. The combination of hypovolemia, acidosis, and electrolyte imbalances will rapidly progress to hypovolemic shock, leading to coma and cardiac and respiratory collapse if left untreated.

4. When should the nurse suspect DKA?

In most cases, patients with a known history of Type I diabetes will report that their blood sugars have been "high" with generalized malaise, polydypsia, and polyuria. Triage vital signs may reveal marked tachycardia, tachypnea, hypothermia, and borderline hypotension (as patients continue to compensate). Patients may also report feeling dizzy, short of breath, and nauseated with mild, diffuse abdominal pain. Objectively they appear pale, cool, dry, distressed, and have a fruity odor of ketones on their breath. Bedside glucose monitoring may indicate glucose levels above 600; however, it is extremely important to note that patients may have DKA with blood glucose levels as low as 250 mg/dl. The metabolic course of DKA is unique to each patient. Therefore the consummate diagnosis is based on laboratory tests that reveal the presence of serum/urine ketones, acidosis, and hyperglycemia.

The following diagnostic lab results are criteria set by the American Diabetes Association (ADA) in assisting the clinician in differentiating DKA from other acidotic conditions:

- Blood sugar greater than 250 mg/dl
- pH less than 7.3
- Bicarbonate less than 15 mEq/L
- Serum osmolality greater than 320 mOsm/kg H_2O

Patients with DKA may present with mild hyperventilation or with Kussmaul's (fast and deep) respirations. Mental status changes may also be reported as patients become volume depleted and acidotic.

Infants and children presenting to the emergency department (ED) in DKA tend to be acutely challenging. Some may present with typical complaints of polydypsia, polyuria, and vomiting and may have new onset diabetes. Be aware, however, that volume depletion caused by osmolar diuresis can progress rapidly. Children can present with altered sensorium to coma, a primary complication of resulting hyperosmolarity (serum osmolarity greater than 320 mOsm/L). Laboratory tests will reveal hyperglycemia (blood sugars greater than 200 mg/dl), hyponatremia, hypokalemia, and acidosis (venous pH less than 7.3). Osmotic diuresis combined with severe electrolyte imbalances can cause acute renal shutdown, seizures, and hypoxia.

5. What is the treatment of DKA?

Attention to airway and work of breathing is the first priority. Institute oxygen via mask or cannula on an awake and cooperative patient. Intravenous (IV) access in one or preferably two sites is required for hydration and medication administration. Simultaneously, draw required labs to include serum ketones and osmolarity, amylase, lipase, cardiac enzymes, and a baseline arterial blood gas (ABG). Consider a serum HCG in women of childbearing age, and obtain a urinalysis with urine drug screen. Frequently the patient is pancultured because sepsis is one of the most common causes of DKA in Type I diabetes. If infection is suspected, initiate appropriate antibiotic therapy as ordered.

It is not uncommon for patients in DKA to receive several liters of normal saline in the first 2 to 3 hours of arrival. Hypovolemia is treated with warmed normal saline fluid boluses to dilute the concentration of glucose and reverse acidosis. Later the solution is switched to half-normal saline, usually with potassium replacement added. An appropriate IV bolus of regular insulin, followed by an insulin drip with hourly bedside glucose monitoring, should be initiated. Recent evidence suggests that insulin via subcutaneous or intramuscular (IM) routes is not beneficial in the presence of DKA. Obtain a 12-lead electrocardiogram (ECG) to assess for signs of hypokalemia, ischemic changes, or other signs of cardiac compromise. Continuous telemetry and pulse oximetry are instituted; placement of an indwelling Foley catheter to monitor urinary output is required to assess for possible signs of renal compromise and allow for assessment of adequate fluid resuscitation and hydration. Frequently assess for fluid overload in patients with histories of congestive heart failure (CHF) or other conditions warranting cautious hydration.

In treating infants and children in DKA, rehydration takes on a new challenge because rapid repletion with fluids can cause irreversible neurological sequelae caused by cerebral edema, a common complication of DKA in this delicate population. Careful weight-based boluses of normal saline followed by half-normal saline, electrolyte monitoring, and insulin therapy (0.1 unit/kg as an infusion) prevents such intracerebral events. The recommended dose for IV hydration is 10 to 20 mg/kg normal saline over 1 or 2 hours. As vital signs, urinary output, capillary refill, and mentation improve, hydration continues over 48 hours using half-normal saline with the addition of potassium. Insulin is given as a continuous drip at 0.1 unit/kg/hr until blood glucose levels return to normal. Phosphate, dextrose, and potassium will also be added to the treatment regimen. Sodium bicarbonate is recommended only for severe acidosis in which the pH is less than 6.9 in the presence of hypotension and cardiac arrhythmias.

Pediatric and adult patients with DKA may stabilize in the ED; however, preparation for transfer to an ICU should be made as soon as possible to monitor for the cascade of metabolic events that can potentially occur.

6. Can DKA mimic other disorders?

Yes. Starvation; alcoholic ketoacidosis; and toxic ingestions of methanol, paraldehyde, antifreeze, salicylates, and metformin can cause varying degrees of acidosis, mental status changes, and electrolyte imbalances. Therefore additional laboratory tests (acetylsalicylic acid [ASA], methanol, ethyl alcohol [ETOH] levels) should be part of the initial treatment when any of the aforementioned are suspected.

7. What can the nurse do to facilitate health promotion in persons with diabetes?

The nurse can educate the patient regarding diabetes and the importance of following the prescribed insulin regimen, especially in the patient with new onset diabetes. To plan for discharge, nutritional consults may be beneficial while patients remain in the hospital. Soliciting family support with diabetic teaching, including recognition of early DKA symptoms, is also vital for prevention of DKA.

Help patients identify and deal with stressors that may contribute to labile glucose levels; encourage them to seek medical attention at the onset of illnesses that may precipitate DKA so their physicians can tailor insulin or oral drugs appropriately. Referring patients to official ADA websites may provide them with additional information, updates, and support groups if needed. For children with diabetes, family and sibling involvement in diabetic education and management are important. For children and adults, the goal is to decrease hospital admissions and long-term complications and to promote a normal, active lifestyle.

8. **What clues indicate that a patient has hyperglycemic hyperosmolar nonketotic syndrome (HHNKS) rather than DKA?**

Objectively, patients with HHNKS present in extremis similar to DKA: hypotensive, tachycardic, tachypneic, flushed, lethargic, or comatose. Two cardinal findings of HHNKS are the absence of serum ketones and acidosis. Whereas DKA may precipitate rapidly, HHNKS is usually associated with Type II diabetes and may occur over a period of several days.

Patients with HHNKS present with extremely high glucose levels (greater than 1500 to 2000 mg/dl) and high serum osmolarity (greater than 350 mOsm/L). Secondary to high osmolarity, profound diuresis causing blood urea nitrogen (BUN) levels to rise as high as 70 mg/dl will occur in conjunction with hypovolemic shock.

9. **How is HHNKS treated?**

After securing a patent airway, initiate IV access, obtain baseline ECG, place patients on continuous telemetry and pulse oximetry, and prepare for IV insulin bolus and drip. Treatment is similar to DKA and is likewise tailored to each patient's needs based on co-morbid conditions and clinical findings.

10. **What is adrenal insufficiency?**

The *inability* of the adrenal glands to secrete cortisol and/or aldosterone secondary to removal, atrophy, neoplasms, autoimmune disturbances, insufficient adrenocorticotropic hormone release (caused by hypothalamic and/or anterior pituitary diseases), and/or chronic exposure to glucocorticoids.

The adrenocortical hormones play a major role in regulating the physiological responses to illness and trauma. Two crucial roles include ensuring adequate circulating glucose for cellular energy and initiating antiinflammatory and immunosuppressive mechanisms; both are vital components in challenging injurious stressors, shock, and sepsis. Other important functions include maintaining systemic vascular tone; inotropic cardiac capabilities; decreasing vascular permeability; and the metabolic breakdown of certain fats, carbohydrates, and protein. Another defining characteristic of adrenal insufficiency is the inability of the kidneys to regulate the absorption of sodium and the excretion of potassium, resulting in critical fluid and electrolyte imbalances.

11. **What are the symptoms of Addison's disease (primary adrenal insufficiency)?**

Subclinical symptoms of Addison's disease include vague complaints of malaise, lethargy, muscle cramping, weight loss, anorexia, and polydypsia.

Until a precipitating event (stressor) occurs, such as syncope from dehydration or an otherwise uncomplicated clinical procedure, patients with Addison's disease may be unaware of their medical condition. The adrenal cortex can effectively function when only 10% of the gland is present. When the adrenal glands have completely failed, patients may present in extremis (e.g., in hypovolemic shock).

An index of suspicion for Addison's disease is laboratory data revealing marked electrolyte disturbances, particularly hyponatremia with low serum cortisol levels. Vital signs reveal marked hypotension (systolic pressure less than 80 mmHg), tachycardia of 120 to 140 beats per minute, and respiratory rates usually normal. Patients appear pale and have delayed capillary refill, decreased skin turgor, and dry mucous membranes. Laboratory findings reveal profound hyponatremia (sodium less than 120 mEq/L), hypochloremia, elevated BUN (some as high as 60), mild hyperkalemia, hypoglycemia, and low cortisol levels (less than 25 mcg/dl) with corresponding high adrenocorticotropin hormone (ACTH) levels (ACTH levels are part of the diagnostic criteria; treatment should not be delayed while waiting for results of this test).

Another finding specific to Addison's disease is hyperpigmentation on various exposed areas of skin. Patients may appear "tan" or have hyperpigmented areas on their upper extremities around the knuckles or particularly in the palmar creases of the hands and axilla. Even the oral mucosa and tongue can be involved.

12. How is Addison's disease treated in the ED?

Depending on the severity of symptoms, fluid resuscitation begins after the airway is protected and/or supplemental oxygen is applied. Baseline labs are drawn to include electrolytes and serum cortisol level. It is not uncommon for these patients to have profound hyponatremia; therefore the IV fluid of choice is normal saline. The patient is placed on continuous telemetry and pulse oximetry until stabilized. Fluid replacement helps stabilize volume status; however, treatment *must* include replenishment of glucocorticoids, typically a bolus of 100 mg of IV hydrocortisone. Additional mineralocorticoid therapy may be added (Florinef) if labile hypotension and hypoglycemia persist.

13. What steps can the nurse take to promote wellness in persons with Addison's disease?

Patients with Addison's disease must understand their disease and the importance of hormonal supplements. To promote adherence with the patient's drug regimen and to prevent frequent emergency visits, the nurse can suggest and reinforce the following:

- Encourage patients to wear medical alert bracelets or carry information that will assist medical personnel in treating their disorder if they are unable to relay the information.
- Advise patients to have on hand a prescribed hydrocortisone emergency injection kit. They should be fully instructed on how and when to use the kit.
- Assist patients in identifying stressors that may require them to seek prophylactic treatment as needed.
- Help patients to understand the emotional or mood swings and other side effects of long-term steroid use (osteoporosis, increase in weight, fluid retention).
- Advise patients not to abruptly stop prescribed medications.

- Ensure that patients follow up with an endocrinologist after discharge.
- Reassure and advise patients to return to the ED at the onset of symptoms that may warrant immediate attention.

14. **What is Grave's disease?**

Grave's disease is an autoimmune hyperthyroid condition that involves oversecretion of T3 and T4 because of circulating antibodies that suppress the thyroid stimulating hormone (TSH) receptors. Antibodies can eventually be measured confirming this condition. The treatment upon presentation to the ED depends on the severity of symptomatology.

15. **What are the presenting complaints for Grave's disease?**

Typically, patients have a known history of Grave's disease. They present with any of the following complaints: palpitations, chest pain, shortness of breath, diarrhea, visual disturbances (diplopia, pain, photophobia), nervousness and tremors, insomnia, muscle weakness, or pruritis. One of the characteristic findings of this disease is exophthalmos (protrusion of the eyes).

16. **What is included in the diagnostic work-up, and what treatments are indicated?**

Vital signs may reveal mild to moderate tachycardia; therefore a baseline ECG and telemetry are warranted and arrhythmias such as atrial fibrillation are treated accordingly. Blood pressure and temperature may also be mildly elevated; however, treatment depends on the severity of symptoms. IV access and labs are obtained, including baseline complete blood count (CBC), electrolytes, and cardiac enzymes with creatinine kinase (CK), TSH, T3, and T4. Additional labs may include blood cultures, urine toxicology screening, and serum HCG. An ABG, spiral computed tomography (CT) scan of the chest, or ventilation-perfusion (VQ) scan may be ordered to rule out pulmonary embolism (PE). Definitive treatment is the administration of thyroid hormone antagonists, such as thiomides and methimazole, with beta blockade for the tachycardia.

17. **Why is a history of pregnancy important when a patient presents to the ED with Grave's disease?**

Generally Grave's disease waxes and wanes in severity. Pregnancy can exacerbate the hyperthyroid effects of Grave's disease. Circulating levels of HCG tend to further stimulate thyroid activity, which can result in thyroid storm (the most severe form of hyperthyroidism). Therefore any woman of childbearing age with Grave's disease should provide an obstetrical history, including antepartum and postpartum complications.

18. **What is thyroid storm?**

Thyroid storm is the *magnified* response to unopposed circulating thyroid hormone. It occurs in patients with known hyperthyroidism (Grave's disease) and can be accelerated by:
- DKA
- Preeclampsia of pregnancy

- Thyroid or other surgeries
- Pituitary tumors
- Infections
- Stress
- Emboli
- Accidental overdose of exogenous thyroid hormone
- Iodine ingestion
- Noncompliance with antithyroid medications

   Although thyroid storm occurs infrequently, it is a life-threatening emergency, often associated with a high mortality rate. Thyroid storm demands prompt recognition and treatment upon presentation.

19. What are the symptoms of thyroid storm?

The clinical symptoms of this disorder are the result of a hypermetabolic/adrenergic state. Patients present in extremis with hyperthermia, tachycardia, hypertension, hyperreflexia, diaphoresis, and an overall appearance of anxiety and irritability. General appearance reveals a typical thin physique, exophthalmos, and an enlarged, nontender thyroid.

20. What is the treatment of thyroid storm?

Thyroid storm is one of the most challenging endocrine emergencies. The hypermetabolic consequences have an effect on every organ system and require aggressive emergency management. The overall goal of treatment is to oppose this life-threatening, hypermetabolic response with supportive management and counteract excessive circulating thyroid hormone.

   Airway management is the priority; oxygen via nasal cannula or mask is given based on patient cooperation and level of irritability or confusion. Patients are placed on telemetry and continuous pulse oximetry with frequent blood pressure monitoring. IV access and labs are obtained to include baseline CBC, electrolytes, cardiac enzymes, ABG, urinalysis, urine toxicology, and HCG. Head CT may be ordered to rule out an intracranial event, because hypertension, widened pulse pressure, and hyperthermia may suggest a thalamus lesion. Propranolol (Inderal) 2 mg via IV is the drug of choice for controlling heart rate and hypertension. Acetaminophen (Tylenol) is given along with the application of cooling blankets for hyperpyrexia. Hydration is begun with D5 half-normal saline. The definitive treatment to control the surge of circulating thyroid hormone is the administration of propylthiouracil (PTU) and methimazole (MMI), which arrest thyroid production.

21. What can the nurse do to help prevent thyroid storm?

- Educate the patient regarding adherence to medication regimen.
- If the patient is female and of childbearing age, reinforce the need to alert her physician so changes in medical regimen may be safely made (e.g., should she become pregnant).
- Review signs and symptoms of exacerbation of hyperthyroid condition.
- Advise the patient to seek medical attention for symptoms.

Key Points

- A history of an endocrine dysfunction is the key to solving the complex cascade of events that follows an endocrine emergency.
- Endocrine disorders can be life threatening; therefore the nurse must be familiar with not only the more common presentations such as DKA and hypoglycemia but also the presentations of thyroid and adrenal disorders that sometimes present in the ED.
- Patients presenting with fever and tachycardia should have a baseline TSH, T3, and T4 drawn to rule out hyperthyroidism. Thyroid storm should be part of the differential diagnosis so that prompt treatment is initiated.
- An infection is one of the most common causes for elevated blood glucose in pediatric and adult patients with diabetes. Check patients in DKA for sources of potential infections, such as pneumonia, gastroenteritis, cellulitis, and tooth or foot infection.
- Children younger than 5 years of age who are in DKA with high serum osmolality are at high risk for cerebral edema. Perform neurological checks before and during hydration. Be alert for early complaints of headache and mental status changes.
- If a patient with adrenal insufficiency presents to the ED for an unrelated endocrine problem, keep in mind that they can tolerate very little exogenous stressors and may need an IV bolus of hydrocortisone for prophylaxis. Research has demonstrated that patients with adrenal insufficiency fare better when hydrocortisone is given early in their hospitalization stay, particularly if they must undergo a surgical procedure.
- Access to hypothermia blankets for patients in thyroid storm should be readily available in the ED. Avoid making the patient shiver; this will increase the already hypermetabolic state.

Internet Resources

American Diabetes Association, Resources for Professionals:
www.diabetes.org/for-health-professionals-and-scientists/resources.jsp

American Thyroid Association, Resources for Professionals:
www.thyroid.org/professionals

Children with Diabetes:
www.childrenwithdiabetes.com

EndocrineWeb.com:
www.endocrineweb.com

Merck Manual of Diagnosis and Therapy, Hyperthyroidism:
www.merck.com/mrkshared/mmanual/section2/chapter8/8d.jsp

National Grave's Disease Foundation:
www.ngdf.org

Society for Endocrinology, Links to Other Sites:
www.endocrinology.org/sfe/gateway.htm

Bibliography

AACE Thyroid Task Force: American association of clinical endocrinologists medical guidelines for clinical practice for the evaluation and treatment of hyperthyroidism and hypothyroidism, *Endocr Pract* 8(6):457-467, 2002.

Agus MSD, Wolfsdorf JI: Diabetic ketoacidosis in children, *Pediatr Clin North Am* 52:1147-1163, 2005.

Chiasson JL et al: Diagnosis and treatment of diabetic ketoacidosis and the hyperglycemic hyperosmolar state, *CMAJ* 168(7):859-866, 2003.

Gillespie GL, Campbell M: Diabetic ketoacidosis: Rapid identification, treatment, and education can improve survival rates, *Am J Nurs* 102:13-16, 2002.

Kronenberg H et al: Principles of endocrinology. In Larsen PR et al: *Williams, textbook of endocrinology,* St Louis, 2003, Mosby.

Malchiodi L: Thyroid storm: Recognizing the signs and symptoms of this life-threatening complication, *Am J Nurs* 102(5):33-35, 2002.

Marik P, Zaloga GP: Adrenal insufficiency in the critically ill: A new look at an old problem, *Chest* 122(5):1784-1796, 2002.

Murphy MB et al: Hyperglycemic crises in diabetes, *Diabetes Care* 27(1):S94-S102, 2004.

Nayback AM: Hyponatremia as a consequence of acute adrenal insufficiency and hypothyroidism, *Emerg Nurs* 26(2):130-133, 2000.

Palmer R: An overview of diabetic ketoacidosis, *Nurs Stand* 19:42-44, 2004.

Sabol VK: Addisonian crisis: This life-threatening condition may be triggered by a variety of stressors, *Am J Nurs* 101(7):24AAA-24DDD, 2001.

Chapter 21

Hematological Emergencies

Krista M. Haugen

1. What constitutes a hematological emergency?

There are a wide variety of disorders that may lead to a hematological emergency. If red blood cells (RBCs), white blood cells (WBCs), platelets, and/or coagulation factors in the blood cannot perform their respective functions, a potentially serious hematological problem exists. All body systems can be adversely affected by hematological disorders. Patients may be at significant risk for bleeding, coagulopathies, infection, infarction, shock, and other complications. Abnormalities in the hematological system are manifestations of underlying diseases, most of which require urgent attention at the very least, and some of which are potentially fatal. These problems may or may not be obvious when the patient presents to the emergency department (ED). To facilitate rapid identification of hematological dysfunction and initiation of treatment, an insightful investigation into the patient's history and current problem is warranted, along with a thorough clinical assessment.

2. What information about the patient's history will be helpful?

Hematological disorders may be chronic, such as sickle cell disease; acute, such as hemorrhage secondary to trauma; or both, as in cases of a patient with hemophilia who may be hemorrhaging secondary to trauma. Some hematological disorders are genetic and therefore inherited, whereas others may be acquired. Patients may already know they have a hematological disorder or that their family history predisposes them to one. In these cases, patients themselves may provide valuable information. Detailed history taking is required for other patients. Is there a family history of blood disorders? Does the patient have any past problems with bleeding associated with minor procedures such as dental work, for instance? Is there a current problem with bleeding? Does the patient take any medication that alters blood cell function? Could the patient be immunosuppressed? Is there a history of alcohol or drug use? Affirmative answers to these and other questions may lead the emergency nurse to suspect a hematological problem. Other cases may be more perplexing because the patient may present with vague complaints necessitating lab studies in addition to an astute clinical assessment to reveal a hematological disorder.

3. What should the assessment of these patients entail?

Disorders of RBCs, WBCs, platelets, and coagulation factors can affect all organ systems. To help guide the assessment of the hematological system, in addition to the general assessment, think of the functions of the main components of the hematological system. The RBC, for example, is responsible for oxygen transport to the tissues. Therefore a patient with RBC dysfunction may exhibit signs and symptoms of inadequate tissue oxygenation. These signs and symptoms may range from quite subtle, such as "not feeling right," to a very obvious altered level of consciousness. Specific functions of WBCs, platelets, and coagulation factors are discussed later in the chapter.

4. System by system, what are some signs and symptoms that might signify or contribute to a hematological disorder?

Patients who present with hematological disorders may exhibit varying degrees of severity. Some may come to the ED by private vehicle and have a subtle presentation; others will arrive by ambulance or an air transport in critical condition. The following table contains some suggested assessment considerations.

Hematological Disorders

System	Assessment Considerations
General appearance	Appears ill, fatigued, chief complaint
Neurological	Level of consciousness, motor function, speech, Glasgow Coma Scale
Cardiovascular	Cardiac rhythm, rate and quality of central and peripheral pulses, blood pressure, orthostatic hypotension, evidence of dehydration, fever, evidence of bleeding, chest pain
Gastrointestinal (GI)	Abdominal pain, nausea, vomiting, diarrhea, blood in stools or vomit, organomegaly, appetite, nutritional status, alcohol consumption
Genitourinary	Pain, flank pain, bleeding, hematuria, priapism (may occur during a vasoocclusive sickle cell crisis)
Musculoskeletal	Pain, swelling, or hematomas in joints or muscles; bone pain; mobility problems; injuries; bleeding
Psychosocial	Adequate coping skills, resources, support systems, stress-management skills; education requirements of patient and family
Respiratory	Dyspnea, tachypnea, shortness of breath at rest or with exertion, work of breathing, lung sounds, evidence of infection, pain, cough, adequate oxygenation/ventilation
Skin	Color, pallor, temperature, rash, bruising, lesions, wounds, bleeding, bleeding with minor procedures, gums bleeding, petechiae or purpura (these reddish-purple nonblanching hemorrhages may occur secondary to blood disorders; petechiae are smaller than 0.5 cm in size; purpura are larger than 0.5 cm)

Additional assessment considerations are presented with the specific blood disorders discussed later in the chapter.

RED BLOOD CELLS

5. **What is normal RBC physiology?**

   The development of blood cells occurs in the bone marrow. The formation of RBCs, otherwise known as erythropoiesis, is regulated by the hormone erythropoietin (EPO). EPO production takes place mostly in the kidneys by cells that respond to changes in tissue oxygenation and metabolism. Vitamin B_{12} and folic acid are also essential to the normal development of RBCs. It takes about 1 week for an RBC to develop, and their life span is approximately 120 days. Once mature, an RBC is able to fully carry out its main function of oxygen transport to the tissues.

6. **How are RBCs measured?**

   Several lab tests evaluate and describe RBC size, shape, color, concentration, and function. Alterations in these lab values may indicate the presence and type of hematological disorder. Patient variables that may affect lab results include age; gender; hydration status; and whether patients smoke, are pregnant, or live at high altitude. The following are definitions of some of the lab tests that evaluate RBCs:
   - **RBC count:** Reflects the number of RBCs in millions per microliter.
   - **Hemoglobin (Hgb):** Measures the concentration of hemoglobin in grams per deciliter.
   - **Hematocrit (HCT):** Measures the percent of RBCs in whole blood.
   - **Mean corpuscular volume (MCV):** Reflects the size of the RBC, which may be microcytic (small), normocytic (normal), or macrocytic (large).
   - **Color:** Described as normochromic (normal color) or hypochromic (pale).
   - **Reticulocytes:** Immature RBCs that usually constitute about 1% of the RBCs in circulation. The measurement of reticulocytes provides information regarding erythrocyte production, function, and ability of the bone marrow to manufacture RBCs to meet the demands of a stressed hematological system. This may also be expressed as a corrected reticulocyte count, which is calculated by a formula and is helpful in distinguishing different types of anemia.

7. **How is oxygen transport accomplished?**

   All cells in the body depend on the adequate delivery of oxygen to function properly. Hemoglobin is the portion of the RBC responsible for oxygen transport. Each hemoglobin molecule contains four iron atoms. Each iron atom binds with one molecule of oxygen for transport to the tissues. How readily the iron atom will let go of the oxygen molecule at the tissue level depends on factors that affect the oxyhemoglobin dissociation curve. Abnormalities in the number, structure, and function of RBCs alter its oxygen-delivering capabilities.

8. **How does the patient's volume status affect lab results?**

   The RBC count, hemoglobin, and hematocrit are expressed as concentrations. Dehydration, overhydration, pregnancy, and fluid shifts, for instance, can all affect red cell concentration. For example, lab results for an anemic patient who is also dehydrated may not reflect anemia because both red cell mass and plasma volume are decreased. After the patient is given intravenous (IV) fluids and the dehydration is corrected, lab results should reflect anemia because the red cell mass is decreased compared with the plasma volume, which has been corrected with IV fluids. Contrarily, patients who are overhydrated may have a relative anemia because the increased plasma volume shifts the RBC-plasma concentration. These factors should be taken into consideration when interpreting lab results, along with the patient's clinical presentation.

9. What are some of the major RBC disorders?

Many of the major RBC disorders fall under the general topic of anemia. Anemia occurs when there is a decrease in circulating RBCs or when there are abnormalities of hemoglobin that interfere with its oxygen-carrying capacity. Anemia can be classified into three main types: (1) decreased RBC production (e.g., iron deficiency; pernicious, aplastic, and other bone-marrow depression diseases); (2) increased RBC destruction, including hemolytic and sickle cell anemia; and, (3) increased blood loss (e.g., hemorrhage, chronic bleeding). A brief review of RBC physiology may be helpful for gaining insight as to the seriousness of each disorder.

10. What types of anemia are related to decreased RBC production?

Iron-deficiency anemia, megaloblastic anemia, and aplastic anemia are anemias of decreased RBC production. Recall the importance of iron in binding and carrying oxygen. If a patient is iron deficient, this directly affects the oxygen-carrying capacity of the RBC, resulting in signs and symptoms of anemia. In addition to general clinical signs of anemia, these patients may also have brittle, concave nails and red, smooth tongues. Iron-deficiency anemia is the most common anemia, and symptoms typically improve with iron therapy.

Megaloblastic (abnormally large RBCs) anemias include pernicious anemia (vitamin B_{12} deficiency) and folic acid deficiency. Vitamin B_{12} deficiency can occur because of poor nutrition or because of problems with absorption. Inadequate B_{12} alters the development of RBCs and WBCs. Pernicious anemia is treatable; however, treatment must continue for life because there is no cure.

Folic acid is also essential to the normal development of RBCs. Folic acid deficiency occurs because of poor nutrition and is common in alcoholics. Treatment includes folate and, depending on the severity of anemia and clinical signs and symptoms, blood transfusions.

Aplastic anemia involves a decrease in production and growth of blood cells. This can lead to pancytopenia, a decreased number of all blood cells. In addition to being anemic, these patients are also at increased risk for bleeding secondary to thrombocytopenia and increased risk for infection secondary to leukopenia.

11. What types of anemia are associated with increased RBC destruction?

Hemolytic anemia exists when RBCs are destroyed too early in their life span. These anemias can be caused by a number of problems, some of which are congenital, but most of which are acquired. Some causes of hemolytic anemias are ABO and/or Rh incompatibility between mothers and babies or transfusion reactions. Other causes include infections such as malaria, toxic chemicals, burns, or trauma inflicted on the RBC by mechanisms such as prosthetic heart valves or as in hemolytic-uremic syndrome (HUS).

12. What is HUS?

HUS is most commonly caused by infection of the GI tract with *Escherichia coli*. This bacteria is found in contaminated meat or vegetables and unpasteurized juices and dairy products. Initial symptoms of *E. coli* infection include bloody diarrhea, abdominal pain, and vomiting. Although most people recover from *E. coli* infection, approximately 10% of children develop HUS; elderly patients are also susceptible. HUS is characterized by microangiopathic hemolytic anemia (MAHA), in which RBCs are damaged or destroyed because of narrowed blood vessels, low platelets, and acute renal failure. As RBCs and platelets are destroyed, signs and symptoms of anemia and thrombocytopenia develop. Fragments of RBCs clog renal vasculature, resulting in signs of renal failure including decreased urine output, hypertension, and edema. Treatment of HUS is supportive, and the majority of patients recover. There is a small percentage of patients, however, that either die in the acute phase or experience serious sequelae. Some require ongoing dialysis or a kidney transplant.

13. What is sickle cell anemia?

Sickle cell anemia is an inherited disease, typically occurring in African Americans, in which an aberrant form of hemoglobin, hemoglobin S, exists. When stressed by various factors such as dehydration, hypoxia, or acidosis, hemoglobin S alters its shape and the RBC becomes sickled in appearance. The oxygen-delivering capability of the sickled RBC is impaired, as is the ability of the RBC to move smoothly through the vasculature. Their long, jagged shape increases the sickled RBCs' tendency to clump and cause vasoocclusion, which can lead to ischemia and organ infarction. In addition, the increase in blood viscosity leads to worsening hypoxia and acidosis, precipitating further sickling. Most sickling can be reversed; however, over time these RBCs become more fragile and may eventually become permanently sickled.

14. What types of sickle cell crises can occur?

There are four types of sickle cell crises: (1) Vasoocclusive crisis, the most common, occurs when the microcirculation is obstructed and blood flow is impaired, resulting in thrombosis or infarction; (2) aplastic crisis exists when the patient's bone marrow is suppressed and the normal compensatory response of the bone marrow to replace hemolyzed RBCs is altered, often because of viral infection; (3) sequestrative crisis occurs when the spleen rapidly sequesters large volumes of blood, and hypovolemic shock can ensue if the spleen ruptures; and (4) hemolytic crisis, the least common type, is manifested by rapid destruction of RBCs, usually related to infection.

Clinical presentations of patients in sickle cell crisis are related to tissue and organ ischemia and infarction. Patients usually experience significant pain. Other signs and symptoms depend on which tissues and organ systems are affected.

15. **How is sickle cell crisis managed in the ED?**

Treatment of sickle cell crisis depends on the severity of the crisis, signs and symptoms, and which tissues and organ systems are involved. Patients generally require supportive care, which may include oxygen if there is evidence of hypoxia, IV hydration, and pain control. A major goal of patient education should be methods of prevention so that the frequency of crises can be reduced. To help keep RBCs adequately oxygenated, patients should be taught to avoid overstressing themselves (both physically and emotionally), to avoid low-oxygen environments such as higher altitudes, and to avoid infections as much as possible. Patients should also be taught to keep hydrated by drinking plenty of fluids and avoiding environments that contribute to dehydration.

Ideally, the care of sickle cell patients should entail a multidisciplinary approach. The physiological, psychosocial, and pain-control issues experienced by this patient population are complex. Coordination between specialties, to include the patient's primary care provider and a case manager, will help to optimally address the challenges faced by people with sickle cell disease.

16. **What accounts for anemia resulting from increased blood loss?**

Blood loss results in a decrease in circulating RBCs. Blood loss can occur acutely, as with a trauma patient or an active GI bleed. Patients can also suffer from chronic bleeding. Whether or not a patient should be transfused should be based on clinical presentation and lab values. An important consideration is the rate of blood loss and whether the patient has had the time and compensatory mechanisms to tolerate anemia. One patient whose lab tests reflect anemia may require a transfusion for signs and symptoms of inadequate tissue perfusion and oxygenation. Another patient with the same lab values may tolerate the anemia and not require a transfusion.

17. **What are some transfusion reactions to look for?**

Although transfusions may be necessary to replenish a blood component, they are not benign and patients should be monitored closely for adverse reactions. Transfusion reactions can occur with infusions of RBCs, platelets, plasma, and coagulation factors.

Febrile nonhemolytic reaction:
- Most frequently encountered transfusion reaction
- Onset approximately 1 to 6 hours after infusion
- Caused by recipient antibodies forming against donor WBCs or platelets
- Symptoms include fever, chills, and possibly shortness of breath
- Although uncomfortable and frightening, it generally has no lasting adverse effects
- Initial symptoms of a febrile nonhemolytic reaction are very similar to those of an acute hemolytic reaction, which has serious sequelae and can be fatal; therefore, transfusions should be stopped immediately until the type of reaction can be determined for certain

Acute hemolytic reaction:
- Occurs when blood products transfused are not ABO compatible with the patient, resulting in an antigen-antibody reaction
- Initial symptoms may vary from fever to hemoglobinuria

- Results in acute intravascular hemolysis that may progress to disseminated intravascular coagulation (DIC), renal failure, and shock
- If symptoms occur, stop the transfusion immediately and expect to provide supportive care

Anaphylactic reaction:
- Occurs in patients with a hereditary IgA deficiency who have developed complement-binding anti-IgA antibodies; anaphylaxis occurs when these anti-IgA antibodies are exposed to donor IgA
- May occur almost immediately after the start of a blood product infusion
- Symptoms may include dyspnea, angioedema, hypotension, and shock
- If symptoms occur, stop the transfusion and expect to treat the anaphylaxis
- Provide supportive care

Urticarial reaction (mild):
- A histamine-related reaction to donor protein
- Manifested by urticaria and pruritis
- Stop the transfusion so that this fairly benign reaction can be distinguished from an anaphylactic reaction
- Generally treated with Benadryl

Transfusion related acute lung injury (TRALI):
- Can occur 2 to 4 hours after a transfusion begins
- Thought to be caused by the interaction between donor antibodies and recipient WBCs
- Symptoms nearly identical to adult respiratory distress syndrome (ARDS): dyspnea, hypoxemia, hypotension, fever, and pulmonary edema
- Unlike ARDS, the prognosis is generally good
- With supportive care, a patient may recover in a matter of days

Other reactions:
- Infection
- Citrate toxicity
- Decreased ionized calcium
- Hyperkalemia/hypokalemia
- Hypothermia
- Volume overload

PLATELETS, THROMBOCYTES, AND CLOTTING DISORDERS

18. How does the clotting cascade function?

The clotting cascade is the means by which fibrin is formed through a sequence of reactions among clotting factors. The cascade consists of two pathways, the intrinsic and extrinsic. These pathways merge together in a final common pathway, and the result is fibrin formation. Each pathway is activated by a specific mechanism.

The prothrombin time (PT) is a test of extrinsic pathway activity. It also measures the body's response to Coumadin and the adequacy of vitamin K. The partial thromboplastin time (PTT) is a test of intrinsic and common pathway activity. It is helpful in monitoring the effectiveness of heparin, and it may be lengthened in hemophilia and von Willebrand's disease. Bleeding time is a test that reflects platelet aggregation and vasoconstriction. It is rarely used and measures the time a small superficial wound takes to stop bleeding. It is lengthened in thrombocytopenia, with aspirin use, and in von Willebrand's disease. In cases of hypercoagulability, the D-dimer is a test generally used as an adjunct to other tests to aid in the assessment of abnormal clotting. This test measures fibrin degradation products that indicate the presence (but not the location) of a clot. It is most often used when deep vein thrombosis (DVT), pulmonary embolism (PE), or DIC is suspected. All of these lab tests help to aid in diagnosis of hemostatic diseases.

19. What is the international normalized ratio (INR)?

Previously, variability in PT results occurred because different labs used different reagents for testing. The INR was developed by the World Health Organization (WHO) to help standardize the PT between different institutions and is particularly helpful for monitoring patients on Coumadin therapy.

20. What are some clotting disorders?

Hemophilia is an inherited coagulation disorder in which clotting factor deficiencies exist. Several types of hemophilia are described. Hemophilia A, also known as classic hemophilia, is a deficiency in Factor VIII. Hemophilia B, also known as Christmas disease, is a deficiency in Factor IX. The PTT in these patients is lengthened, whereas the PT and platelets are normal. Von Willebrand's disease is a form of hemophilia in which there is a Factor VIII deficiency as well as platelet dysfunction. Clinical signs and symptoms vary but are generally not as serious as hemophilia A and B.

Bleeding may occur either spontaneously or after minor injury in hemophilia patients. Joints and muscles are common sites of bleeding. The severity of bleeding depends on the degree of deficiency of clotting factors as well as the severity of injury.

21. How is hemophilia managed in the ED?

Treatment of hemophilia revolves around replacing clotting factors, stopping the bleeding, and pain control. The dosage of factor replacement is calculated by a formula. The goal is to restore clotting factor levels to the point where hemostasis can be maintained.

22. When should fresh frozen plasma (FFP) be transfused?

FFP contains coagulation factors but no RBCs, leukocytes, or platelets. FFP may be indicated for patients who have other coagulation factor deficiencies and are actively bleeding. It may also be indicated for patients undergoing a massive transfusion. A further use is to reverse the effects of Coumadin, if indicated, or for patients with vitamin K deficiency. FFP is *not* the first-line treatment for diseases for which specific factors are available to correct deficiencies, such as hemophilia A and B.

23. What is disseminated intravascular coagulation (DIC)?

DIC is a thrombohemorrhagic complication of a number of different illnesses or injuries such as trauma, malignancies, obstetrical problems, snakebites, infection, sepsis, and transfusion of incompatible blood products. DIC is thought to initially involve a massive activation of clotting factors, consuming them faster than they can be restored. With an inadequate supply of clotting factors in the circulation, hemorrhage ensues. Of note, injured brain tissue releases thromboplastin, which may initiate the coagulation cascade even though no significant hemorrhage has occurred.

Assessment may reveal bleeding from venipuncture sites, IV sites, and invasive monitoring sites. Petechiae, purpura, and bruising may be present. The condition may progress to multiple organ dysfunction syndrome (MODS), shock, intracranial bleeding, and other internal bleeding. Susceptibility to infection may increase as well.

24. How is DIC treated?

The underlying disease thought to have precipitated the DIC needs to be treated, and clotting factors should be replaced. Metabolic, hemodynamic, and ventilatory problems should also be corrected because they contribute to the perpetuation of clotting cascade dysfunction.

25. What are thrombocytes?

The function of thrombocytes, or platelets, in hemostasis is to form platelet plugs to help stop bleeding. When platelets are activated they change their shape to facilitate clumping. The resultant platelet plug is then reinforced by fibrin and, ideally, the bleeding is stopped.

26. What are some platelet disorders?

Thrombocytopenia occurs when there is a decrease in the number of platelets in circulation. This predisposes a patient to bleeding. Normal platelet counts are generally considered between 150,000 and 400,000 units/L. Thrombocytopenia exists when the platelet count drops below 100,000. It is recommended that patients with a platelet count of less than 50,000 be placed on bleeding precautions (e.g., limiting the number of IV sticks or other invasive procedures). Platelet counts of less than 20,000 can result in spontaneous bleeding.

27. What causes thrombocytopenia?

Thrombocytes are actually fragments of megakaryocytes, which are large cells that develop from stem cells and are mostly found in bone marrow. Diseases that alter production of megakaryocytes can cause thrombocytopenia. Examples include diseases of the bone marrow, megaloblastic anemia, and iron-deficiency anemia. Destruction of platelets can also result in thrombocytopenia. A variety of drugs can destroy platelets or alter platelet function; heparin is the biggest offender. Some other potential causes of platelet destruction include snake venom, malaria, sepsis, or autoimmune problems. Diseases that cause increased consumption of platelets can also result in thrombocytopenia. Idiopathic thrombocytopenia purpura (ITP) is the most common cause in this category. Patients may present with petechiae, purpura, nosebleeds, or other bleeding issues.

28. When should platelets be transfused?

Platelets may be indicated in thrombocytopenia to prevent bleeding or in cases of abnormal platelet function.

WHITE BLOOD CELLS

29. What are leukocytes?

Leukocytes, or WBCs, are the cells responsible for defending the body against infection. They accomplish this by phagocytosis, which basically means they eat cells, including bacteria, and cell debris. Polymorphonuclear granulocytes (PMNs) make up the majority of WBCs. PMNs can be further described as neutrophils, basophils, and eosinophils, each of which has a specific function. Neutrophils constitute the majority of PMNs and can be identified in three different cell forms. A mature neutrophil is classified as a segmented neutrophil, or "seg." A less mature neutrophil is called a "band." And finally, a totally immature neutrophil is known as a "metamyelocyte."

30. What does the phrase "shift to the left" mean?

Picture cellular development as a process or scale that occurs from left to right, with immature cells on the far left and fully mature cells on the far right. When an infectious process is present in the body, the neutrophils are called into action. This leads to an increased demand in production from the bone marrow. If the bone marrow cannot fully meet this demand, it resorts to releasing immature cells, the bands. This is known as a "shift to the left" because on the cellular development scale, bands fall farther left given their immaturity. The bands are identified in the WBC differential (which identifies the type of WBCs present as percentages). If an elevated WBC count is present during the shift to the left, this generally represents a normal bone marrow response to infection. However, if there is a shift to the left without an elevated WBC count, this may indicate that the bone marrow is overwhelmed.

31. What are some disorders of leukocytes?

Leukocytosis, or an abnormally high WBC count, occurs in response to several different stressors as a defense mechanism. It occurs most commonly in response to infection but may also be secondary to malignancies or blood disorders. Leukopenia, or an abnormally low WBC count, can result in significantly increased risk for serious infections. Leukopenia can be caused by cancer treatments such as chemotherapy and radiation, and by other diseases that cause bone marrow depression.

32. What is leukemia?

Leukemia exists when immature WBC proliferation is out of control, resulting in an overabundance in the blood and overcrowding in the bone marrow, which further inhibits production and development of other blood cells. Pancytopenia (decreased RBCs, WBCs, and platelets) can result, as can MODS, DIC, sepsis, and other major complications. The clinical presentation of patients with leukemia may include signs and symptoms of pancytopenia, including infection, fever, bleeding, and the sequelae from malignant cells invading organs.

33. What is a blast crisis?

A blast cell is an undifferentiated cell in the bone marrow that, in some stages of leukemia, may proliferate unchecked and accumulate in the bone marrow and blood, causing a "blast crisis." Some forms of leukemia can produce a massive leukocytosis with WBCs numbering more than 100,000. This constitutes an emergency because this degree of leukocytosis can bring about leukostasis, in which circulation becomes congested and impaired, usually affecting the lungs and brain. A blast crisis can also precipitate leukostasis. Management includes fluid resuscitation and correction of electrolyte imbalances and coagulation abnormalities. Chemotherapy and leukapheresis may be warranted, and efforts should be made to prevent tumor lysis syndrome.

34. What is tumor lysis syndrome?

Tumor lysis syndrome is a potentially life-threatening problem that may occur when blast cells or other cancer-related cells die and spill intracellular contents, causing metabolic abnormalities and electrolyte disturbances. Hyperkalemia, hyperuricemia, hyperphosphatemia, and hypocalcemia may result, leading to renal failure. Multiple organ failure is a potential complication and coagulopathies may also be an issue. Treatment includes IV hydration, correction of metabolic abnormalities and electrolyte disturbances, and prevention of potential sequelae.

35. What is neutropenia?

Neutrophils are the key players in the inflammatory response. As with anemia, the causes of neutropenia can be considered in the categories of increased destruction, inadequate production, or overwhelming demand. If neutropenia exists, patients are increasingly susceptible to infection even from their own normal flora. The normal response to infection, however, is altered in the neutropenic patient. Neutrophils are unable to mount their usual lines of defense that constitute signs and symptoms of infection, especially that of pus production, a common clinical indicator of infection. Therefore, a moderately or severely neutropenic patient may not fit the clinical presentation that is anticipated for a particular infection. A patient may present with a chief complaint of fever. Because the normal response is altered, fever may be the only clue that a patient has an infection. A fever above 100° F in a patient with neutropenia should be considered an emergent problem.

Neutropenia can be classified as mild, moderate, or severe. In the complete blood count (CBC), the neutrophils are expressed as a percentage. The absolute neutrophil count (ANC) expresses the total number of neutrophils in the blood and is calculated by the following formula:

$$(\% \text{ neutrophils} + \% \text{ bands}) \times \text{total WBC} = \text{ANC}$$

Mild neutropenia is generally defined as an ANC from 1000 to 1500/microL. An ANC between 500 and 1000/microL is considered to be moderate and the risk for infection begins to rise. Severe neutropenia exists when the ANC is less than 500/microL and is considered life threatening.

36. **What should nursing care of patients with WBC dysfunction entail?**

Normal defense mechanisms are compromised in many of these patients, making them highly susceptible to infection and sepsis. These patients are also at significant risk for bleeding, MODS, DIC, and other major complications. Recognizing the potentially emergent nature of the patient's problem is paramount. These patients should be taken to a treatment room and evaluated immediately because immunosuppression may require isolation, and sepsis may develop rapidly. Prompt antibiotic therapy is usually also warranted. Whether the ED staff wears isolation gowns and masks or the patient is placed in a mask (if tolerated) varies between institutions. In any case, steps should be taken to prevent nosocomial infections. Strict aseptic technique for invasive procedures should be followed. Patients with WBC dysfunction may also be thrombocytopenic so bleeding precautions such as limiting invasive procedures if possible, monitoring for bleeding, and preventing injury should be taken.

37. **What are the emotional effects of hematological disorders?**

Patients with hematological problems, whether acute or chronic, may experience a high degree of fear, anxiety, frustration, and pain because of the nature of these life-altering and often life-threatening disorders. Their coping skills, as well as those of their families, should be assessed and assistance should be provided if necessary. Educating patients about their hematological disorder can ease their fear and help maximize their quality of life. Counseling, pastoral services, social services, and support groups may also be helpful for patients and their families.

 Key Points

- Hematological abnormalities are manifestations of underlying diseases or problems.
- There are a wide variety of different hematological disorders that may involve any or all of the components of the hematological system.
- Disorders of RBCs, WBCs, platelets, and/or coagulation factors can affect all body systems adversely.
- Clinical presentation of hematological disorders may be subtle, yet can rapidly become life threatening if not recognized and treated early.
- Lab results, although important, should be interpreted within the context of the patient's clinical picture.
- Transfusions, although life saving for some patients, are not benign. Hospital policies and procedures should be followed and patients should be closely monitored for transfusion reactions.
- If a patient exhibits signs or symptoms of a possible transfusion reaction, the transfusion should be stopped immediately and the physician should be notified. Preparations should be made to manage the type of reaction the patient may be experiencing.
- The psychological and emotional toll of blood disorders, whether chronic or acute, can be extreme. Care should be taken to provide resources for education and psychosocial support.

Internet Resources

Centers for Disease Control and Prevention, Hereditary Bleeding Disorders:
www.cdc.gov/ncbddd/hbd/hemophilia.htm

Puget Sound Blood Center, Blood Components Reference Manual:
www.psbc.org/bcrm/03_index.htm

UpToDate:
www.uptodateonline.com

U.S. National Library of Medicine, Genetics Home Reference, Sickle cell anemia:
www.ghr.nlm.nih.gov/condition=sicklecellanemia

Bibliography

Baehner R: *Congenital neutropenia*, UpToDate, 2004. Available at www.uptodateonline.com.

Drews R: *Approach to the patient with a bleeding diathesis*, UpToDate, 2004. Available at www.uptodateonline.com.

George J: *Drug-induced thrombocytopenia*, UpToDate, 2003. Available at www.uptodateonline.com.

Landaw S: *Approach to the patient with thrombocytopenia*, UpToDate, 2004. Available at www.uptodateonline.com.

Leung L: *Pathogenesis and etiology of disseminated intravascular coagulation*, UpToDate, 2004. Available at www.uptodateonline.com.

Majhail N, Lichtin A: Acute leukemia with a very high leukocyte count: Confronting a medical emergency, *Cleve Clin J Med* 71:8, 2004.

Mansen T, McCance K: Alterations of hematologic function. In Huether S, McCance K, editors: *Understanding pathophysiology*, ed 3, St Louis, 2004, Mosby.

May A, Kauder D: *Use of blood products in the intensive care unit*, UpToDate, 2004. Available at www.uptodateonline.com.

McCance K: Structure and function of the hematologic system. In Huether S, McCance K, editors: *Understanding pathophysiology*, ed 3, St Louis, 2004, Mosby.

McCormick D: Immunology and hematology. In Ahrens T, Prentice D, editors: *Critical care certification, preparation, review, and practice exams*, ed 4, Stamford, Conn, 1998, Appleton & Lange.

Rogers R: *Emergencies in hematology and oncology*, EmedHome.com, 2005. Available at www.emedhome.com.

Sacher R, McPherson R, Campos J: *Widmann's clinical interpretation of laboratory tests*, ed 11, Philadelphia, 2000, FA Davis.

Schrier S: *Aplastic anemia: Pathogenesis; clinical manifestations; and diagnosis*, UpToDate, 2005. Available at www.uptodateonline.com.

Schrier S: *Approach to the patient with anemia*, UpToDate, 2004. Available at www.uptodateonline.com.

Silvergleid A: *Immunologic blood transfusion reactions*, UpToDate, 2004. Available at www.uptodateonline.com.

Silvergleid A: *Transfusion of plasma components*, UpToDate, 2004. Available at www.uptodateonline.com.

Wagner K: Acute hematologic dysfunction. In Kidd P, Wagner K, editors: *High acuity nursing*, ed 3, Upper Saddle River, NJ, 2001, Prentice-Hall.

Wallas C, May A, Kauder D: *Indications for red cell transfusion*, UpToDate, 2004. Available at www.uptodateonline.com.

Wanke C: *Diarrheagenic* Escherichia coli, UpToDate, 2005. Available at www.uptodateonline.com.

Nonurgent Problems

Joann M. Sorrentino

1. In assessing a patient, what is an easy way to make sure that an adequate history of the patient's complaint was obtained?

A mnemonic that works well is **OLD CART:**

O	Onset
L	Location
D	Duration
C	Characteristics
A	Alleviating factors
R	Related signs and symptoms
T	Treatment measures

2. What is a dry socket, and how is it treated?

Dry socket is local alveolar osteitis and occurs in approximately 5% of all tooth extractions. It is seen more commonly with the removal of an impacted third molar (wisdom tooth). Patients describe intense pain 2 to 3 days after an extraction. The pain is caused by irritation of the sensory nerves in the dry, exposed bony socket, often after a blood clot dislodges at the site of extraction. Pain management with oral narcotics or nonsteroidal antiinflammatory drugs (NSAIDs) and referral to the dentist are indicated. The socket reepithelializes in approximately 10 days.

3. What is a simple remedy for dental pain secondary to dental caries, with visible decay of the tooth, or a broken tooth until the patient can see the dentist?

Oil of clove on a cotton ball placed directly over the tooth with the dental caries can provide temporary pain relief. Application can be every 1 to 2 hours or when the pain recurs. Dental wax can also be used by the patient to cover the painful or broken tooth and temporarily decrease discomfort.

4. What is the proper treatment for a permanent tooth avulsed by trauma?

Ideally all teeth should be reimplanted immediately. The root portion of the tooth should not be touched; it should be handled by the crown only. Rinse the tooth thoroughly with tap water. Do not scrub. If it is not possible for the tooth to be reimplanted at the scene, place the tooth under the injured person's tongue. If the injured person is not responsible because of age or degree of injury, wrap the tooth in moist gauze and place it in a cup of saline solution, saliva, milk, a specifically prepared tooth saver solution, or Hank's solution. A tooth reimplanted within 30 minutes has a good prognosis for long-term retention.

5. What are conjunctivitis and keratitis? What are the common pathogens and treatment modalities?

Conjunctivitis is the inflammation of the mucous membrane that covers the anterior sclera and inner eyelids. **Keratitis** is inflammation of the cornea. Common viral pathogens include adenoviruses, herpes simplex, and herpes zoster. Infection starts in one eye and may become bilateral with a significant watery discharge. Herpes simplex conjunctivitis presents with conjunctival hyperemia and clear discharge. Lid vesicles and ulcerations may spread rapidly to the cornea, resulting in a dendritic ulcer. Herpes zoster ophthalmicus should be suspected if the nasociliary branch of the fifth cranial nerve is involved. Bacterial pathogens include staphylococci; pneumococci; diphtheroids; *Neisseria gonorrhoeae;* and *Haemophilus, Pseudomonas, Proteus,* and *Moraxella* species. The onset is often acute and unilateral with crusting of the lids. True "pinkeye" is epidemic keratoconjunctivitis. Treatment for both conjunctivitis and keratitis is with a topical antibiotic (eye ointments or eyedrops).

6. What is the difference between periorbital or preseptal cellulitis and orbital or postseptal cellulitis?

Lid edema, swelling of the conjunctivae, and facial swelling are often caused by allergic or contact reactions and do *not* involve the deeper or retrobulbar or postseptal soft tissues. Periorbital cellulitis involves swelling, erythema, and tenderness but does not involve changes in extraocular motion or pupillary findings. Periorbital cellulitis does not traverse the orbital septum. As a result visual acuity, pupillary reaction, and ocular motility are preserved.

Orbital cellulitis is a true ophthalmological emergency progressing rapidly with pain with eye movement, swelling, erythema, and conjunctival infection. Extension from infected sinuses is a common cause of orbital cellulitis. Immediate evaluation should include high-resolution computed tomography (CT) scan of the orbit and paranasal sinuses to establish the presence or absence of a retroorbital abscess. Aggressive treatment should be considered, including parenteral antibiotics and possible hospitalization and drainage of the abscess.

7. What are key findings of otitis media when examining the tympanic membrane?

There are five findings used in diagnosing an ear infection (acute otitis media—AOM) that are obtained when using an otoscope and insufflator.

Diagnosing an Ear Infection

Findings	Normal Eardrum	AOM
Color	Gray or pink	Red, yellow, or cloudy
Position	Neutral position	Bulging or full position
Translucency	Clear	Opaque
Mobility	Fully mobile with pneumatic otoscopy	Reduced mobility
Ancillary findings		Effusion present

Mobility is a key finding. In children, a red eardrum can often result simply from persistent crying during the examination.

8. **What are some key concepts needed to evaluate and educate a patient with a complaint of a sore throat?**

Acute pharyngitis is one of the most common conditions encountered in office practice and emergency departments (EDs). However, group A *Streptococcus* (GAS) is the cause of only approximately 10% of adults seeking medical care for this problem. Rhinoviruses, coronaviruses, adenoviruses, parainfluenza virus, and influenza virus account for approximately 40% of pharyngitis complaints.

Patients who present with the following four clinical manifestations have a 40% to 60% chance of having GAS: (1) tonsillar exudates, (2) tender anterior cervical adenopathy, (3) history of a fever, and (4) absence of a cough.

Throat cultures have always been the "gold standard" for diagnosing streptococcal pharyngitis. The rapid antigen test (RAT) shows a sensitivity of 80% to 90% and specificity of 90% to 100%.

Treatment for GAS is based on two major strategies:

- Clinical prediction rules: Treat those with all four clinical criteria; perform RAT on those with two or three criteria and use antibiotics only if RAT results are positive.
- Results of RAT combined with clinical symptoms: Patients with a negative RAT should get a throat culture with final results in 24 to 48 hours.

Patient education about symptomatic treatment of pharyngitis that is negative for GAS is essential. Treatment includes antipyretics, fluids, and gargles. Lozenges and herbal teas may relieve irritation. Irritants such as cigarettes should be avoided.

9. **What is the significance of earwax (cerumen) in the ear canal, and when is intervention indicated?**

Cerumen is a protective covering in the ear canal. It protects the skin of the external canal from water damage, infection, and trauma, and it traps foreign particles and aids in elimination of bacteria.

The main reasons cerumen accumulates in the ear canal are:

- Obstruction of cerumen elimination by ear canal disease
- Narrowing of the ear canal

- Failure of skin migration (glands of early canal atrophy in aging process, producing a harder, less fluid cerumen that migrates more slowly)
- Overproduction

Inappropriate attempts at removal are the most common reason for cerumen accumulation. Cotton-tipped swabs tend to push cerumen deeper in the ear canal and over time can cause complete obstruction in some individuals. Hearing aids, earplugs and swim molds also obstruct the ear canal.

Cerumen needs to be removed to visualize the ear canal and tympanic membrane in the setting of otological complaints. Examples of such complaints include hearing loss, ear pain, ear fullness, unexplained fever, facial paralysis, and dizziness.

Removal methods include ear curettes, lavage, and ceruminolytics. Curettes are generally most effective for removing cerumen in the lateral third of the ear canal.

Lavage can be accomplished using a 20-ml syringe or Water Pik and a combination of warm water and hydrogen peroxide. Lavage should not be performed if the patient reports drainage from the ear, which may indicate a perforation of the tympanic membrane. Periodic evaluation during the lavage should be performed to assess the removal of wax.

Ceruminolytics are safe to use in patients with no history of infections, perforations, or otological surgery. Common ceruminolytics are preparations of mineral oil and hydrogen peroxide. Other preparations include mineral oil and liquid docusate sodium. Ceruminolytics can be used by the patient safely at home. Using two drops weekly can help prevent accumulation of cerumen.

10. **What is otitis externa, and how is it managed?**

Otitis externa, commonly called "swimmer's ear," is most often related to water retention in the external canal followed by an overgrowth of bacteria. *Pseudomonas* is the usual organism. Diagnosis is suggested when pain is elicited by pulling on the pinna or by pushing on the tragus and is confirmed by visualizing a swollen, red external ear canal, often with a purulent drainage.

Treatment is topical because otitis externa is a topical infection. An antibiotic eardrop can be administered to eradicate the bacterial infection (e.g., gentamicin, polymyxin, neomycin, Floxin, Cipro HC). Because the bacteria causing otitis externa are acid-labile, an acidic eardrop (e.g., VoSol Otic solution, four drops four times per day) is usually an effective agent. Patients should refrain from swimming during treatment, which is usually 3 to 5 days.

11. **How should the nurse respond when a parent asks how high a fever can get before it causes concern?**

Tell the parent that fever usually is defined as a rectal temperature higher than 100.4° F (38° C) or oral temperature higher than 100° F (37.8° C). In most cases fever indicates that an illness is present. Fever by itself is not harmful; in fact, it may help the body fight infections more effectively. Teething can cause a low-grade fever as high as 100° F. Body temperature also can be above normal when an infant is overdressed or in a room that is too warm. Children tend to run higher fevers than adults. Convulsions from fever occur only occasionally. Febrile convulsions occur in children who have had a *rapid* rise in temperature.

The degree of the fever is not always related to the severity of the infection. How the child looks and acts is a better guide than the thermometer. Generally, if a child older than age 3 is comfortable, leave the fever alone. If the child is uncomfortable, give acetaminophen or ibuprofen.

Contact a health professional if:

- An infant younger than 3 months of age develops a fever higher than 101° F (38.3° C)
- A child 3 months to 3 years of age has a fever of 103° F (39.4° C) or higher for 24 hours
- A child has other complaints that may be causing the fever, such as ear pain; painful urination; respiratory symptoms; joint pain; unexplained skin rash; or vomiting, diarrhea, and stomach pain

12. At what age can an accurate oral temperature be obtained on a child?

Children under the age of 2½ tend to bite down on the thermometer. However, at about the age of 2½, a child understands the concept of "making a kiss." Therefore, it is possible to insert the thermometer under the child's tongue and have the child make a kiss. It is not wise to try this with a glass thermometer because obtaining an accurate temperature with a glass thermometer requires the thermometer to be under the tongue for at least 3 minutes.

13. What is the difference between laryngitis, pharyngotonsillitis, peritonsillar abscess, and retropharyngeal abscess?

Differences Between Laryngitis, Pharyngotonsillitis, Peritonsillar Abscess, and Retropharyngeal Abscess

Diagnosis	Etiology	Signs and Symptoms
Laryngitis	Viral, upper respiratory infection	Hoarseness, caused by swelling of the vocal cords
Peritonsillar abscess	Complication of tonsillitis, frequently seen in teenagers and young adults	Facial swelling on affected side with unilateral erythema extending onto soft palate; trismus (inability to open mouth fully)
Pharyngotonsillitis	Bacteria, virus, or fungus	Fever, headache, dehydration, difficulty swallowing; soft palate, tonsils, and pharyngeal mucosa are erythematous; white or yellow exudates may be present on tonsils
Retropharyngeal abscess	Infection of space between fascia adherent to paraspinal muscles and posterior pharyngeal mucosa	Fever, neck pain, sore throat, dysphagia, and drooling; airway maintenance is of great concern

14. **What is the significance and seriousness of human bites, cat bites, and dog bites?**

Human bites or "closed fist bites" that occur to the hands carry a high rate of infection and potential for loss of function. These bites always need to be treated with antibiotics and often require examination under anesthesia to evaluate the extent of the injury and perform extensive wound irrigation. Aggressive use of antibiotics for 10 to 14 days is necessary.

Cat bites account for 10% to 18% of reported animal bites. These often occur on the fingers, hands, and forearms. Because the cat's teeth are sharp and small, they cause deep puncture wounds and are associated with a high rate of infection. The major pathogen is *Pasteurella multocida*, which results in a rapidly developing inflammatory response with pain, swelling, and minimal discharge. These wounds should be aggressively cleaned, dressed, and splinted.

Dog bites are responsible for 90% of reported animal bites. Although dog bites carry a lower rate of infection, they still require irrigation and treatment with antibiotics. Closure of these wounds is often delayed 3 to 4 days unless they are on the face.

15. **What factors determine whether a laceration is sutured?**

Indications for sutures include deep cuts that have jagged edges or gape open; deep lacerations over a joint (i.e., elbow, knuckle, knee); lacerations on the palm side of the hand or fingers; lacerations on the face, eyelids, or lips; lacerations in an area where scarring is a concern; and lacerations that extend into the muscle or bone. There is a 6- to 10-hour window of time following an injury when a laceration can be repaired. After that time, the risk of infection rises sharply.

16. **What factors should be considered when evaluating extremity injuries?**

- Mechanism of injury. Falling on an outstretched arm is associated with wrist fractures. Hyperextension of the elbow is associated with supracondylar fracture of the distal humerus.
- Anatomical and radiological evaluation of the extremity. It is important to remove clothing and jewelry from the injured part. Inspect the extremity for deformity, swelling, and bruising. Palpate the extremity to identify the most tender spot. This is important in identifying what x-ray to order.
- Neurovascular status distal to the injury should be included in the initial exam and after splinting, especially if there is a fracture. The radial nerve is tested in the web space between the thumb and index finger. The median nerve is tested at the tip of the index finger. The ulnar nerve can be tested at the small finger.

17. **What acronym is used to evaluate fractures of a long bone when viewing an x-ray?**

LARD

L   Length: Is the bone lengthened or shortened?

A   Angulation: Angulation is often described in terms of the distal fragment (i.e., a distal radius fracture may have a dorsally angulated distal fragment [apex volar]).

R   Rotation: Are bone fragments rotated? Look at the bone fragment edges and see if they line up.

D   Displacement: Is the fracture displaced? This is usually described as a percentage.

18. What is plantar fasciitis?

The plantar fascia arises from the calcaneus bone in the foot and inserts into the forefoot at the metatarsal heads. This band of fascia supports the internal convex arch of the metatarsal bones.

Plantar fasciitis is an inflammatory condition that presents as tenderness at the medial portion of the calcaneus and in the bottom of the foot medially. Common symptoms are pain in the heel, particularly with walking, on arising, and when barefoot.

Initial treatment includes ice to the area, NSAIDs, stretches of the Achilles' tendons, heel pads or orthotics, physical therapy, and possibly steroid injections.

19. What is the difference between a sprain and a strain?

A sprain is a ligamentous injury. Ligaments connect bones to bones. Common sprains involve the ankle.

A strain is a pulled muscle. Tendons connect muscles to bones. Common strains involve the muscles of the upper back and the hamstring of the lower leg.

20. What are the Ottawa ankle rules?

They are indicators for obtaining an x-ray for an acute ankle injury to rule out a fracture.
- Tenderness on palpation at the (posterior) tip of the lateral malleolus.
- Tenderness on palpation at the (posterior) tip of the medial malleolus.
- Inability to bear weight (four steps) at the time of injury or at the time of physical exam.

Physician discretion dictates the use of the rules when treating an ankle injury.

21. Why and when are women more prone to urinary tract infections (UTIs)? What is the pathogenesis?

The female anatomy, specifically the shorter length of the female urethra compared with the male, predisposes women to UTIs. Symptomatic lower UTIs are more common during pregnancy and with the onset of sexual activity.

The pathogenesis of UTIs in women is related most commonly to the ascent of gram-negative aerobic bacilli in the urethra. The vast majority of these are *Escherichia coli* (90% of first episodes). Staphylococci, saprophytic, and species of *Klebsiella, Proteus, Enterobacter,* and *Pseudomonas* may also cause infection.

Also consider other infections with similar symptoms, such as vaginitis, pelvic inflammatory disease (PID), and sexually transmitted infections (STIs) as differential diagnoses.

22. **What is the best way to identify and manage croup?**

Croup is a respiratory problem most common in children 2 to 4 years old. It usually accompanies a viral infection, such as a cold. The main symptom is a harsh cough that sounds like a seal's bark. A fever from 100° to 101° F (37.7° to 38.3° C) is common. Croup usually worsens at night and may last several days. Immediate home treatment is cool moist air. Going out into the cool fresh air at night or using a cool mist vaporizer are helpful, but advise parents to keep the child dressed warmly. Another option for moist air is to sit with the child in the bathroom with hot water running and the door closed.

Assessing the degree of respiratory distress is essential. Immediate medical care is needed if the child has stridor, a squeaky or raspy sound on inhalation; costal retractions; flaring of the nostrils; inability to talk or walk because of shortness of breath; or drooling or breathing with the chin jutting out and the mouth open. Steroids may be prescribed to treat croup.

23. **What can a patient do to manage a common viral upper respiratory infection?**

Educating the general population that there are more than 200 viruses causing infection, many of which present with upper respiratory symptoms such as the common cold, is an ongoing challenge. Symptoms of the common cold include runny nose, red eyes, sneezing, sore throat, dry cough, headache, and general body aches. As the disease progresses, the sore throat lessens and nasal drainage may thicken. Symptoms usually last 1 to 2 weeks.

Treatment focuses on alleviating the symptoms. A decongestant such as pseudoephedrine helps to relieve the nasal stuffiness. A cough suppressant containing dextromethorphan helps to control a nagging cough. Acetaminophen or ibuprofen lessens general body aches and low-grade fever. Teaching the patient that antibiotics will not cure a viral infection is essential. If, however, the symptoms worsen over the course of a viral infection, including a change in the color of the sputum, increasing shortness of breath, tightness in the chest, persistent fever, localized sinus pain, or a cough that lingers more than 10 to 14 days, the patient should be evaluated for a possible secondary bacterial infection.

24. **What are some key facts about back pain?**

Back pain affects 90% of the population at some time. It is second only to only upper respiratory infection as a symptom-related reason for visits to the primary care doctor or an urgent care clinic. The following table summarizes "red flags" in the history and physical examination that signal potentially serious back conditions.

Serious Back Conditions

Red Flag	Possible Cause
Duration longer than 6 weeks	Tumor, infection, rheumatological problem
Age younger than 18 years	Congenital defect, tumor, infection
Age older than 50 years	Tumor, abdominal aortic aneurysm, infection
Major trauma	Fracture
Cancer history	Tumor
Fever, chills, night sweats	Tumor, infection
Weight loss	Tumor, infection
Injection drug use	Infection
Immunocompromised status	Infection
Recent GI or GU procedure	Infection
Night pain	Tumor, infection
Unremitting pain, even when supine	Tumor, infection, abdominal aortic aneurysm, nephrolithiasis
Pain worsened by coughing	Herniated disk
Saddle anesthesia	Cauda equina syndrome

GI, gastrointestinal; *GU*, genitourinary.

25. **What symptoms should alert the clinician to a serious back problem requiring emergent management?**

    - Unexpected anal sphincter laxity
    - Perianal or perineal sensory loss (saddle anesthesia)
    - Major motor weakness
    - Point tenderness to percussion
    - Positive straight leg raise test result with radiation of pain below knee

26. **Which disc is most commonly involved in low back pain?**

    L4 to L5—the L5 nerve root

27. **What is paronychia, and how is it treated?**

    Paronychia is an infection of the soft tissue surrounding the nail bed. These infections usually begin from a hangnail or splintered nail penetrating the adjacent soft tissue. *Staphylococcus aureus* is the most common infecting organism. Symptoms include unilateral redness, swelling, and tenderness. Treatment involves drainage of the fluctuant area by advancing a scalpel away from the nail bed. The patient should also be placed on an antibiotic for several days.

28. **How should the nurse approach patients with common complaints such as headache and back pain?**

    Common complaints often trigger personal biases among staff. Leave these biases at home; do not let them cloud decision making or prevent listening to the patient and performing a proper assessment. Be aware that patients' underlying problems are often "hidden" from the medically oriented chief complaint. Try asking patients to tell the story of what brought them to the ED.

Key Points

- Musculoskeletal injuries are common nonurgent problems. They require careful assessment to identify specific injuries and differentiate more serious injuries requiring emergent care.

- Nonurgent problems are often issues that do not require a visit to an ED but also cannot wait 1 to 2 weeks to be evaluated at a regular office visit. Dental and ear, nose, or throat (ENT) complaints are common and require management.

- Careful questioning when obtaining the history will help identify a more serious or emergent problem.

- Good assessment skills include careful examination (e.g., assessing the ears or throat, palpating an injured extremity).

- Patient teaching regarding medical problems is a key component in helping patients understand their illness and its management.

Internet Resources

American Academy of Family Physicians, familydoctor.org, Urinary Tract Infections
www.familydoctor.org/190.xml

WebMD, Understanding Otitis Media:
www.webmd.com/content/article/54/61540.htm

Bibliography

Barker LR et al: *Principles of ambulatory medicine,* ed 6, Baltimore, 2002, Lippincott Williams & Wilkins.

Biros M, Sterner S, Vogel E: *Handbook of urgent care medicine,* ed 2, Philadelphia, 2002, Hanley & Belfus.

Della-Giustina D, Kilcline B: Acute low back pain: Recognizing the "red flags" in the workup, *Consultant* 1277, 2002.

Edwards T, Mayer T: *Urgent care medicine,* New York, 2002, McGraw-Hill.

Heikkinen T, Jarvinen A: The common cold, *Lancet* 361(9351):51-59, 2003.

Henry G: Medical practice risk assessment: An introduction to emergency medicine risk management, continuing medical education lecture, attended February 7, 2005.

Pichichero ME: Acute otitis media: Part I. Improving diagnostic accuracy, *Am Fam Physician* 61: 2051-2056, 2000.

Schroeder M: Describing fractures, *Clin Advis* 76, January 2001.

Section III

Trauma Care

Mechanism of Injury

Debra Cason and Karen M. Pickard

1. What does "mechanism of injury" mean?

"Mechanism of injury" refers to how a traumatic event occurred, the injuring agent, and information about the type and amount of energy exchanged during the event.

2. Why is the mechanism of injury important to emergency nurses?

Knowledge of how a traumatic event occurred assists in the early identification and management of injuries that may not be apparent on initial assessment. Overlooked injuries can be devastating, particularly when they become apparent only after the body has exhausted compensatory mechanisms. In addition, knowledge of mechanism-of-injury patterns can assist the emergency nurse in injury prevention and patient teaching during the "teachable moment."

3. How is information about mechanism of injury collected?

The patient is a great source of information if he or she is verbal and recollects the incident. Otherwise, do not let prehospital personnel leave without obtaining information about the scene, vehicle damage (if a vehicle was involved), assailant (if one exists), and other valuable information that they may have. Police or family members also may provide helpful information. In the case of vehicle crashes, many prehospital personnel units take pictures of the car and are able to bring the pictures to the hospital with the patient. These pictures can provide additional clues to potential injuries.

4. What types of questions should be asked?

In general, the main questions are, "What happened?" and "How was the patient injured?" Depending on the injuring agent, the following pieces of information may be vital:
Vehicle collisions:
- Type of crash
- Location in the vehicle
- Type of seat belts worn (lap belt or three-point restraints)
- Presence and deployment of air bags (frontal, side impact)
- Whether a helmet was worn (motorcycle or bicycle collision)
- Speed of the vehicle at impact
- Whether rapid deceleration occurred

- What was hit
- Interior and exterior damage to the vehicle, including a spider type configuration on the windshield from the inside
- Intrusion into the passenger compartment of the vehicle
- Whether the patient hit the steering wheel, dashboard, or windshield
- Condition of the steering wheel, dashboard (bent, indented), and windshield
- Evidence of vehicle rollover, and if so, approximately how many times

Gunshot wounds or stabs:
- Type of weapon (type of knife or firearm)
- Caliber of bullet
- Length of knife
- Position of patient when event occurred

Falls:
- Height of fall
- What the patient landed on
- Impacted body part(s)

5. **How do the type of energy and amount of energy affect the patient?**

Energy comes in various forms. Most of the trauma seen in the emergency department (ED) is from mechanical energy or motion that transfers energy to the body during either blunt trauma (vehicle collisions, falls, aggravated assaults, contact sports) or penetrating trauma (gunshot wounds or stabs). As Newton's Law of Conservation of Energy states, energy cannot be created or destroyed—it can only be changed in form. Thus, when a vehicle in motion stops, the energy must be changed to another form. Hopefully, for the sake of the driver and passengers, the energy is changed into thermal (heat) energy from friction of the brakes, and a safe stop occurs. However, if a vehicle crashes into a wall, the energy is distributed to the vehicle and the persons in it, causing vehicle damage and bodily injury.

6. **What are likely mechanisms of injury in vehicle crashes?**

A compression or crushing type of injury is experienced in automobile crashes because of the three types of collisions:
- **Machine collision:** The vehicle impacts another stationary or moving object, and mechanical energy may cause direct contact injury to the driver or passenger.
- **Body collision:** The victim hits parts of the vehicle, such as the windshield and steering wheel.
- **Organ collision:** The supporting body structures, such as cranium, ribs, or spine, collide with movable organs, such as the brain, heart, liver, or spleen.

7. **What injuries should the nurse anticipate in a sudden deceleration event?**

Sudden deceleration injuries can result from vehicle crashes or falls. As the collision occurs, fixed vessels and organs shear away from their attachments as one organ continues its forward motion and another organ stops abruptly. Common deceleration injuries include tears (partial or complete) of the descending thoracic aorta, stretching or tearing of the renal artery from the renal pedicle, intestinal and spleen attachment tears, and liver lacerations.

8. What are common types of vehicle crashes?

- Head-on collision (frontal impact)
- T-bone or lateral impact collision
- Rear-end collision
- Rollover

9. What injuries commonly result from a head-on collision?

In a head-on collision, the energy transfer to the body can be tremendous and causes multiple injuries. The unrestrained person is likely to strike the windshield, steering column, or dashboard. Injuries to anticipate from the windshield include injuries to the head and cervical spine, larynx, and trachea. Injuries to anticipate from the steering wheel include laryngeal and tracheal injuries; pulmonary contusions; myocardial contusions; rib fractures with pneumothorax, hemothorax, or flail chest; abdominal organ lacerations and rupture; diaphragm rupture; and shearing injuries at the aortic arch, liver, spleen, or kidneys. The dashboard injury should arouse suspicion for injuries to the head, face, cervical spine, hip, pelvis, and knees.

10. What injuries commonly result from a T-bone or lateral impact collision?

When the side of the vehicle is impacted, a similar mechanism occurs as in a head-on collision except that additional lateral energy is involved. Commonly the head is struck, causing direct injury to the impacted side plus injury to the opposite side when the brain collides against the cranium (coup-contrecoup injury). The neck may sustain both lateral flexion and rotation of the cervical spine, leading to severe injury. The humerus or clavicle can sustain a fracture on the side of impact. Depending on the degree of displaced energy, thoracic injuries may include rib fractures, pulmonary contusion, pneumothorax, hemothorax, and aortic injury. Lateral impact can also cause abdominal organ tears, pelvic injuries, and lower extremity injuries depending on the level of the impact. If a right-side occupant is struck, consider liver injury; if a left-side occupant is stuck, consider spleen injury.

11. What injuries should the nurse suspect in the patient involved in a rear-end collision?

If the car is struck by a vehicle traveling at a high speed, the sudden acceleration can cause hyperextension of the cervical spine if the headrest is not properly adjusted. Deceleration injuries also should be suspected. A subsequent frontal collision may occur if the vehicle has been projected forward.

12. Can the nurse predict injuries sustained in a rollover collision?

Not really. Rollover collisions involve the potential for significant injury, but any of a wide variety of injuries may occur. It is important to remember that there is a potential for impact of the patient with the vehicle every time the vehicle rolls over. Ejection of an unrestrained occupant is more likely in a rollover collision and is associated with a high mortality rate.

13. **What restraint system provides the best protection against injury in a vehicle collision?**

The three-point system of a lap and shoulder belt is the most effective method of restraint. When worn properly, the diagonal belt stops forward movement of the upper body, usually preventing dashboard, windshield, and steering wheel impact. Proper use means that the lap belt is worn below the anterior/superior iliac spines of the pelvis and above the femur. In addition, the belt must not be loose and should secure the occupant to the vehicle frame during collision. The shoulder-belt component should fit snugly across the shoulder, clavicle, and rib cage. Shoulder restraints worn alone can result in neck injuries, torsion, and even decapitation.

14. **Do air bags minimize injury?**

Air bags are supplemental protective devices and do not replace seat belts. Air bags reduce fatalities in frontal crashes by about 30% but are not beneficial in some types of crashes. Air bags do not provide protection if a second impact occurs, nor do they provide protection in rollover or rear-end collisions. Side air bag systems are now in use in some vehicles, as are some under-the-dash air bags.

Deployment of air bags does not guarantee an injury-free occupant. A false sense of security concerning the patient protected by an air bag may result in delayed identification of significant injuries. EMS personnel should be instructed to lift and look under the air bag to ascertain steering wheel condition. It should also be noted that steering wheel air bags do not prevent injuries that can occur as the driver is forced down and under the steering wheel and pushed against the lower dash.

15. **Do air bags cause injuries?**

Air bags frequently produce minor abrasions or burns to the arms, chest, eyes, and face, as well as injury from the occupant's eyeglasses. Air bags have caused approximately 100 deaths since their introduction in 1986. In each death the air bag was extremely close to the victim. The victims have been (1) unrestrained young children, (2) infants in rear-facing child seats who ride with their heads extremely close to the passenger air bag, and (3) drivers (especially unrestrained ones) who sit extremely close to the steering wheel. For this reason, children and infants should ride restrained in the back seat. In addition, vehicle manufacturers can install manual on/off switches for passenger air bags in vehicles without appropriate rear seats for children or for people who are short in stature and therefore must sit within 10 inches of the steering wheel. Ten inches is considered to be the minimum required distance for prevention of air bag injuries.

16. **What injuries should be anticipated in the pedestrian struck by a motor vehicle?**

Typically there are three impacts in the adult pedestrian struck by a motor vehicle:
- The vehicle's front bumper collides with the adult's legs and pelvis.
- The torso and head hit the vehicle's hood and windshield.
- The victim falls off the vehicle and either hits the ground or another object. Head and spine injuries are likely during this phase.

17. Children constitute a large percentage of pedestrian-vehicle collisions. Is the mechanism of injury different in children and adults?

Yes. Compared with adults, children are shorter, lighter, and more likely to be facing the oncoming vehicle (adults tend to be struck in the side as they attempt to get out of the way). Impacts in the child pedestrian struck by a motor vehicle include:
- The vehicle's front bumper collides with the child's anterior pelvis or torso.
- The child's head or face collides with either the ground or the vehicle's hood.
- The child may be dragged by the car or run over by a front wheel. Children are less likely than adults to be thrown clear of the car.

18. What are the important factors in falls?

- **Distance (height) of the fall**. As a general rule, a fall of three times a person's height can cause severe injury. Low-level falls (less than 20 feet) are underappreciated as a mechanism of injury and also cause significant injuries, most commonly to the head and spine. Deceleration type injuries also occur.
- **Area of the body hitting bottom**. If the fall is feet first and the energy is transferred to a small area (even if the victim wears size 13 shoes), heel, femur, hip, and pelvis fractures should be suspected, as well as vertebral compression fractures. If a larger portion of the body hits the surface (e.g., the back), the energy is dissipated over more surface area and the injuries are likely to be less severe.
- **Type of surface struck**. If the surface struck is soft ground, the injuries may be less severe than if the surface is hard or irregular, such as stadium seating or a concrete sidewalk.

19. How is the mechanism of injury in falls altered in older patients?

The mechanism of injury does not vary in older patients. However, a simple fall can cause significant injury. People older than 65 have a lower injury rate than people younger than 50, but they are much more likely to die from their injuries. Falls are the leading cause of accidental deaths in older persons and a major cause of disability. Older persons are predisposed to falls because of their general loss of agility and proprioception (position sense) in the lower extremities, as well as loss of vestibular function and visual sensory input. Underlying medical problems and medications also may predispose older adults to falls. Musculoskeletal injuries are most common. Extremity fractures account for the majority of fractures, followed by face, rib, spine, and skull fractures.

20. How are penetrating weapons classified?

The energy produced by a bullet or knife depends mostly on velocity; consequently weapons are classified as high, medium, or low velocity. Low-velocity weapons such as knives are much less destructive than medium-velocity weapons (handguns and some types of rifles) or high-velocity weapons (assault weapons, hunting rifles). Low-velocity weapons, however, certainly can cause fatal injuries, depending on the body part struck.

21. **How do the physical characteristics of the bullet affect injury to the patient?**

   - The larger the size of the impact surface area (i.e., the larger the bullet), the greater the damage.
   - A hollow-point bullet widens when it hits tissues, causing a wider path of destruction.
   - The bullet that tumbles around damages more tissue.
   - Soft-nose bullets or bullets with vertical cuts in the nose break apart on impact, spreading fragments in a wider path and causing more tissue and organ damage. A shotgun blast also causes fragmentation.

22. **How does an entrance wound differ from an exit wound?**

   An entrance wound is typically round or oval with a small black or red area around the wound. Powder wounds may be present if the injury was sustained at close range. An exit wound is usually ragged and irregular because the tissue splits as the bullet exits the body. However, nursing documentation should not identify wounds as "entrance" or "exit." Simply document the location and appearance of the wounds and let forensic experts determine which wound is which.

23. **After an entrance and an exit wound have been identified, can the nurse accurately trace the path of the bullet and consequently identify the likely organs injured?**

   Yes and no. Because the characteristics of missiles and the density and elasticity of body tissue are variable, the path of damage may not coincide with a line drawn from entrance wound to exit wound. For example, a bullet that encounters bone at a certain angle may follow the curvature of the bone. However, in many cases the missile follows the predicted path, damaging surrounding tissue and organs up to 14 times the diameter of the missile.

24. **A patient who has been stabbed in the chest at the nipple line may sustain injury to which organs?**

   Because the diaphragm can rise as high as the nipple line with deep inspiration, a stab wound to the nipple line can injure not only intrathoracic structures but also abdominal structures and organs.

25. **Which abdominal organs are most likely to be damaged by penetrating trauma?**

   The small and large intestines, liver, and stomach are the most likely abdominal organs to be affected by a penetrating injury.

26. **In-line skaters (roller bladers) appear in the ED frequently. What are their typical injuries?**

   In-line skaters primarily sustain upper limb injuries, usually radial fractures close to the wrist. The site of the initial impact when an in-line skater falls is most often the hands and wrists. The second most likely location for injury is the lower extremity. In addition, use of wrist guards and other protective gear is not common among in-line skaters.

27. **People with car radiator burns often appear in the ED during the summer months. What types of injuries should be anticipated?**

The most common types of injuries that occur with car radiators are scald burns to the face, head, and upper torso with car radiator fluid. These injuries can include blindness and disfiguring burns to the upper torso and upper extremities.

28. **Trampolines have become increasingly popular. What types of injuries should be anticipated from them?**

Although trampoline injuries are on the increase, they still rank behind bicycle, baseball, and softball injuries in children. However, there are still large numbers of trampoline injuries. Extremity injuries are the most common trampoline injury, but cervical spine injuries also occur. Landing on the head from a jump high into the air can result in lower cervical spine injury. Extremity injuries may include knee dislocations from landing on hyperextended legs.

29. **What are some of the mechanisms of injury in crush syndrome?**

A common scenario is patients being crushed under heavy objects for a period of time, such as in structural collapse. In structural collapse the entire body is often involved and the outcome is usually poor. Other types of injuries in which crush injuries occur are limbs that are caught in machinery, or when a single limb is caught under an immovable object for a prolonged period of time.

30. **Are there other things to consider with a crushed limb besides the obvious trauma?**

Yes. It is important to consider the entrapment time, or the time that the limb has been immovable. The crushed and torn tissue and the resultant hemorrhage are part of the obvious injury, but the anoxia and absent circulation to the crushed tissue must also be evaluated. Tissue ischemia and muscle destruction create rhabdomyolysis, which in turn causes a release of myoglobin. Ultimately the myoglobin will be toxic to the renal tubules, causing renal failure, electrolyte imbalances, acid-base imbalances, cardiac arrhythmias, and death. Some prehospital agencies have protocols regarding extrication from prolonged crush scenarios that are intended to protect the patient from the sudden release of myoglobin into the systemic circulation.

Key Points

- Injuries may not be obvious upon initial assessment; knowledge of mechanism will assist in early identification of nonapparent injuries.

- Understanding energy exchange during traumatic events assists in determining the types of injuries to anticipate. If, for example, a vehicle comes to a sudden stop, the nurse will benefit from knowing whether the patient was restrained and whether the vehicle stopped with no further movement, causing the patient to absorb all of the energy from the collision.

- Important factors to consider after a fall include the distance of the fall compared with the person's height, the part of the body hitting the surface, and the type of surface struck.

- Mechanism of injury principles do not vary for falls in older adults, but the injuries sustained can have longer lasting, more disabling effects. They also have an associated high mortality rate.

- Crush syndrome is a critical, yet often underestimated effect of injury that leads to renal failure and death if not recognized and treated rapidly.

Internet Resources

Department of Transportation, National Highway Traffic Safety Administration, Federal Motor Vehicle Safety Standards; Occupant Crash Protection:
www.nhtsa.dot.gov/cars/rules/rulings/Anton_FRNov16.html

National Highway Traffic Safety Administration:
www.nhtsa.gov

Bibliography

Atwell SL: Trauma in the elderly. In McQuillan K et al, editors: *Trauma nursing from resuscitation through rehabilitation*, ed 3, Philadelphia, 2002, WB Saunders.

Bledsoe BE, Porter RS, Cherry RA: *Paramedic care principles and practice: Trauma emergencies*, vol 4, ed 2, Upper Saddle River, NJ, 2005, Pearson Education.

Campbell JA, editor: *Basic trauma life support*, ed 5, Upper Saddle River, NJ, 2004, Pearson Education.

Creel JH: Scene sizeup. In Campbell JE, editor: *Basic trauma life support*, Englewood Cliffs, NJ, 2004, Brady.

Esposito PW: Trampoline injuries, *Clin Orthop* 409:43-52, 2003.

Grange JT, Corbett SW, Cotton A: Street bikes versus dirt bikes: A comparison of injuries among motorcyclists presenting to a regional trauma center, *J Trauma* 57(3):591-594, 2004.

Grossman M: Patterns of blunt injury. In Pleitzman AB et al, editors: *The trauma manual*, Philadelphia, 2002, Lippincott Williams & Wilkins.

Hubble MW, Hubble JP: *Principles of advanced trauma care*, Albany, NY, 2002, Delmar.

Johnston JJ, McGovern SJ: Alcohol related falls: An interesting pattern of injuries, *Emerg Med J* 21(2): 185-188, 2004.

Keall M, Frith W: Adjusting for car occupant injury liability in relation to age, speed limit, and gender specific driver crash involvement risk, *Traffic Inj Prev* 5(4):336-342, 2004.

Rabbitts A et al: Car radiator burns: A prevention issue, *J Burn Care Rehabil* 25(5):452-455, 2004.

Rowe SA et al: Pelvic ring fractures: Implications of vehicle design, crash type, and occupant characteristics, *Surgery* 135(4):842-847, 2004.

Sanders MJ, McKenna K, editors: Trauma systems and mechanism of injury. In Sanders MJ: *Paramedic textbook*, ed 3, St Louis, 2005, Mosby.

Walsh CR: Musculoskeletal injuries. In McQuillan KA et al, editors: *Trauma nursing from resuscitation through rehabilitation*, ed 3, Philadelphia, 2002, WB Saunders.

Weigelt JA, Klein JD: Mechanism of injury. In McQuillan KA et al, editors: *Trauma nursing from resuscitation through rehabilitation*, ed 3, Philadelphia, 2002, WB Saunders.

Shock

Sharon Saunderson Cohen

1. **What is shock?**

   Shock is inadequate tissue perfusion resulting in oxygen debt at the cellular level. Shock may be due to failure of one of three components of the body that affects the delivery of oxygen and nutrients to the cells: the heart (pump), the vascular system (vessels), or the circulating blood volume. Ultimately, shock leads to organ failure and death if not reversed.

2. **What are the four types of shock?**

   - Hypovolemic (a result of blood [hemorrhagic] or fluid loss)
   - Cardiogenic
   - Distributive (also known as vasogenic, which includes septic, anaphylactic, and neurogenic causes of shock)
   - Obstructive (caused by pericardial tamponade and tension pneumothorax)

3. **What are the endpoints of resuscitation?**

   Normalization of heart rate (HR), blood pressure (BP), and pulse pressure; improved mentation; and adequate tissue perfusion and urine output are indicators of a stabilized patient. Because stability may be transient, continued evaluation and close monitoring of the patient are necessary.

4. **How is cardiac output (CO) calculated? What is the normal value? Why is it important?**

$$CO = \text{stroke volume (SV)} \times HR$$

   The normal value of CO in adults is 3 L/min. CO serves as the primary compensatory mechanism for increasing oxygen delivery to the tissues when needed.

HYPOVOLEMIC SHOCK

5. **What is hypovolemic shock?**

   Hypovolemic shock results from acute blood loss (hemorrhagic shock) or the loss of plasma and extracellular fluids with reduction of intravascular volume.

6. What are the most common causes of hypovolemic shock?

Causes of hypovolemic shock include gastrointestinal (GI) bleeding; ruptured ectopic pregnancy; severe burns; and dehydration resulting from vomiting, diarrhea, profuse diaphoresis, or nasogastric suctioning. In trauma, it is the most common form of shock and results from acute blood loss (overt and covert).

7. What are the common signs and symptoms of *early* hypovolemic shock?

Altered level of consciousness. This simple but consistent sign in the awake patient is one of the earliest indicators of shock. In particular, restlessness, agitation, and central nervous system depression are key indicators. In addition to a change in level of consciousness, other signs and symptoms such as cold, clammy skin; orthostatic hypotension; mild tachycardia; and vasoconstriction may be present. These indicate that compensatory mechanisms such as vasoconstriction and catecholamine release are attempting to optimize blood flow to vital organs.

8. What are the common signs and symptoms of *late* hypovolemic shock?

Late signs of shock include a marked change in mental status (including coma), hypotension, and marked tachycardia.

Caution: In hemorrhagic hypovolemic shock, the otherwise healthy adult does not become hypotensive until as much as 30% of the blood volume is lost. Impending shock should be treated as quickly as possible, before the patient becomes hypotensive.

9. Why does tachycardia occur in hypovolemic shock?

Tachycardia occurs as an early compensatory mechanism to maintain or increase CO and to improve perfusion to the vital organs and tissues. If SV decreases, HR increases to maintain CO.

10. Do all patients in hypovolemic shock experience tachycardia?

No. Often elderly patients or patients with a known history of myocardial infarction (MI) are taking beta blockers, which block the compensatory mechanism of tachycardia. When an elderly trauma patient arrives in the emergency department (ED) with obvious blood loss, a HR of 80 beats per minute, and decreasing BP, think of beta blockade. Even more complex is the patient who has a concomitant spinal cord injury and therefore cannot increase HR in response to blood loss and hypotension.

11. What is the best way to manage hypovolemic shock before or in addition to treating the underlying cause?

Warmed intravenous (IV) fluids and blood.

12. In traumatic hemorrhage, is it necessary to treat hypovolemic shock with IV fluids and blood?

Yes. But IV fluids and blood only buy time to get the patient to the operating room (OR) for surgical correction of the bleeding (if bleeding is the cause). The greater the hemodynamic stability at the time of surgery, the better the outcome.

A controversial study by Bickell et al (1994) demonstrated improved outcomes when aggressive administration of IV fluids to hypotensive patients with penetrating injuries to the torso was delayed until the time of operative intervention. More data are needed before substantial practice changes can be recommended.

13. **What is the preferred initial fluid for the resuscitation of patients in hypovolemic shock?**

Initially an isotonic crystalloid solution, such as lactated Ringer's (LR), should be infused. Normal saline (NS) is an acceptable alternative but may produce metabolic acidosis with prolonged administration. The preferred fluid for resuscitation is controversial: either a crystalloid or colloid solution. Weinstein and Doerfler (1992) describe complications with crystalloid fluid resuscitation, whereas Schierhout and Roberts (1998) identify complications with colloid fluid resuscitation. Schierhout and Roberts acknowledge that neither fluid has been associated with better outcomes in any randomized trial. Because colloids are considerably more expensive than crystalloids, crystalloid fluids usually are recommended.

14. **When should blood transfusions be started in patients with hypovolemic shock?**

Studies examining the time to begin blood resuscitation report varying results. As a general rule, most trauma centers initially infuse 2 to 3 liters of LR or NS, then begin blood if the patient remains symptomatic. During the administration of the crystalloid infusion, the patient should be type and cross matched so that type-specific blood can be administered.

15. **If type-specific blood is not available, what is the blood type of choice for emergency transfusion?**

Type-specific blood is preferred, but when time is of the essence and the patient is in shock, the universal donor type O, Rh-negative is given. In men and women beyond childbearing age, O, Rh-positive blood often is administered until type-specific blood is available.

16. **What compound, found in circulating blood, is missing from crystalloid solutions and banked blood?**

Banked blood (older than a few days) and crystalloids lack 2,3-diphosphoglyceric acid (2,3-DPG). This lack causes an increase in hemoglobin-oxygen affinity, which means that the blood molecule does not easily release the oxygen molecule to the tissues.

17. **Are there any new treatment modalities on the horizon for the treatment of hemorrhagic shock?**

The optimal type and amount of fluid for resuscitation of injured patients in hemorrhagic hypovolemic shock remains controversial. Use of HS-DFO (Hespan [hydroxyethyl starch—HS], a colloid plasma expander, and deferoxamine [DFO], an iron chelator and oxygen-free radical scavenger) was recently studied in animal models (Waheed, 2002). The data from these studies show promise in the use of HS-DFO conjugate as a resuscitative adjuvant for hemorrhagic hypovolemic shock.

18. What is the shock index (SI)?

$$SI = HR \div \text{systolic BP}$$

SI may be a useful marker of acute critical illness. The normal value is 0.5 to 0.7. Values above 0.9 have been associated with injury or illness requiring immediate intervention.

19. Are orthostatic vital signs helpful to diagnose hypovolemia?

Current literature indicates that the most helpful physical findings associated with blood loss are severe postural dizziness (which prevents measurement of upright vital signs) or a postural pulse change of 30 beats per minute or more (Bench, 2004).

To obtain orthostatic vital signs, take the pulse and BP after the patient has been supine for 2 minutes. Then have the patient assume an upright standing position, and note any symptoms of hypotension (e.g., dizziness, lightheadedness, feelings of near syncope). Standing vital signs should be obtained after 1 minute; counting the pulse for 30 seconds and doubling the result is more accurate than counting for 15 seconds. Orthostatic hypotension generally is defined as a decline of 20 mmHg or more in systolic pressure on assuming an upright standing position *along with* clinical signs and symptoms.

20. What central venous pressure (CVP) value may indicate hypovolemic shock?

CVP is determined by four components: blood volume, intrathoracic pressure, right ventricular (RV) function, and venomotor tone. Normal values are 6 to 12 cmH$_2$O. A CVP below 6 cmH$_2$O generally indicates hypovolemia. An elevated CVP, however, does not rule out hypovolemia. Certain pathologies, such as RV infarction or pulmonary embolism (PE), can produce a high CVP, yet the patient has a low left ventricular (LV) filling pressure and needs volume infusions. Like most numbers, the trend in CVP readings with volume challenges is more helpful than absolute numbers.

21. How can one tell whether fluid resuscitation is adequate or more fluid is needed?

Follow the CVP measurement trend. For example, if CVP is low and volume challenge results in minimal change in CVP, the patient is significantly hypovolemic and further aggressive crystalloid fluids are needed. If CVP is normal, however, and volume challenge results in a rapid increase in CVP with no improvement or deterioration in hemodynamic status, the cause of the shock state is pump dysfunction and further volume infusion is not indicated. In all patients, especially those who are very young or elderly and those with renal impairment or poor cardiac pump, fluid resuscitation carries the risk of fluid overload. Frequent patient reassessment is key to successful fluid resuscitation.

22. Are there any endpoints to resuscitation?

Several factors may be considered as endpoints in shock resuscitation. Obviously adequate oxygenation on the cellular level is required. The multitude of factors that play into oxygenation and the definition of "optimal" are all considered in the predictive outcome of a patient in shock. To look at global endpoints, oxygen delivery and the timeliness of return to supranormal oxygen delivery are important. Hemodynamic stability and urine output are also considerations; however, the practitioner must keep in mind the physiological state of the patient, including age, (the young and elderly carry more risk for fluid imbalances and complications such as fluid overload), premorbid conditions, and length of time in a shock state. Several endpoints have been discussed by Tisherman et al (2003), including mixed venous oxygen saturation, invasive hemodynamic monitoring and interpretation, arterial base deficit, arterial lactate, end-tidal carbon dioxide levels, gastric tonometry, and physical examination.

23. Are military antishock trousers (MASTs; also known as pneumatic antishock garments or PASGs) indicated for control of hemorrhage?

In the trauma setting MASTs do *not* improve survival, and their application must not delay transport or fluid resuscitation. Currently recommended indications for use include stabilization of pelvic and lower extremity fractures and control of associated hemorrhage.

CARDIOGENIC SHOCK

24. What is cardiogenic shock?

Cardiogenic shock results when the pump or heart becomes inefficient, resulting in decreased CO and inadequate tissue perfusion. The mortality rate is as high as 70% to 90% without aggressive and highly technical care. Classic cardiogenic shock is related to systolic dysfunction or inability of the heart to pump blood. The result is a decrease in SV and, therefore, a decrease in CO.

25. What are the common causes of cardiogenic shock?

The heart can become inefficient for various reasons, including MI (in particular, any significant loss of LV myocardium, especially in patients with ischemic heart disease) and blunt cardiac injury.

26. What are the clinical symptoms of cardiogenic shock?

Symptoms vary with the cause of pump failure. Because of reduced CO, stimulation of the sympathetic nervous system, and decreased peripheral perfusion, nonspecific findings include cool and clammy skin, decreased pulse pressure with weak peripheral pulses, fatigue, weakness, and hypotension. Changes in level of consciousness may be seen, including anxiousness, restlessness, and confusion. Pulmonary vascular congestion is frequently present and may manifest as dyspnea, labored respirations, rales (particularly in the lung bases), tachypnea, distended neck veins, and high CVP readings (above 15 cmH$_2$O). In more severe cases, frothy sputum or cyanosis may occur.

27. Do all patients in severe cardiogenic shock present with pulmonary congestion?

Initially the answer may be yes, until it is considered that the patient may have suffered an RV infarction. Such patients may present in cardiogenic shock with clear lung fields.

28. What cardiac sound may be heard in patients presenting with cardiogenic shock?

Typically auscultation of heart sounds is abnormal in patients in cardiogenic shock. A prominent S_4 indicates decreased ventricular compliance and, if accompanied by chest pain, suggests myocardial ischemia. An S_3 indicates increased ventricular diastolic pressure and congestive heart failure (CHF). In addition, a holosystolic murmur may be heard if mitral regurgitation is present. A systolic thrill and holosystolic murmur, heard best at the lower left sternal border, are indicative of ventricular septal rupture.

29. What interventions may be expected in the resuscitation of patients in cardiogenic shock?

Always begin with the ABCs (airway, breathing, circulation). Allow the alert, normotensive patient to sit upright to facilitate breathing. Consider endotracheal intubation if the airway is compromised or respiratory parameters are poor. Attach a cardiac monitor and immediately treat cardiac arrhythmias that may contribute to the shock state according to advanced cardiac life-support guidelines. Prepare for pharmacological therapy to support hemodynamic function and maximize cardiac function. Additional medications may include dopamine and analgesia for chest pain. If pharmacological therapy fails to support cardiac status, external or transvenous pacing may be necessary.

DISTRIBUTIVE (VASOGENIC) SHOCK

30. What is distributive or vasogenic shock?

Distributive shock occurs when the blood vessels dilate. Distributive shock states include septic shock, neurogenic shock, and anaphylactic shock.

31. What causes distributive shock?

In septic shock, massive infection results in endotoxin release that causes vasodilation. In anaphylactic shock, a severe allergic reaction results in the following cascade: histamine release, increased capillary permeability, and dilation of arterioles and venules. Neurogenic shock occurs after a spinal cord injury disrupts the sympathetic pathways and results in arteriole and venule dilation.

32. With so many causes of distributive shock, are all clinical presentations the same?

Some symptoms are similar, but others are vastly different. Typical clinical presentations for distributive shock are outlined in the following table.

Clinical Presentations for Distributive Shock

Shock State	Heart Rate	Blood Pressure	Specific Findings
Septic shock	Increased	Decreased	Temperature may or may not be elevated
Anaphylactic shock	Increased	Decreased	Respiratory difficulty
Neurogenic shock	Decreased	Decreased	Plegia from spinal cord injury or injury to medulla

33. What is the difference between high-output and low-output stages in septic shock?

The high-output stage refers to increased CO and decreased systemic vascular resistance, resulting in a hyperdynamic state (or early shock). Conversely, the low-output stage (or late shock) is a hypodynamic state in which the CO is decreased and systemic vascular resistance is increased. Whether patients can in fact be divided into one of these two groups is controversial, and it may be more appropriate to view the two processes as a continuum rather than distinct stages.

34. What is a common symptom of septic shock?

Because the signs and symptoms of sepsis can occur without infection, the concept of systemic inflammatory response syndrome (SIRS) was created. Sepsis is SIRS with documented infection. Septic shock is sepsis with organ dysfunction (hypotension or hypoperfusion).

35. Do all patients presenting with septic shock have an elevated temperature?

No. Temperature elevation or hypothermia may or may not be present in patients with septic shock. In neonates, immunosuppressed patients, or elderly patients, a subnormal temperature reading often is noted.

36. What is the immediate treatment for patients in septic shock?

Airway management, IV fluids, pressors, and antibiotics are the initial priorities for patients in septic shock. Broad-spectrum antibiotics should be started until specific culture results are available.

37. What new treatments are available to treat sepsis in hopes of avoiding septic shock?

In the PROWESS trial, recombinant human-activated protein C (rhAPC; drotrecogin alfa—Xigris) was administered to patients who had early sepsis including SIRS, with a reduction in the relative risk of death of 19% and an absolute reduction in the risk of death of 6% (Dhainaut, 2003). Similar to treatment of any shock state, early recognition and treatment improve the probability of a favorable outcome. In addition, no treatment is a "cure all."

38. What does rhAPC do in the septic phase to prohibit (when effective) septic shock from occurring?

It inhibits several pathways associated with mediation of cytokine, interleukin-1, tumor necrosis factor (TNF), and other antigenic components from releasing or causing increased inflammation leading to progressive SIRS and septic shock.

39. Can steroids be used as a treatment for septic shock?

Use of corticosteroids in the treatment of septic shock has been controversial. Numerous studies in the 1980s and 1990s generally showed no significant improvement with corticosteroid therapy. More recently, investigations have focused on use of more modest doses of corticosteroids in patients with refractory shock despite adequate resuscitation. One recent study has shown a trend toward improved survival rates (Abraham, 2002). The data in this area is limited, but these and other results suggest that corticosteroids may be beneficial in a subset of patients with refractory shock.

40. Is there a role for methylene blue (Methblue 65, Urolene Blue) in the treatment of septic shock?

Methylene blue has been shown to improve mean arterial pressure in patients with septic shock. Nitric oxide, which is released from endothelial cells, contributes to vasodilation and cardiac depression. Inhibition of nitric oxide synthesis by methylene blue may improve patient outcomes.

41. What is the usual treatment of anaphylactic shock?

Definitive therapy for anaphylactic shock is directed at identification and removal of the antigen responsible for the allergic reaction. If a blood transfusion is the causative factor, the transfusion should be stopped. If the causative factor is exposure to a chemical or substance, removal of the chemical or substance is necessary. Treatment of symptoms includes maintaining a patent airway, effective breathing, and circulation. High-flow oxygen and IV administration of epinephrine, 0.1 to 0.5 ml of 1:10,000 solution, repeated every 5 to 15 minutes, are indicated for profound shock. Antihistamines, such as diphenhydramine (Benadryl) and cimetidine (Tagamet), and/or bronchodilators, such as albuterol, also may be necessary.

42. Are neurogenic shock and hypovolemic shock treated with similar techniques of fluid resuscitation?

Unlike hypovolemic shock, which is a volume problem, neurogenic shock is a problem of arteriolar and venous dilation. The volume is present, but it flows through very dilated vasculature, which results in venous and arterial pooling and hypotension. Treatment begins with spinal cord stabilization concomitantly with the ABCs. Specific treatment may include maintaining a flat position and IV fluids, but often IV vasopressors are required to help constrict the vasculature and increase the BP.

OBSTRUCTIVE SHOCK

(See Chapter 26, Thoracic and Neck Trauma, for management of pericardial tamponade and tension pneumothorax, the primary causes of obstructive shock.)

43. What ethical dilemmas arise when an exsanguinating, competent adult who is a Jehovah's Witness refuses blood transfusions?

No ethical dilemma is associated with this scenario. Patient autonomy is the dominant ethical principle guiding the actions of healthcare providers. Respect for autonomy ensures the patient's right to choose actions that are consistent with his or her personal values and life plans, even when the choices are not consistent with healthcare providers' values of preserving life. Nonetheless, such a scenario can be morally troublesome for ED clinicians. It is important to uphold professional duties of respect and beneficence (do no harm), but when individual values are not aligned, this goal can be difficult. Open discussion of the issues and sharing one's feelings and perceptions often help to deal with morally challenging situations.

Key Points

- Regardless of the precipitating cause, shock leads to decreased perfusion that is inadequate to meet the needs of the tissues.
- Early symptoms of shock are often subtle and require extra vigilance by nursing staff to avoid them being overlooked.
- All patients in shock are at risk of deterioration and therefore require prompt intervention, often involving the use of oxygen, fluid, and/or inotropic/vasopressor pharmacological therapy.
- For nurses to care for a patient in shock safely, they must understand the pathophysiology of different etiologies of shock.

Internet Resources

American Association of Critical-Care Nurses:
www.aacn.org

Ed Friedlander, Fluid and Hemodynamic Derangements:
www.pathguy.com/lectures/fluids.htm

HealthCentral.com:
www.healthcentral.com

Internet Journal of Rescue and Disaster Medicine, *Analysis of an Emergency Department's Experience:*
www.ispub.com/ostia/index.php?xmlFilePath=journals/ijrdm/vol4n2/
emergency.xml

Virtual Naval Hospital, Standard First Aid Course, Chapter 4: Shock:
www.brooksidepress.org/Products/OperationalMedicine/DATA/operationalmed/Manuals/
Standard1stAid/chapter4.html

Bibliography

Abboud CR et al: Trends in cardiogenic shock: Report from the SHOCK study, *Eur Heart J* 22:472-478, 2001.

Abraham E, Evans, T: Corticosteroids and septic shock, *JAMA* 886-887, 2002.

Alderson P et al: Colloids versus crystalloids for fluid resuscitation in critically ill patients, *Cochrane Database Syst Rev* 4, 2004.

Bench S: Clinical skills: Assessing and treating shock: A nursing perspective, *Br J Nurs* 13(12):715-721, 2004.

Bickell WH et al: Immediate versus delayed fluid resuscitation for hypotensive patients with penetrating torso injuries, *N Engl J Med* 331(17):1105-1109, 1994.

Blackbourne LH: *Surgical recall*, ed 3, Baltimore, 2003, Williams & Wilkins.

Cohen SS: *Trauma nursing secrets*, Philadelphia, 2002, Hanley & Belfus.

Dhainaut JF et al: The clinical evaluation committee in a large multicenter phase 3 trial of drotrecogin alfa (activated) in patients with severe sepsis (PROWESS): role, methodology, and results, *Crit Care Med* 31(9):2291-301, 2003.

Emergency Nurses Association: *Course in advanced trauma nursing II: A conceptual approach to injury and illness*, Park Ridge, Ill, 2003, Emergency Nurses Association.

McGee S, Abernethy W, Simel D: Is this patient hypovolemic? *JAMA* 281:1022-1029, 1999.

Newberry L, editor: *Sheehy's emergency nursing principles and practice*, ed 4, St Louis, 2003, Mosby.

Schierhout G, Roberts I: Fluid resuscitation with colloid or crystalloid solutions in critically ill patients: A systemic review of randomized trials, *BMJ* 316:961-964, 1998.

Schulman C: Is your patient fully resuscitated? *Nurs Manage* 34(7):44-47, 2003.

Tisherman SA et al: *Clinical practice guideline: Endpoints of resuscitation*, Winston-Salem, NC, 2003, Eastern Association for the Surgery of Trauma.

Waheed RM et al: Deferoxamine and Hespan complex as a resuscitative adjuvant in hemorrhagic shock Rat model, *Shock* 17(4):339-342, 2002.

Weinstein PD, Doerfler ME: Systemic complications of fluid resuscitation, *Crit Care Clin* 8:439-447, 1992.

Chapter 25

Head and Face Trauma

Pamela W. Bourg

1. **Why is knowledge of head and face trauma important to emergency nurses?**

   Two million head injuries occur each year in the United States. One and a half million are mild injuries treated on an outpatient basis, whereas 500,000 are severe enough to require hospitalization. These numbers predict that the likelihood of emergency nurses encountering head-injured patients is high. Brain injury is the leading single-organ cause of death related to trauma. Head injury is the cause of 50% of all deaths resulting from motor vehicle crashes. Young people, 15 to 24 years old, have the highest incidence of head injuries. Older persons are the next highest group. As the aging population of the United States grows, the number of patients with head injuries will increase.

   Emergency nurses must be able to adequately assess and initiate care for head-injured patients. Although the nurse's role in prevention programs is important, the role in recognizing and caring for brain injury is critical.

2. **What is the major cause of death in brain and craniofacial trauma?**

   Airway obstruction caused by occlusion by the tongue, accumulation of secretions or blood, and/or facial edema.

3. **What are the key elements of the assessment for traumatic brain injury (TBI)?**

   - Initial assessment: airway with cervical spine control, breathing, and circulation
   - Level of consciousness: AVPU assessment (A = alert, V = responsive to verbal stimuli, P = responsive to painful stimuli, and U = unresponsive)
   - Assessment of vital signs
   - Mini-neurological exam: Glasgow Coma Scale, pupillary size and response, and motor function
   - History of injury

4. **What happens to intracranial contents when acceleration-deceleration forces are encountered?**

   When the head strikes a solid object, the impact may result in bony deformity and injury to cranial contents. A pressure wave generated at the point of impact then travels across cranial contents and eventually dissipates. Both the initial impact and the pressure wave can cause lacerations, local injury, skull fractures, and contusion of the brain within the cranial vault.

5. What is the difference between primary and secondary brain injury?

Primary brain injury is mechanical injury to the brain and occurs at the moment of impact (i.e., contusion or concussion). Secondary injury occurs within seconds, hours, or days after the primary injury. Causes of secondary injury include hypoxemia, systemic hypotension, cerebral edema, and sustained increased intracranial pressure (ICP). Secondary injury also includes cellular or microscopic injury. Causes of microscopic injury include free radicals and inflammatory response.

6. What is cerebral perfusion pressure (CPP)? How is it calculated?

CPP is defined as the difference between the mean arterial pressure (MAP) and the ICP:

$$CPP = MAP - ICP$$

For example, if the MAP is 90 mmHg and the ICP is 25 mmHg, the CPP is 65 mmHg. Normal CPP is 50 to 130 mmHg. CPP is an important parameter to follow. The brain can survive CPPs in the 50s, but neurological outcome is much improved if CPP is in the 60s for adults and 40s for children. Lower values are consistent with ischemia.

7. What is the significance of hypotension and tachycardia in patients with TBI?

Neither is normal. Usually they are attributable to bleeding associated with concurrent injury in the thoracic, abdominal, or pelvic cavity. Hypotension (systolic blood pressure less than 90 for adults) is correlated with worse outcomes with head injury.

8. What are the three components of the Glasgow Coma Scale?

Eye opening, best motor response, and best verbal response. The highest score possible is 15; patients with score below 8 have sustained a severe head injury. Other conditions, such as hypothermia, hypotension, and alcohol or drug abuse, may artificially lower the score. The trend of the score may be more helpful than the actual number; as always, it needs to be interpreted in conjunction with other clinical assessment findings.

Glasgow Coma Scale

Eye Opening

Spontaneously	4
To verbal command	3
To pain	2
No response	1
S = Eyes swollen shut, unable to evaluate	

Continued

Glasgow Coma Scale—cont'd

Best Motor Response

Obeys commands	6
Localizes pain	5
Withdraws from pain	4
Abnormal flexion	3
Abnormal extension	2
No response	1
IP = Chemically paralyzed	

Best Verbal Response

Oriented	5
Confused	4
Inappropriate words	3
Incomprehensible sounds	2
No response	1
IT = Intubated	

| **Total** | **3-15** |

9. What is the significance of a large, nonreactive pupil in patients with TBI?

The nonreactive pupil, usually on the side of the expanding mass lesion, is caused by compression of the third cranial (oculomotor) nerve. It is usually a sign of uncal herniation. Rarely is a nonreactive pupil the only symptom; other physical findings include changes in mental status (confusion, agitation, coma) or motor weakness contralateral to the mass lesion.

10. Injuries to the brain may cause damage to which structures? What are the types of injuries and the associated mechanism?

Brain Injuries: Signs and Symptoms

Structures	Types of Injuries	Usual Mechanism	Associated Symptoms
Brain	Concussion/diffuse injury Mild without loss of consciousness and memory loss	Acceleration/deceleration (shearing stress on reticular formation)	Nausea and vomiting, confusion, dizziness, memory loss

Brain Injuries: Signs and Symptoms—cont'd

Structures	Types of Injuries	Usual Mechanism	Associated Symptoms
	Classic with loss of consciousness and memory loss		
	Contusion Bruising and damage in a localized area	Direct impact of acceleration/deceleration usually located where brain impacts bony protuberances of the skull	Inappropriate behavior and cognitive deficits Contusion can cause secondary edema and increase ICP
Covering structures (intracranial)	Epidural: collection of blood between skull and dura Associated with fractures of temporal or parietal bone that lacerate the middle meningeal artery	Direct impact	Patient classically loses consciousness, then has a lucid interval, then rapid deterioration— papillary signs (ipsilateral) Seen more often in children
	Subdural: tear in bridging veins occurs	Acceleration/deceleration: can be acute or chronic after trauma	Increase in local edema leading to increase in ICP and gradual deterioration in level of consciousness
	Subarachnoid or intraventricular hemorrhage		Often indicates severity of trauma; nuchal rigidity, and ipsilateral dilated pupil
	Intracerebral hematoma: collection of blood greater than 5 ml; tends to occur in frontal and temporal lobes	Acceleration/deceleration	Unconsciousness at onset of bleeding, headache, decreased level of consciousness, and hemiplegia on contralateral side
Skull	Fractures	Impact	Pain, bleeding, swelling
Nerve cells	Diffuse axonal injuries	Acceleration/deceleration forces producing shearing or tensile stress	Immediate unconsciousness, hypertension, hyperthermia, decortica- tion or decerebration, and initial low ICP

11. **Patients with TBI often require sedation for agitation, restlessness, mechanical ventilation, or painful interventions. What drugs are used?**

Benzodiazepines are used most commonly. Specifically, lorazepam (Ativan) or midazolam (Versed) minimally affects ICP, cerebral oxygen demand, or cerebral blood flow. Propofol is another common sedative. For analgesia, fentanyl or morphine in conventional doses is administered. Don't forget that sedated patients often still need analgesia. Patients should be as lightly sedated as possible.

12. **Are corticosteroids effective in managing TBI?**

Steroids are no longer considered effective because they are thought to increase the risk of death when given to head-injured patients.

13. **In what instances can hyperventilation be used in the emergency department (ED) to treat acute elevation of ICP or sudden neurological deterioration (blown pupil)?**

Hyperventilation is indicated for brief periods only if first-tier therapies (cerebrospinal fluid [CSF] drainage, paralysis, sedation, osmotic diuretics) fail.

Prophylactic or chronic hyperventilation should be avoided because it reduces cerebral blood flow without consistently reducing ICP. Autoregulation may be interrupted and causes further compromise of blood flow to the injured area. If hyperventilation is used, the target level for partial pressure of carbon dioxide (P_{CO_2}) is 30 to 35 mmHg.

14. **Are basiliar skull fractures more serious than cranial vault fractures?**

Yes. Basilar skull fractures can cause leakage of CSF through the dural tear. The CSF will leak from the nose or ears. Continued leakage of CSF can lead to meningitis or abscesses.

15. **What is the clinical significance of periorbital ecchymosis or raccoon's eyes?**

Basilar skull fractures may be accompanied by bleeding into the anterior fossa fracture, which causes the appearance of bruising and swelling around both eyes.

16. **What signs and symptoms are commonly seen in basilar skull fractures?**
   - Headache
   - Ecchymosis
   - Altered levels of consciousness
   - CSF rhinorrhea or otorrhea

17. **Why is it important to position the head in the midline when patients have sustained craniofacial trauma?**

Positioning the head into the midline facilitates venous drainage. Rotation of the head may compress the neck veins and result in both venous engorgement and decreased drainage from the brain, which increases ICP and decreases CPP.

18. How are avulsed tissue or organs from the face managed?

All tissue and organs should be recovered. If possible, irrigate with normal saline and transport in soaked gauze sponge.

19. Can repair of clean facial wounds be delayed?

Yes. Repair may be delayed as long as 24 hours. Clean facial wounds should be irrigated and the edges kept moist with saline dressings. The exception is bites (animal and human). Because of the gross contamination of the wound, bites should be treated as soon as possible.

20. What is the drug of choice for patients with TBI who present to the ED with generalized tonic-clonic seizures?

Benzodiazepines (lorazepam is common) usually are given first to terminate the seizure, followed by phenytoin (Dilantin) for prevention of further tonic-clonic seizures and temporal lobe seizures. Phenytoin works on the motor cortex, where spread of seizure activity is inhibited. Phenytoin is given by slow intravenous (IV) push at no more than 50 mg per minute through a filter. The maximum dose is 18 mg/kg. Cardiac status should be monitored during the infusion.

21. What instructions are appropriate for a patient discharged with a mild TBI (concussion)?

It is important for the family and patient to recognize signs and symptoms of changes in neurological status. Patients should be given the following information and be able to verbalize an understanding to seek medical attention as necessary.

Mild head injuries in adults and children:
Mild head injuries, also known as concussions, are caused by striking the head against an object or by a blow to the head. Car crashes and falls are often the cause. Symptoms may include:
- Headache
- Nausea
- Vomiting
- Depression
- Memory loss
- Ringing in ears
- Slight dizziness
- Increased sleepiness
- Blurry vision

Instructions for patients:
- You were examined at the time of your injury, and no serious brain or skull injuries were noted. However, it is possible for more serious symptoms to develop later. If possible, have someone stay with you for 24 hours after the injury. This person should wake you every 4 hours and look for the symptoms listed below.
- You may take acetaminophen every 4 hours to relieve pain. *Do not take aspirin or ibuprofen.* Take only medications prescribed for you at this time.
- A clear liquid diet for 12 to 24 hours is recommended.

- *No* alcoholic beverages for 24 hours.
- Rest for the next 24 hours.
- Do not drive, operate machinery, or make important legal decisions.

Contact your physician if you experience any of the following symptoms in the next few weeks:

- Inability to answer simple questions, such as, "What day is it?" or "What happened to you?"
- Increased headache or the inability to wake up completely
- Nausea and vomiting or vomiting three or more times
- Problems with walking or stumbling (or problems with coordination)
- Slurred speech
- Seizures or convulsions
- Weakness of the arms and legs

You or someone with you should dial 911 for an ambulance if you have any of these symptoms.

Normal reactions to head injuries may be experienced for some time; however, if these symptoms persist or increase in severity, contact your physician:

- Are you having trouble remembering things?
- Do you have trouble with concentrating?
- Trouble with your eyes? Double or blurred vision?
- Are you more irritable or easily agitated? Have trouble concentrating?
- Are you having problems with depression since the accident?
- Weakness or fatigue? Dizziness?
- Difficulty sleeping or a noticeable change in the number of hours you are sleeping?
- Are you experiencing difficulty in performing your normal daily activities?

22. When is a skull fracture considered open?

If there is an overlying scalp laceration, the fracture is considered open.

23. Maxillary fractures are classified by the Le Fort system, named after French surgeon Renée Le Fort at the turn of the century. What are the three types of Le Fort fractures? What facial bones are involved?

Le Fort I: Transverse maxillary fracture above the level of teeth, resulting in a separation of teeth from rest of maxilla.

Le Fort II: Pyramidal fracture through or above the nasal bridge, with separation involving the maxillary segment of zygomatic, nasal, and orbital bones of the midface. It is characterized by obvious fracture of nasal bones, and a CSF leak is possible.

Le Fort III: A complete maxillary fracture involving separation of the midface from the cranium and/or mandible. This fracture may cause diplopia.

In addition, most facial fractures do not occur in isolation and frequently are accompanied by other significant head and multisystem trauma. The most frequent fractures affect the zygomatic arch: maxillary, mandible, and orbital floor wall.

24. Why must patients with multiple facial fractures be kept under constant observation?

Edema and clot formation may occur, causing airway obstruction. A cricothyrotomy tray should be in close proximity until the patient is out of danger. The face is highly vascular and obtains its blood supply from two branches of the external carotids (the facial and maxillary arteries). Injuries to these vessels can result in massive hemorrhage. There is also the risk of airway obstruction from loose teeth, bridges, crowns, dentures, bone fragments, dirt, and debris (including food and gum).

25. What are the major effects of head injuries inflicted by guns and bullets?

Cerebral contusions and lacerations, focal tissue damage, and hemorrhage caused by tearing of blood vessels. Hemorrhage and edema may produce increased ICP and possible herniation associated with rapid expansion during impact and in response to a space-occupying lesion. Impalement injuries involve piercing of the scalp, skull, or brain by a foreign object, such as an ice pick; such injuries can be missed on exam if the object was removed and only a puncture wound remains.

26. What lab studies and diagnostic tests are typically done during initial resuscitation and treatment of the brain-injured patient with a Glasgow Coma Scale score of 8 or less?

- Complete blood count (CBC)
- Arterial blood gases (ABGs)
- Electrolytes, glucose
- Creatinine, blood urea nitrogen (BUN)
- International normalized ratio (INR)
- Prothrombin time (PT) and partial thromboplastin time (PTT)
- Drug screen
- Chest radiograph
- Cervical spine films (to rule out cervical fractures or unstable vertebral column); computed tomography (CT) scans of the neck have replaced standard cervical spine films at some centers
- CT scan as soon as possible (gold standard for head injury diagnosis; should be done immediately when the patient is stabilized)

27. How is corneal reflex tested?

In a conscious or unconscious patient, touch each cornea with a wisp of cotton and observe for blinking. If the reflex is intact, the eye will blink. Corneal reflex is mediated by cranial nerves V (trigeminal) and VII (facial).

28. What are the various modalities to reduce ICP?

- Evacuation of mass lesions (epidural hematoma, subdural hematoma, intracranial hemorrhage)
- Head position at 30 degrees elevation if spinal films are cleared and the patient is hemodynamically stable; note that this is somewhat controversial because elevating the head may also decrease CPP

- Mannitol, 1 gm/kg by IV push; use filter; dose can be repeated
- Sedation/paralysis
- Hyperventilation with ICP monitor in place
- CSF drainage (ventriculostomy, spinal drain)
- Pentobarbital coma

29. What is the desired action of mannitol in a patient with TBI?

In hemodynamically stable patients, an osmotic diuretic such as mannitol can be given. Mannitol promotes diuresis by forming an osmotic gradient between the extravascular intraparenchymal space and the intravascular space. This gradient promotes fluid movement from the parenchymal space into the vascular space, which decreases cerebral edema and ICP. Mannitol also decreases hematocrit and blood viscosity, which improves cerebral blood flow and oxygen delivery. Serum sodium levels should be maintained at 145 to 150 and serum osmolarities at 290 to 300.

30. What are the nursing responsibilities for patients with a ventriculostomy and ICP monitor in the ED?

- Explain to the patient and/or family the need for monitoring.
- Gather and assemble equipment.
- Flush the lines and calibrate equipment.
- Perform neurological assessment.
- Administer light sedation/analgesia.
- Place head of bed at 30 degrees (if prescribed in a hemodynamically stable patient).
- Prepare operative site, establish sterile field, and assist physician as needed.
- Connect monitoring catheter to transducer or monitor.
- Observe the numerical readings and wave patterns; adjust characteristics to obtain visual reading.
- Cover site with sterile dressing.
- Adjust alarm system to unit parameters.
- Obtain frequent checks of neurological status and patency of system; irrigate system using sterile technique to maintain patency according to unit policy.

31. What are the current controversies in management of a patient suffering from TBI?

Many clinicians still advocate fluid restrictions or small volume resuscitations if TBI is present. However, there is mounting experimental and clinical evidence that suggests secondary brain insults can be avoided with aggressive fluid resuscitation.

Mild hypothermia has been advocated in TBI but remains controversial. Human trials have been complicated by hypothermia effects of coagulopathy, infection, and myocardial performance. In selected paralysis some patients who were hypothermic on arrival at the hospital did better if not warmed aggressively. More clinical research is needed.

32. What does the future hold in the management of TBI?

There continues to be a search for serum markers of brain damage (e.g., troponin for heart damage) that could be measured quickly and may partially replace expensive and tedious neurological imaging procedures. None have been established, but ongoing trials continue.

More research is needed in posttraumatic brain extracellular lactate accumulation. Some studies suggest that lactate may be an alternative for neurons during the acute postinjury phase.

Key Points

- Airway obstruction continues to be a major cause of death and disability in patients with TBI and/or craniofacial injury.
- The Glasgow Coma Scale is an effective tool for determining the severity of TBI. A score of 15 to 13 is minor, 12 to 9 is moderate, and below 8 is major.
- Motor exam results that differ between the patient's right and left side, progressive deterioration, or posturing of any sort indicate a lesion that may require immediate surgical intervention.
- Discharge education after TBI is critical for patients. Minor TBI is a common injury. Potential for deterioration always exists.
- Patients with altered levels of consciousness should have reversible conditions such as hypoxia, hypertension, and hypoglycemia corrected as soon as they are identified.

Internet Resources

Brain Injury Association of America:
www.BIAUSA.org

Brain Trauma Foundation:
www.braintrauma.org

Coma Waiting Page:
www.waiting.com

National Guideline Clearinghouse:
www.guideline.gov

National Institute of Neurological Disorders and Stroke (NINDS) Traumatic Brain Injury Information:
www.ninds.nih.gov/health_and_medical/disorders/TBI_doc.htm

Traumatic Brain Injury Survival Guide:
www.tbiguide.com

Bibliography

Biros M, Heegaard W: Brain resuscitation. In Marx JA, Hockberger RS, Walls RM, editors: *Rosen's emergency medicine: Concepts and clinical practice*, ed 5, St Louis, 2002, Mosby.

Brain Trauma Foundation; American Association of Neurological Surgeons, Joint Section on Neurotrauma and Critical Care: *Management and prognosis of severe traumatic brain injury*, New York, 2000, Brain Trauma Foundation. Available at www2.braintrauma.org/guidelines/downloads/btf_guidelines_management.pdf.

Cantrill SV: Face. In Marx JA, Hockberger RS, Walls RM, editors: *Rosen's emergency medicine: Concepts and clinical practice*, ed 5, St Louis, 2002, Mosby.

Gunnarsson T, Fehlings M: Acute neurosurgical management of traumatic brain injury and spinal cord injury, *Curr Opin Neurol* 16(6):717, 2003.

Longhi L, Stocchetti N: Hyperoxia head injury: Therapeutic tool? *Curr Opin Crit Care* 10(2):105, 2004.

McQuillan KA, Mitchell P: Traumatic brain injuries. In McQuillan KA et al, editors: *Trauma nursing*, ed 3, Philadelphia, 2002, WB Saunders.

Reilly PL, Bullock R, editors: *Head injury: Pathophysiology and management*, ed 2, London, 2005, Hodder Arnold.

Valadka A: Injury to cranium. In Moore EE, Feliciano D, Mattox K, editors: *Trauma*, ed 5, New York, 2004, McGraw-Hill.

York J et al: Fluid resuscitation and severe closed head injury: Experience with aggressive fluid resuscitation strategy, *J Trauma* 48(3):376, 2000.

Thoracic and Neck Trauma

Margaret J. Neff and Janet A. Neff

1. **What is the thorax?**

   The thorax, or chest, includes both the chest wall structures and thoracic viscera. Its contents are responsible for breathing and circulation. It is a critical region where injuries can quickly become life threatening.

   The thorax is closely linked to the airway and is in close proximity to the abdomen. At the root of the neck is the cervicothoracic inlet, where vital structures such as the trachea, major vessels, and esophagus cross boundaries into the thorax. More distally, the thorax interfaces with the abdominal cavity. Clearly, abdominal organs such as the liver, spleen, and stomach are within the structure of the lower rib cage, and the diaphragm lowers significantly during inspiration.

RIB FRACTURES

2. **Which ribs are injured most frequently?**

   The third to tenth ribs tend to be injured most frequently because they have limited protection. Fracture of the scapula or first rib indicates a high-energy mechanism of injury and is associated with a high risk for vascular injury. Lower rib fractures may be associated with concurrent spleen, liver, and kidney injuries.

3. **When a patient asks, "How many ribs did I break?" can a reliable answer be given?**

   Although the patient can be told the number of rib fractures clearly seen on chest radiograph or computed tomography (CT) scan, most radiographs do not clearly show all rib fractures, nor is injury to the cartilage evident radiographically. Some centers perform oblique films to try to identify all fractures. Although they do not add to the clinical treatment plan in the acute setting, they may sometimes be done to validate the patient's pain and assist with issues regarding return to work.

4. **Is the patient's concern about pain important?**

   Yes. Pain limits the patient's ability to perform activities of daily living. Simple acts such as raising an arm can be exquisitely painful. Rib pain with deep breathing potentiates the risk of atelectasis and pneumonia. It is important to evaluate respiratory rate and depth. Shallow respirations indicate guarding or splinting efforts. In patients with multiple rib fractures, epidural analgesia (when possible) should be considered because it has been shown to decrease the rate of hospital-acquired pneumonia and to shorten the length of time on the ventilator in critically ill patients. The impact of rib fractures, even just one fracture, is of significant concern in the elderly who have twice the mortality of younger patients with similar injuries. Recognizing this increased risk may lead to earlier intervention and more intensive monitoring of this high-risk group.

When the patient is discharged home from the emergency department (ED) with a diagnosis of rib fractures, demonstration of deep breathing and holding or pausing at the end of inspiration is essential to keep the alveoli open. Motivate the patient and, if indicated, suggest a device such as an incentive spirometer. Ambulation, as clinically appropriate, is one of the best ways to prevent atelectasis. Medications such as nonsteroidal antiinflammatory drugs (NSAIDs) can help with bone and cartilage pain. Stronger medication such as acetaminophen with codeine may be needed in the early injury phase to promote comfort.

5. When do rib fractures tend to heal?

Callus starts to form at the fracture site within 10 to 14 days after injury. The ribs typically heal within 3 to 6 weeks unless comminuted fractures or major displacement is present.

6. Are children's ribs as likely to break as those of adults?

No. Young ribs deform more easily and have resilient cartilage. This does not mean the child has less thoracic trauma. The underlying viscera may have sustained a significant force without an overlying rib fracture to alert injury.

7. What term is used when two or more adjacent ribs are broken in two or more places, creating a free-floating segment?

Flail chest.

8. How is flail chest detected without a radiograph?

Through careful inspection of spontaneous respiratory movement, a section of the chest wall moving opposite to the rest of the chest during breathing may be noticeable. Generally, the flail segment moves inward on inspiration as the diaphragm descends and outward during expiration. This pattern is called paradoxical motion. Normal respiratory mechanics depend on a rigid chest wall against which the lungs can develop negative intrathoracic pressure and a resultant inspiratory breath. With a flail segment, the rigid chest wall is compromised, resulting in increased work of breathing. It may be necessary to look at the patient's chest movement from the foot of the bed at stretcher height to visualize the uneven paradoxical movement; when standing directly to the patient's side, it is harder to notice. If the patient is splinting because of pain, abnormal movement may not be noticed until he or she becomes fatigued. It is much harder to detect posterior flail because the musculature is heavier and the patient usually is lying supine during the initial examination. Pain and crepitus, a crunchy, crackly feeling on palpation over the ribs, are present over the site. If the patient is receiving positive pressure ventilation from a bag-valve-mask or ventilator, the paradoxical chest wall motion is not present.

9. How is the patient with a flail chest managed?

Monitor oxygen saturation and arterial blood gases (ABGs) continuously. If the patient is intubated, also monitor continuous end-tidal carbon dioxide. The patient who becomes fatigued, hypoxic, or dyspneic may need assisted ventilation. Adequate pain control, which may include epidural analgesia or a regional block, is essential. In the ED, rapid but short-acting analgesia such as fentanyl may be optimal to address issues of pain while monitoring ventilation and fatigue level. Maximize gas exchange by positioning the patient in an upright position after the spine is cleared. Binding the ribs and compressing with packs are not recommended because both further reduce tidal volume and increase the risk of atelectasis and hypoxia.

10. What medical therapy may be needed in the patient who is not tolerating the flail chest?

Noninvasive positive pressure support via bilevel positive airway pressure (BiPAP) or continuous positive airway pressure (CPAP) mask, or potentially endotracheal intubation and positive pressure ventilation, may be necessary. Positive pressure helps the lung to expand and maintains normal motion of the flail segment during inspiration. Pain control can be optimized after airway management has been established.

11. What factor other than the flail segment and pain may cause pulmonary compromise with a flail chest?

The force required to create a flail segment frequently injures the lung tissue, resulting in a pulmonary contusion. Always suspect it in the presence of flail chest or multiple rib fractures.

PULMONARY CONTUSIONS

12. What is a pulmonary contusion?

A contusion is a parenchymal injury to the lung. It often results in some degree of hemorrhage and edema with an inflammatory process extending beyond the site of injury. The result is a ventilation-perfusion mismatch, which leads to hypoxia.

13. How does a pulmonary contusion occur?

Pulmonary contusions result from blunt thoracic trauma with multiple rib fractures, flail chest, rapid deceleration forces, extreme concussive impact, or blast force. Pulmonary contusions are common findings in victims of motor vehicle collisions.

14. How is a pulmonary contusion diagnosed?

There may be evidence of chest wall tenderness and ecchymosis from blunt contact with an object such as a steering wheel. Chest radiograph may show an infiltrate. Sometimes the contusion is not evident on radiograph for as long as 12 to 24 hours. A CT scan shows evidence of the contusion earlier. The patient has impaired pulmonary function, which, if severe, may progress to Acute Lung Injury (ALI).

15. How is a pulmonary contusion treated?

Despite the relatively high mortality associated with a pulmonary contusion (10% to 40%), there are no known therapies other than supportive and expectant care. Supportive care includes managing pain and encouraging incentive spirometry to minimize atelectasis and the development of pneumonia. Anticipatory care involves recognizing the risk for evolution to ALI. If ALI is diagnosed, current management recommendations include a low tidal volume strategy of mechanical ventilation, which should be initiated as soon as the patient is no longer in shock or profoundly hypoxemic.

PLEURAL INJURIES

16. What is a pneumothorax?

A pneumothorax is air in the pleural space. It may result from traumatic injury to the lung (as with a fractured rib or stab wound) or occur spontaneously, with or without underlying lung disease. Inflation of the lung depends on negative pressure in the pleural space. When air is introduced into the pleural space, the negative pressure is lost, and the lung collapses, either partially or completely. The severity of symptoms depends on the extent of collapse, the patient's underlying lung function, and the body's demands on the respiratory system.

17. What mechanism of injury is associated with a pneumothorax?

With traumatic injuries, the force is typically applied laterally, and the rib often fractures toward the lung parenchyma. In contrast, during anterior-posterior chest wall compression, such as a direct blow to the chest or impact with a steering wheel, ribs may fracture but usually in an outward fashion with less likelihood of a resultant pneumothorax. A sudden increase in intrathoracic pressure (e.g., from a compressive force while the glottis is closed), which creates high airway pressure and may rupture alveoli, also may result in a pneumothorax. Although rare, this injury may occur with breath holding out of fear or in an attempt to brace oneself for a crash or fall. A penetrating injury creates an open pneumothorax. Iatrogenic pneumothorax may occur during central line placement (subclavian or jugular sites). Pneumothoraces are seen in up to 30% of patients with thoracic trauma.

18. How is pneumothorax detected clinically?

Auscultation of the lung usually reflects decreased breath sounds over the affected lung, and percussion usually reveals hyperresonance. The patient may be mildly or acutely dyspneic. Subcutaneous emphysema may result from air that dissects into the tissues and creates a light, crunchy feeling within distended, puffy tissue.

A pneumothorax usually can be identified by plain chest radiography. With supine films, the only radiographic evidence of a pneumothorax may be a deep sulcus sign, which is caused by air in the pleural space anterior to the diaphragm and looks like a "finger" of air running laterally and inferiorly to the lung. Chest CT is the most sensitive test for identifying air and may detect pneumothoraces not appreciated on chest radiograph. It may be surprising to find a pneumothorax during an abdominal CT; this scan includes cuts of the lower thorax that may identify a pneumothorax.

19. How should a traumatic pneumothorax be treated?

Treatment depends on clinical findings and other planned patient therapy. If the pneumothorax is small (less than 20%), with no fluid accumulation, no ventilation problems, and no plan for positive pressure ventilation, the patient may be observed. Otherwise, a chest tube is indicated.

20. What is a sucking chest wound? What is the immediate treatment?

When a thoracic wound communicates through the pleural space (an open chest wound), air is "sucked" into the thorax through the wound during inspiration. A gauze dressing is placed over an open chest wound to limit the amount of air entering the chest cavity during inspiration. Tape only three sides of this dressing, allowing the fourth edge to "flutter" so that air can be released during expiration to prevent a tension pneumothorax. Close observation for a tension pneumothorax is essential, and chest tube insertion should be accomplished promptly.

21. What is a tension pneumothorax?

A tension pneumothorax is a life-threatening event that results when air accumulates in the pleural space and causes an increase in intrathoracic pressure. The air accumulation results when air continues to leak into the pleural space but cannot escape. This scenario can occur in blunt trauma when air enters from the lung or bronchial tree or through an open chest wall injury. The increased pressure forces the thoracic contents to shift away from the injured side. The heart and other vital structures are compressed as the mediastinal shift occurs. Venous return to the heart is compromised, and cardiac function is impaired.

22. What symptoms are associated with a tension pneumothorax?

Dyspnea, hypoxia, and hypotension. Auscultation reveals decreased breath sounds over the affected lung; percussion usually reveals hyperresonance. These findings often are difficult to appreciate because of noise in the resuscitation room and transmitted sounds from within the thorax. Neck and upper extremity vein distention may be noted if the patient's blood volume is adequate. The trachea deviates away from the affected side but may be difficult to observe, especially with a cervical collar in place. A conscious patient is usually very dyspneic and may be frantic from the sensation of suffocation.

23. What is the immediate treatment of a tension pneumothorax?

A tension pneumothorax requires immediate decompression. Needle thoracostomy should not be delayed for a confirmatory chest radiograph.

24. Where is a needle thoracostomy performed?

Typically in the second intercostal space, at the midclavicular line on the side of the chest with no breath sounds (the trachea is deviated away from the side with the tension pneumothorax). The needle should be inserted over the rib to avoid the neurovascular bundle. A 14- or 16-gauge, 2 inch (or longer) catheter is commonly used. Heavily muscled chests might require a spinal needle for greater length to evacuate the air. If a tension pneumothorax exists, air is released rapidly when the needle reaches the level of the air accumulation. Immediate patient improvement usually is noted. Needle thoracostomy is a temporizing procedure. The needle is removed, and the catheter can remain in place until chest tube insertion is accomplished.

25. What is a hemothorax?

A hemothorax is an accumulation of blood in the pleural space. It is easiest to detect on an upright chest radiograph or CT scan because the fluid layers out when the patient is supine. However, most trauma patients must follow cervical spine precautions and cannot sit up; clinicians rely on the initial chest radiograph to determine findings. The radiograph on the side of a hemothorax often shows a diffuse opacity in the lung fields that must be distinguished from pulmonary contusion. Blood most commonly comes from an intercostal vessel injury but also may stem from a major pulmonary hemorrhage, the heart, or the aorta.

26. Is there any risk to placing a chest tube in a patient with a hemothorax?

Yes. In a patient with a large hemothorax, the initial chest drainage may release the protective tamponade effect within the thorax. Significant hemorrhage may ensue.

27. What actions are indicated for massive chest tube output?

- Autotransfusion. Each autotransfusion system works differently. Be familiar with them because acting fast is crucial. Some centers use an anticoagulant such as citrate phosphate dextrose (CPD) or anticoagulant citrate dextrose (ACD) to help avoid development of clots; others use none because the free blood within the thorax is defibrinated and therefore should not clot. If the department uses an anticoagulant, try to distribute it through the interior filter so that blood passes through it.
- Be certain that the transfusion department has a patient blood sample and is alerted to the situation.
- Infuse fluid and blood products through a rapid infusion/warming system because hypothermia can cause coagulopathy. Autotransfused blood from a chest tube drainage system does not usually need to be warmed.
- Be ready for possible ED thoracotomy or rapid departure to the operating room (OR).

28. What are the maximal and minimal amounts of autotransfused blood that should be administered?

Most trauma centers recommend stopping after 1500 ml of blood have been infused. Intraoperative systems such as cell savers have sophisticated systems to wash the blood, which reduce some of the complications associated with massive autotransfusion, including obstruction caused by clot formation, contamination, hypothermia, and citrate toxicity. Cell washing for intraoperative cell salvage can result in coagulopathy from clotting factor loss. Generally, no less than 400 to 500 ml is retransfused to an adult because the procedure is not warranted physiologically with smaller amounts of blood loss.

29. What are the nursing priorities associated with chest tube insertion?

- **Pain control**. When possible, the physician should inject the insertion site with lidocaine and allow time for it to take effect. If the patient is stable, intravenous (IV) analgesics should be administered. If the patient's condition is critical, distraction techniques and psychosocial support are appropriate.
- **Proper size chest tube**. For major trauma, a 36- to 40-French chest tube is used in adults. *Forensic tip:* The physician should avoid placing the chest tube through the site of the penetrating injury (i.e., stab or gunshot wound). If the case involves a violent crime, law enforcement officials and clinical forensic specialists will want to examine the entrance and exit wounds.
- **Set-up and management of chest drainage device and suction**. Be familiar with wet and dry systems in terms of the seal that prevents air from entering the chest and how the amount of suction is controlled. If the physician quickly places the tube and needs the drainage system immediately, fill the water seal with fluid before connecting the tubing. The water seal is essential for patient safety. The suction chamber can be filled after the chest tube is connected. Excessive bubbling will just cause noise and quicker evaporation of the water. Some units use a "dry" system, thereby avoiding the need for fluid in water seal and/or suction chambers.
- **Applying a dressing**. Most commonly, Vaseline-impregnated gauze is used around the insertion site to help provide an occlusive dressing with additional absorbent gauze on top to manage drainage from the site. Some institutions have gone to dry gauze to avoid maceration of the skin. A secure tape job over the dressing, tube, and tubing connections is important. The tube itself should be taped to the body, away from the dressing site, so that an unexpected tug does not dislodge the tube.
- **Chest radiograph**. This should follow chest tube insertion to determine correct placement and improvement of pneumothorax or hemothorax.
- **Safe transport procedures**. Do *not* clamp the chest tube. A tension pneumothorax may develop. Continue to mark output levels with times, and closely watch for sudden changes in drainage or changes in air leak patterns. Some patients with air leaks need suction to help remove air. In the CT scan suite or other locations, be sure to reconnect the suction. Keep fluid-filled chest drainage units upright.

30. What body location is used most often for emergent chest tube placement?

Most chest tubes are placed at the fifth intercostal space anterior to the midaxillary line. This site allows drainage of blood and air. A higher or anterior placement is designed only for a known small pneumothorax. A lower position risks entry into the liver or spleen.

31. What amount of blood drainage from a chest tube should cause concern?

More than 1500 ml initially and more than 250 ml/hr over 3 to 4 hours.

32. What finding indicates a worrisome air leak? How should this be evaluated?

Any air leak that is constant (i.e., present during inspiration and expiration) is of concern. Check the system to ensure that the leak does not stem from a loose connection or a cracked collection device. Check the patient for a dislodged tube or a chest tube drain hole outside the body under a dressing that is not airtight. If the leak persists, assume that the leak is within the patient, and notify the physician. Intervention may include placement of a second chest tube or evaluation of a bronchopleural fistula (BPF).

33. What is a BPF?

In the setting of trauma, a BPF can result from tracheal or direct lung injury. A BPF is essentially persistent communication between the large airways, alveoli (air sacs), and the pleura. It may be suspected when there is a persistent air leak from existing chest tubes or persistent or worsening pneumothorax or subcutaneous air. Most tracheobronchial injuries occur within 2 cm of the carina, at the point where there is maximum shear force between the fixed trachea and more mobile bronchial tree. Pulmonary lacerations result in disruption or tearing of the lung parenchyma. In both mechanisms, gas exchange may be significantly affected, precipitating further bronchoscopic and/or surgical evaluation and treatment. A child with significant BPF may benefit from extracorporeal membrane oxygenation (ECMO).

BLUNT CARDIAC INJURIES

34. What is a blunt cardiac injury (often referred to as cardiac contusion)?

The heart sits behind the sternum, rib cage, and chest musculature, which help to protect the heart from harm. But with significant blunt trauma the heart may be contused or bruised by these structures. A significant contusion can result in compromised heart function.

35. Should a monitored bed automatically be requested for a patient admitted with the diagnosis of cardiac contusion?

No. Studies have shown that unless conduction abnormalities are seen on electrocardiogram (ECG) or arrhythmias are documented during the initial ED presentation, the likelihood of future significant arrhythmia or cardiac injury is very low. However, if the patient is unstable, echocardiography is appropriate. In this setting or in the event of arrhythmias or conduction abnormalities, 48 hours or more of monitoring is suggested.

CARDIAC TAMPONADE

36. What unique findings help to make the diagnosis of cardiac tamponade?

The clinical features of cardiac tamponade include tachycardia, hypotension, muffled or "silent" heart sounds, and distended neck veins (indicating increased jugular venous pressure). As in the case of tension pneumothorax, venous distention may be difficult to observe, even in a supine patient. Pulsus paradoxus (an exaggerated decrease in systolic pressure occurring during inspiration) is another finding that signifies unexpected changes in venous pressure. Echocardiography can confirm the presence of an effusion into the fibrous pericardial sac and aids in assessing the hemodynamic impact of the tamponade. The heart sounds are muffled because the fluid surrounding the heart decreases the transmission of heart tones.

Some trauma centers have introduced surgeon-performed cardiac ultrasound to diagnose hemopericardium, thereby reducing the need for empiric pericardiocentesis.

37. Is cardiac tamponade more common in blunt or penetrating trauma?

Tamponade occurs most commonly with penetrating injury to the heart when blood leaks from the heart into the pericardial sac. If the wound to the pericardial sac seals over, the blood remains in the sac, creating a constricting fluid-filled sac.

38. How is cardiac tamponade treated emergently?

A pericardiocentesis may be performed. A 6-inch, 16-gauge needle is inserted under the xiphoid process, directed toward the apex of the heart. The needle may be attached to a 12-lead ECG via alligator clamps to help determine when the needle touches the heart. Significant ST elevation and a sharp deflection appear on the ECG pattern. Pericardiocentesis is associated with a significant false-positive rate, because the clinician may actually be drawing blood from the right ventricle itself. A general rule that may guide decision making is that blood from the pericardial sac usually does not clot, whereas blood from inside the heart should clot. At best, pericardiocentesis is a temporizing measure, performed to improve cardiac function pending surgical intervention. Emergent thoracotomy may be necessary, either in the ED or the OR. In some centers, pericardial windows are performed emergently in the ED by surgical or cardiothoracic physicians.

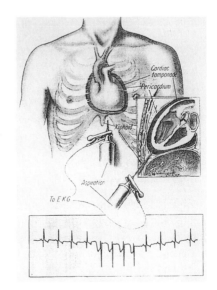

Technique of pericardiocentesis. Negative deflection of the QRS complex indicates contact with the epicardium. *(From Ebert P: The pericardium. In Sabiston DC, Spencer FC, editors: Gibbon's surgery of the chest, ed 4, Philadelphia, 1997, WB Saunders, with permission.)*

BLUNT TRAUMATIC AORTIC INJURIES

39. What is being measured in the widened mediastinum?

The width of the mediastinal shadow is measured on the chest radiograph at the aortic knob. A measurement larger than 8 cm is considered abnormal. Widening usually is caused by hemorrhage or hematoma in the vicinity of the aorta. Other findings on the chest radiograph are obliteration of the aortic knob and a pleural cap. A supine film can distort the mediastinum to appear wider than it is, and anteroposterior views can artificially widen the mediastinum, especially if the x-ray tube is placed too close to the patient when the radiograph is taken.

40. Why does the aorta tear?

Aortic tear is associated with a major deceleration force that is distributed unequally along the aorta because of its attachment to internal structures. The ligamentum arteriosum "fixes" the aorta at its proximal point, whereas the lower portion of the aorta is mobile. Deceleration forces cause stress at this fixed point, just distal to the branch of the left subclavian artery, and the intimal lining of the aorta can tear. If the adventitial layer remains intact, a contained hematoma prevents exsanguination. Sudden increases in pressure can weaken the adventitia, and at any time the patient may hemorrhage into the mediastinum.

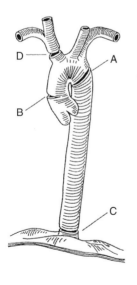

Sites of aortic rupture in order of frequency. *A*, Distal to left subclavian artery at the level of the ligamentum arteriosum. *B*, Ascending aorta. *C*, Lower thoracic aorta above diaphragm. *D*, Avulsion of innominate artery from aortic arch. *(Reprinted with permission from Frey C: Initial management of the trauma patient, Philadelphia, 1976, Lea & Febiger.)*

41. What additional symptoms may be reported?

Pain radiating to the back, hoarseness caused by pressure on the laryngeal nerve by the hematoma, and dyspnea and dysphagia are frequently reported symptoms. Depending on the location of the tear, variations in blood pressure between the left and right arm may be noted.

42. If the OR is not clearly indicated at this point, where should the patient be transported?

To the angiography suite for an arch aortogram or to the CT suite if a rapid spiral chest CT is diagnostically indicated. (Transesophageal echocardiography, another potential diagnostic modality, would often be performed at bedside.) A protocol is needed to guide the diagnostic process so that the patient does not undergo two ionic dye loads, one for CT and one for the angiogram. Full resuscitative support must be available in the angiography suite, requiring appropriate staff, close monitoring, and easily accessible trauma equipment and supplies.

43. What is the management strategy for blunt traumatic aortic injuries (BTAIs)?

While the patient with suspected BTAI is being evaluated and surgical options considered, a main goal of medical therapy should be to reduce aortic wall tension and thus minimize further shear forces. This is usually achieved by maintaining tight blood pressure and heart rate control, usually with a beta blocker. A short-acting drip such as esmolol allows for better control in patients who may still be unstable from other injuries. In general, early surgical intervention for BTAI is preferred. However, some patients may have other life-threatening injuries or be too unstable for surgery, resulting in delayed management. Endovascular stent-grafts may ultimately provide the trauma surgeon with additional therapeutic options for specific patient populations.

44. What new procedure can repair some aortic injuries without surgical intervention?

Endovascular stent-grafts can be placed during angiographic study through the left femoral artery. The stent is inserted, guided retrograde up the aorta, and released at the exact site of the aorta to cover the defect, ballooning open in response to aortic blood flow. A second stent-graft can be placed to overlap with the first if coverage is inadequate. However, a missed deployment that kinks or occludes vascular outflow from the aorta can be problematic. In contrast to abdominal aortic aneurysms where stent-grafts have been used extensively in select patients, the use of stent-grafts for thoracic injuries is still under investigation.

RESUSCITATIVE THORACOTOMY

45. What is ED resuscitative thoracotomy (EDRT)?

In extreme cases, when the patient has no signs of life, a thoracotomy may be done in the ED resuscitation room. This procedure is called an EDRT. It is an aggressive procedure performed for emergent management of exsanguinating hemorrhage.

46. What are the indications for EDRT?

Clear indications for EDRT include a victim of penetrating chest trauma who arrests in the ED or en route to the hospital or who has arrested at the scene and has recovered some signs of life (pulse, respirations, or reactive pupils).

EDRT has no role in the blunt trauma patient in pulseless arrest. Controversial issues include the following:

- The time frame for loss of vital signs is inconsistent in the literature.
- Children may benefit more than adults. Should the indications be expanded?
- Should any resuscitation occur if EDRT is not indicated?
- Should invasive procedures be performed for "practice"?

47. What is the best way to prepare for EDRT?

At the time of prehospital notification, ED staff mobilize the preassigned trauma team and prepare the resuscitation room. The room should be warm, with full lighting, and the stretcher should be draped with absorbent pads. Trauma team personnel should wear all necessary protective clothing, including face and eye protection. The thoracotomy tray should be opened or at least in close proximity to the stretcher. IV access trays, additional fluid lines, and type O blood should be available. The fluid warmer should be flushed and warming. Warm saline to pour over the heart should be available, and suction should be functional. Assemble the internal defibrillation paddles, in pediatric or adult size, and review the correct joules to use. The OR should be notified before the patient's arrival, and security should be notified of the potential need for quick access to the OR. Have oxygen and IV poles on the stretcher to facilitate quick transport to the OR if indicated. All staff should be familiar with the equipment on the thoracotomy tray and know where to find back-up supplies.

NONSKELETAL NECK TRAUMA

48. What is the function of the larynx?

The primary function of the larynx is respiration. It is also essential for phonation in verbal communication and protects the airway during swallowing.

49. How can the airway be compromised with neck trauma?

Swelling of the neck or tongue, hemorrhage into the throat, hematoma pressing against the larynx, or instability from thyroid or cricoid cartilage fracture can result in airway compromise. Simple injuries such as small lacerations to the tongue can evolve into large hematomas that block the airway. Close assessment of patients with facial or neck trauma is essential.

50. What signs and symptoms may be present with laryngeal injury?

Stridor, dyspnea, severe restlessness, altered voice quality, hoarseness, pain on palpation, and difficulty swallowing. Cervical subcutaneous emphysema may develop and extend to the mediastinum if pharyngeal or esophageal injuries are present.

51. If intubation is considered hazardous because of significant neck disruption, what procedure may be indicated?

Cricothyrotomy is the preferred surgical procedure. Assistance may be needed to position the mandible properly for temporary stabilization in cases associated with massive facial fractures. Be certain to be familiar with difficult airway supplies and know where the appropriate specialty trays are located and the types of tubes that may be placed after obtaining access to the airway. Carefully secure the tube in place; it may be the only chance for airway management. Tracheostomy is rarely indicated in the ED and is a more difficult, higher-risk procedure than cricothyrotomy. It is best performed in the OR.

52. **What diagnostic studies are most common in neck trauma?**

CT scan is the examination of choice for the larynx, along with fiberoptic laryngoscopy to examine soft tissue structures of the neck. Angiography or Doppler imaging is indicated in penetrating injury to the neck to evaluate for any vascular injury. Esophagrams, endoscopy, and/or operative examination should be used to evaluate possible injury to the esophagus. Nearly one-half of patients with a penetrating injury to the trachea also have an injury to the esophagus. Leakage from the esophagus into the mediastinum can be life threatening when undetected.

53. **How are neurological symptoms related to neck trauma?**

Carotid artery injuries are caused by penetrating injuries in over 95% of cases. Penetrating injuries can cause significant hemorrhage and symptoms of shock or may result in lack of proper carotid arterial flow leading to stroke. Blunt trauma, in particular motor vehicle collisions, can also cause significant neurological injury (e.g., stroke), particularly if not identified early. Mechanisms of injury include hyperextension and rotation, direct injury (e.g., a high-riding shoulder belt), facial injury, and basilar skull fracture. Although absolute screening protocols are still being standardized, CT or angiography is generally recommended in patients who are either symptomatic or have a high-risk mechanism of injury: C-spine fracture, basilar skull fracture, or major midface or mandibular fracture. Potential injuries include intimal tears, dissection, or pseudoaneurysms of both the carotid and vertebral arteries. Depending on the findings, therapy may include antiplatelet agents, heparin, or even stenting. Emboli monitoring and follow-up angiogram at 7 to 10 days are also generally recommended. A high index of suspicion and early screening can make a substantial difference in overall outcome.

Key Points

- Fractures of the scapula or first rib indicate a high-energy mechanism of injury and are often associated with vascular injuries. Similarly, lower rib fractures should raise the possibility of abdominal injuries.

- A tension pneumothorax is a life-threatening event where air continues to enter the pleural space but has no exit. Immediate therapy requires needle decompression, followed by chest tube placement.

- Hemothorax is blood in the pleural space and may appear as a diffuse opacity on chest x-ray. Therapy includes chest tube placement. More than 1500 ml initial output or more than 250 ml/hr for 3 to 4 hours raises the concern of significant thoracic vascular injury and may necessitate operative intervention.

- Blunt cardiac injury may result from blunt trauma to the chest. Conduction abnormalities or arrhythmias should trigger cardiac monitoring for the patient.

- Cardiac tamponade may occur with blunt or penetrating trauma and may be identified by tachycardia, hypotension, muffled heart sounds, and jugular venous distention. Diagnosis may be made by ultrasound, and emergent therapy is by pericardiocentesis or pericardial window.

- A widened mediastinum might indicate a BTAI, a type of injury associated with a major decelerating force. Medical management should target blood pressure and heart rate control to minimize shear stresses on the aorta.

- Blunt carotid (or vertebral) artery injuries may be suspected in certain high-risk mechanisms of injury such as C-spine fracture, basilar skull fracture, or midface/mandibular fractures. Early screening can help identify injuries and initiate appropriate therapy, thus minimizing the risk of subsequent embolic stroke.

Internet Resources

American College of Surgeons:

Managing Life-Threatening Thoracic Injuries:
www.facs.org/trauma/publications/thoracic.pdf

Thoracotomy in the Emergency Department:
www.facs.org/trauma/publications/thoracotomy.pdf

Eastern Association for the Surgery of Trauma:

Guidelines for the Diagnosis and Management of Blunt Aortic Trauma:
www.east.org/tpg/chap8.pdf

Pain Management in Blunt Thoracic Trauma (BTT): An Evidence-Based Outcome Evaluation:
www.east.org/tpg/painchest.pdf

Practice Management Guidelines for Screening of Blunt Cardiac Injury:
www.east.org/tpg/chap2.pdf

Trauma.org, Thoracic Trauma:
www.trauma.org/thoracic

Bibliography

The Acute Respiratory Distress Syndrome Network: Ventilation with lower tidal volumes as compared with traditional tidal volumes for acute lung injury and the acute respiratory distress syndrome, *N Engl J Med* 342:1301-1308, 2000.

American College of Surgeons: *Advanced trauma life support (ATLS) student manual*, Chicago, 2004, American College of Surgeons.

Asensio JA et al: Penetrating cardiac injuries: A prospective study of variables predicting outcomes, *J Am Coll Surg* 186:24-34, 1998.

Asensio JA et al: Penetrating esophageal injuries: Multicenter study of the American Association for the Surgery of Trauma, *J Trauma* 50(2):289-296, 2001.

Biffl WL et al: Treatment-related outcomes from blunt cerebrovascular injuries: Importance of routine follow-up arteriography, *Ann Surg* 235(5):699-707, 2002.

Bulger E et al: Epidural analgesia improves outcome after multiple rib fractures, *Surgery* 136:426-430, 2004.

Bulger E et al: Rib fractures in the elderly, *J Trauma* 48(6):1040-1047, 2000.

Dong Xu S et al: Treating aortic dissection and penetrating aortic ulcer with stent graft: Thirty cases, *Ann Thorac Surg* 80:864-868, 2005.

Ebert P: The pericardium. In Sabiston DC, Spencer FC, editors: *Gibbon's surgery of the chest*, ed 4, Philadelphia, 1997, WB Saunders.

Frey C: *Initial management of the trauma patient*, Philadelphia, 1976, Lea & Febiger.

Karmy-Jones R et al: Endovascular stent grafts and aortic rupture: A case series, *J Trauma* 55(5):805-810, 2003.

Karmy-Jones R, Nathens A, Stern E, editors: *Thoracic trauma and critical care*, Boston, 2002, Kluwer Academic.

Keough V, Pudelek B: Blunt chest trauma: Review of selected pulmonary injuries focusing on pulmonary contusion, *AACN Clin Issues* 12(2):270-281, 2001.

Mattox KL, Wall MJ: Historical review of blunt injury to the thoracic aorta, *Chest Surg Clin N Am* 10(1): 167-182, 2000.

Miller PR et al: ARDS after pulmonary contusion: Accurate measurement of contusion volume identifies high-risk patients, *J Trauma* 51(2):223-230, 2001.

Ott MC et al: Management of blunt thoracic aortic injuries: Endovascular stents versus open repair, *J Trauma* 56(3):565-570, 2004.

Seaton A, Seaton D, Leitch AG, editors: *Crofton and Douglas's respiratory diseases*, vol 2, ed 5, Oxford, 2000, Blackwell Science.

Sherry E, Trieu L, Templeton J, editors: *Trauma*, Oxford, England, 2003, Oxford University Press.

Vidhani K, Kause J, Parr M: Should we follow ATLS guidelines for the management of traumatic pulmonary contusion: The role of non-invasive ventilatory support, *Resuscitation* 52(3):265-268, 2002.

Wellons ED et al: Stent-graft repair of traumatic thoracic aortic disruptions, *J Vasc Surg* 40(6):1095-1100, 2004.

Abdominal Trauma

Kathleen Flarity

1. **What are the three regions of the abdomen, and what is contained in each region?**

   The peritoneal cavity, the pelvic cavity, and the retroperitoneal cavity.

Organs by Abdominal Region

Peritoneal Cavity
Upper abdomen: diaphragm, liver, spleen, stomach, transverse colon
Lower abdomen: small bowel, sigmoid colon

Pelvic Cavity
Rectum, bladder, iliac vessels, internal genitalia (women)

Retroperitoneal Cavity
Abdominal aorta, inferior vena cava, most of the duodenum, pancreas, kidneys, ureters, ascending and descending colons

---

2. **What is the most common mechanism of injury associated with abdominal trauma?**

   Motor vehicle crashes account for the majority of abdominal trauma, including admissions in both rural and urban trauma centers.

3. **What are the biomechanics associated with blunt abdominal trauma?**

   Blunt injuries result from motor vehicle and pedestrian crashes, assaults, and falls. Blunt abdominal injuries result from mechanical energy that includes external forces (deceleration and acceleration) and internal forces (stress and strain). The aorta is a good example. Deceleration (external forces) make fixed anatomical structures such as the descending thoracic aorta susceptible to injury, and shearing stress (internal forces) results in tearing of the aorta.

4. Which organs are most commonly injured as a result of blunt abdominal trauma?

The spleen (40% to 55%) and liver (35% to 45%).

5. What mechanism of injury is associated with penetrating trauma to the abdomen?

Penetrating trauma may result from stabs, gunshot wounds, or impalements. In the case of stab wounds, the injury is related to the length and shape of the instrument, the angle of the entry, and the velocity at which the force is applied. Organ and tissue damage resulting from missiles is related to projectile mass and shape, missile velocity, fragmentation, and tissue transversed. As many as 96% to 98% of gunshot wounds that penetrate the abdomen produce significant intraabdominal injury.

6. When should the clinician consider a patient to have an abdominal injury from penetrating trauma?

The abdomen extends from the nipples to the groin crease anteriorly and from the scapular to gluteal fold posteriorly. Any penetrating injury that may have entered this region should be evaluated for abdominal trauma.

7. Which organs are most commonly injured as a result of penetrating trauma?

Stab wounds transverse adjacent abdominal structures and most commonly result in injuries to the following organs:
- Liver (40%)
- Small bowel (30%)
- Diaphragm (20%)
- Colon (15%)

Gunshot wounds typically cause more intraabdominal injuries and commonly involve the following organs:
- Small bowel (50%)
- Colon (40%)
- Liver (30%)
- Abdominal vascular structures (25%)

8. What common injury patterns are associated with blunt abdominal trauma?

Blunt Abdominal Trauma Injury Patterns

Musculoskeletal Injury	Underlying Organ Injury
Right lower rib fractures	Liver
Left lower rib fractures	Spleen
Anterior pelvic fractures	Bladder, urethra
Lumbar (Chance) fractures	Small bowel or colon

9. What physical findings are indicative of intraabdominal injury?

Evaluation of the abdomen is one of the most critical components of the initial assessment. Unrecognized abdominal injuries are a major cause of preventable deaths after trauma. Any patient with significant mechanism must be assumed to have an abdominal injury until proven otherwise.

Physical Findings Indicative of Intraabdominal Injury

Finding	Sign	Implications
Periumbilical ecchymosis	Cullen's sign	Peritoneal bleeding
Ecchymosis of flank	Grey Turner's sign	Retroperitoneal bleeding
LUQ pain radiating to left shoulder	Kehr's sign	Splenic or diaphragm injury
Ecchymosis of perineum, scrotum, or labia	Coopernail's sign	Pelvic fracture
Fixed area of dullness in percussion of LUQ	Balance's sign	Splenic hematoma

LUQ, left upper quadrant.

10. What techniques should be employed for examination of the abdomen?

The physical examination is the most informative portion of the diagnostic evaluation. Abdominal injury may be insidious and requires a close systematic assessment by emergency department (ED) personnel to facilitate early diagnosis and intervention. The sequence of abdominal examination is as follows:
- Inspection
- Auscultation
- Percussion
- Palpation (begin in a quadrant where the patient has not complained of pain)

11. Which diagnostic tools are used for the initial evaluation of blunt abdominal trauma?

The most common diagnostic modalities are diagnostic peritoneal lavage (DPL), computed tomography (CT), and ultrasonography (i.e., focused abdominal sonography for trauma—FAST—scan).

12. What is a FAST scan?

The FAST scan is a limited ultrasound procedure used on trauma patients to detect free fluid in the abdomen or pericardium. In the hands of an experienced operator the average time to perform a FAST scan is 2 to 3 minutes. Indications for the FAST scan include all cases of suspected intraabdominal injury from trauma. It is especially useful in hemodynamically unstable patients or patients who are not ideal candidates for CT scan.

13. What are the advantages and disadvantages of CT, DPL, and FAST scan in the evaluation of abdominal trauma?

Advantages and Disadvantages of Tests

Test	Advantages	Disadvantages
CT	Noninvasive; most specific for injury: 92%-98% accurate	Cost and time, including transport time; misses bowel tract, diaphragm, and some pancreas injuries
DPL	Quick, early diagnosis; sensitive: 98% accurate	Invasive; misses injury to diaphragm and retroperitoneum
FAST	Quick, early diagnosis; noninvasive and easily repeated; sensitivity of 97.6% and specificity of 98.7% with experienced operator	Operator-dependent; bowel gas and subcutaneous air distortion; misses diaphragm, bowel, and some pancreas injuries; requires approximately 200 ml of fluid for visualization, so may be negative if performed early

14. What four areas of the abdomen are examined with ultrasound for the detection of free fluid? What is seen in each area?

Ultrasound Detection Areas

Abdominal Area	Visualizes
RUQ abdomen (Morison's pouch)	Subhepatic fluid collections and upper pole of kidney; right lobe of liver; lesions of right kidney or retroperitoneal space; costophrenic intrathoracic fluid
Subxiphoid (pericardial) area	Lesions of pancreas; left lobe of liver; pericardial fluid
LUQ	Lesions of spleen and perisplenic fluid; fluid in pericolic gutter
Pelvis (Douglas's pouch)	Fluid in anterior pelvis; can visualize bladder, prostate, or uterus and lateral pelvic walls

RUQ, right upper quadrant; *LUQ,* left upper quadrant.

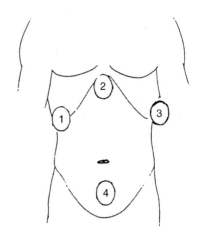

Areas of ultrasound evaluation and sequence. *1*, RUQ abdomen (Morison's pouch); *2*, subxiphoid (pericardial) area; *3*, LUQ; *4*, pelvis (Douglas's pouch). *(Adapted from Rozycki GS et al: Surgeon-performed ultrasound for the assessment of truncal injuries, Ann Surg 228:557, 1998.)*

15. What does a positive FAST scan indicate?

If blood is found in any of the sites with the FAST scan, it is presumed that the patient has a hemoperitoneum and should undergo abdominal surgical exploration. However, if the FAST scan is negative (no blood identified in the sites), but there is a high clinical suspicion of injury, consider additional testing such as a CT scan.

16. What are the criteria for a positive DPL result?

In blunt trauma:
- 10 ml or more of gross blood with initial aspiration. Otherwise, 1 L of warm saline or lactated Ringer's solution is infused and drained back out and sent for analysis. If the returned fluid contains:
  - 100,000 or more red blood cells (RBCs)/mm^3
  - 500 or more white blood cells (WBCs)/mm^3
  - Presence of bile, bacteria, or fibers

In penetrating trauma:
- 10 ml or more of gross blood with initial aspiration
- 50,000 or more RBCs/mm^3 in the returned fluid

17. What are the general indications for exploratory laparotomy in adults?

- Blunt abdominal trauma with positive DPL or ultrasound
- Blunt abdominal trauma with recurrent hypotension despite adequate resuscitation
- Penetrating abdominal wound with hypotension
- Penetrating trauma with blood from the stomach, rectum, or genitourinary tract
- Evisceration of abdominal contents
- Gunshot wounds transversing the peritoneal cavity
- Evidence of peritonitis

18. Do all patients with solid organ injuries go to surgery?

The management of injuries of the abdominal solid organs (liver, spleen, kidney, and pancreas) has evolved from routine operative exploration to cautious observation for most injuries in hemodynamically stable patients—adult and pediatric. Solid organ pathways and classifications have been developed by institutions and organizations such as the American Association for the Surgery of Trauma (AAST) to aid in injury management.

DIAPHRAGM INJURIES

19. Which area of the diaphragm is more likely to be injured by blunt trauma? Why?

Approximately two thirds of diaphragm injuries involve the left hemidiaphragm for the following possible reasons:
- It is thought that the left hemidiaphragm is less resistant to high abdominal pressures.
- The esophagus passes through an opening in the left hemidiaphragm.
- The liver protects the right diaphragm.

20. What is the incidence of associated injuries related to diaphragmatic trauma?

Penetrating trauma to the diaphragm is associated with other injuries in approximately 75% to 80% of cases. Isolated diaphragm injuries are extremely rare in blunt trauma but may occur with mechanisms involving severe compression of the abdomen. Blunt trauma generally produces a significant number of extraabdominal thoracic injuries.

21. What organ injuries are commonly seen in patients with diaphragmatic injury?

The lung is the most commonly injured organ in conjunction with blunt or penetrating diaphragmatic trauma. Approximately 60% of patients have a pneumothorax or hemothorax. Injuries to the liver, stomach, spleen, and lungs are also common with penetrating trauma. Most patients with blunt diaphragmatic injuries also have orthopedic injuries, particularly pelvic fractures, neurological injuries, and a variety of solid viscous injuries.

22. What diagnostic modalities are used in detecting diaphragm rupture?

Chest radiograph is the most useful noninvasive tool for diagnosis of diaphragm injury. A nasogastric tube placement will allow decompression of the stomach and may help diagnose the diaphragm injury on chest x-ray. A contrast study of the gastrointestinal (GI) tract is the most accurate radiological test for diaphragmatic rupture. Contrast material delivered through an indwelling nasogastric tube clearly demonstrates displacement of the stomach in the chest. Although CT scan is a useful adjunct, few specific CT findings relate to diaphragm injuries. Laparoscopy is also a reliable modality but is invasive and requires a trip to the OR.

DPL is also unreliable in diagnosing isolated diaphragm injury; positive results are usually because of associated intraabdominal organ injury. A negative DPL does not rule out a diaphragm injury. Magnetic resonance imaging (MRI) can provide accurate recognition of diaphragmatic defects and visceral herniation; however, this may not be practical in patients with multisystem trauma.

23. Do all diaphragmatic lacerations require surgical repair?

Yes. All acute diaphragm injuries should be repaired, because complications may develop at any time. Complications include herniation, viscerothorax, intestinal obstruction, bowel strangulation, hemothorax, or pneumothorax. Herniation of the stomach or bowel may occur hours or years after the initial injury and can cause life-threatening respiratory distress.

LIVER INJURIES

24. What mechanism of injury is associated with liver damage?

Penetrating trauma (stab and gunshot wounds) accounts for the majority of liver injuries. Motor vehicle crashes are the major cause of liver injuries caused by blunt trauma.

25. How common are liver injuries in blunt trauma? What are the associated injuries?

The liver is the second most commonly injured solid organ (after the spleen) in blunt trauma. Approximately 90% of blunt hepatic injuries are associated with injuries to other intraabdominal organs, especially the spleen, intestines, and kidneys. Chest trauma is also common with liver injury—especially the right lower chest.

26. What tools are used to diagnose liver injuries?

- The FAST scan is preferred to DPL in most centers in the United States, Europe, and Japan. It is accurate in detecting hemoperitoneum but lacks the specificity of CT scan. It provides a rapid assessment of intraabdominal fluid.
- CT scan is advocated for stable trauma patients and is useful in diagnosing specific organ injury. It also can be useful in grading the severity of liver injury, thus enabling the surgeon to determine operative versus nonoperative management.
- DPL is extremely useful in patients with suspected intraabdominal injury and has a 90% to 98% accuracy rate in detecting blood in the peritoneal cavity. DPL can be performed quickly in hemodynamically unstable trauma patients.

27. What are the physical indications of potential liver injury?

- Trauma to the right upper quadrant (RUQ) of the abdomen or right lower chest
- Right-sided rib fractures
- Penetrating injury at or below the right fourth intercostal space
- Referred pain to the right shoulder

28. How are liver injuries classified?

Liver injuries may be classified anatomically by the AAST Organ Injury Scaling Committee guidelines. The six-grade system is based on the size and length of the hematoma or laceration and the presence of vascular injury. The scale is from grades I (hematoma) to VI (hepatic avulsion).

Liver Injury Scale

Grade*	Injury	Description
I	Hematoma	Subcapsular, less than 10% surface area
	Laceration	Capsular tear, less than 1 cm parenchymal depth
II	Hematoma	Subcapsular, 10%-50% surface area
		Intraparenchymal, less than 10 cm in diameter
	Laceration	1-3 cm parenchymal depth; less than 10 cm in length
III	Hematoma	Subcapsular, more than 50% surface area or expanding ruptured subcapsular or parenchymal hematoma
		Intraparenchymal hematoma larger than 10 cm or expanding
	Laceration	More than 3 cm parenchymal depth
IV	Laceration	Parenchymal disruption involving 25%-75% of hepatic lobe or one to three Couinaud's segments within a single lobe
V	Laceration	Parenchymal disruption involving more than 75% of lobe or more than three Couinaud's segments within a single lobe
	Vascular	Juxtahepatic venous injuries (i.e., retrohepatic vena cava/central major hepatic veins)
VI	Vascular	Hepatic avulsion

*Advance one grade for multiple injuries, up to grade III.
Modified from Moore EE et al: Organ injury scaling: Spleen and liver (1994 revision), *J Trauma* 33:323-324, 1995.

29. What is the mortality rate for patients sustaining liver injury?

Because most liver injuries are grade I or II, the overall mortality rate is low (about 10%) for liver injuries. Most immediate deaths are caused by exsanguination; later, postoperative deaths are usually attributable to sepsis.

SPLEEN INJURIES

30. What solid organ is the most commonly injured in blunt trauma?

The spleen is the most commonly injured intraabdominal organ, with mortality rates ranging from 3% to 23%. The spleen is the most vascular organ and holds approximately 1 L of blood.

31. **What physical findings indicate a possible splenic injury from blunt trauma?**

Compared with other injuries, blunt injury to the spleen has a more subtle and varied presentation. Abdominal tenderness and distention are present in only 50% of patients with a splenic injury. Hypotension is a presenting symptom in 25% to 30% of the patients. Some patients are asymptomatic and others are hemodynamically unstable. Some findings suggestive of splenic injuries include:
- Trauma or ecchymosis over the left lower chest wall or left upper abdomen
- Abdominal pain or tenderness, especially in the left upper quadrant (LUQ)
- Left ninth, tenth, and eleventh rib fractures (left lower rib fracture is present in 44% of patients with splenic rupture)
- Referred pain to the left shoulder from diaphragmatic irritation (Kehr's sign)
- Signs of shock, such as tachycardia and hypotension

32. **What chest radiographic findings signal the clinician to suspect splenic injury?**

- Left pleural effusion
- Elevated left hemidiaphragm
- Left lower lobe pulmonary contusion
- Fractures of ninth, tenth, and eleventh ribs of the left chest
- Medial displacement of the gastric bubble and inferior displacement of the splenic flexure gas pattern

33. **What other diagnostic tools are used to identify splenic injuries?**

Abdominal CT with intravenous (IV) contrast to maximize density differences between the splenic parenchyma and hematomas is the study of choice for identifying splenic injuries in stable patients. CT with contrast also gives the advantage of simultaneously imaging all organs for injury. The disadvantage is the motion artifact if the patient cannot remain still. DPL and the FAST scan may be useful in unstable patients.

34. **How are splenic injuries classified?**

Splenic injuries have been classified anatomically into five grades based on the size and length of the fracture and the presence of vascular injury by the AAST Organ Injury Scaling Committee. The range is from grade I for hematomas to grade V for the devascularized spleen.

Spleen Injury Scale

Grade*	Injury	Description
I	Hematoma	Subcapsular, less than 10% surface area
	Laceration	Capsular tear, less than 1 cm parenchymal depth
II	Hematoma	Subcapsular, 10%-50% surface area
		Intraparenchymal, less than 10 cm in diameter
	Laceration	1-3 cm parenchymal depth, which does not involve a trabecular vessel
III	Hematoma	Subcapsular, more than 50% surface area or expanding
		Ruptured subcapsular or parenchymal hematoma
		Intraparenchymal hematoma larger than 5 cm or expanding
	Laceration	More than 3 cm parenchymal depth or involving trabecular vessels
IV	Laceration	Laceration involving segmental or hilar vessels producing major devascularization (more than 25% of spleen)
V	Laceration	Completely shattered spleen
	Vascular	Hilar vascular injury that devascularizes spleen

*Advance one grade for multiple injuries, up to grade III.
Modified from Moore EE et al: Organ injury scaling: Spleen and liver (1994 revision), *J Trauma* 33:323-324, 1995.

35. What are the management options for patients with splenic injury?

Most patients with penetrating splenic injury have associated injuries that require surgical intervention, thereby justifying the universal consensus that penetrating trauma requires operative intervention. Patients with grades I to III blunt splenic injuries without evidence of active bleeding may be managed nonoperatively. All others require surgical intervention.

36. What criteria must be met for nonoperative management of splenic injuries?

- Hemodynamic stability
- Isolated splenic injury
- No signs or symptoms of bleeding
- No evidence of hypovolemia or hypotension
- Neurologically intact patient
- No evidence of coagulopathy

GASTRIC AND SMALL BOWEL INJURIES

37. What organs are injured most frequently in penetrating abdominal trauma?

The stomach and small bowel combined are the most commonly injured organs in penetrating abdominal trauma. Eighty percent of small bowel injuries are caused by gunshot wounds.

38. How often does injury to the stomach and small bowel occur in blunt abdominal trauma?

The incidence of gastric injury is low (estimated at 1% to 2%). The incidence of small bowel injury caused by blunt trauma ranges from 5% to 15%.

39. What is the significance of a Chance fracture in blunt abdominal trauma?

A Chance fracture is a fracture of the lower thoracic or lumbar spine, transversely through the vertebral body. It is produced by a flexion-distraction mechanism of injury, which often involves a safety belt. Chance fractures are a particularly important indicator of the possible presence of blunt intestinal injury.

40. Are stomach injuries fairly easy to diagnose on physical exam?

Yes. The acidity inside the stomach produces peritoneal signs and symptoms (abdominal pain or tenderness, rigidity, fever, chills, decreased bowel sounds) that are more acute and severe than with other hollow viscus injuries. Bloody nasogastric returns also may indicate a gastric injury.

41. What laboratory studies are helpful in diagnosing gastric and small bowel injuries?

No laboratory studies are specific for gastric or small bowel injury. A rising WBC count may be indicative of GI injury.

42. What is the most reliable method for detecting hollow visceral injury?

DPL is probably the most reliable test for detecting hollow visceral injury. An increased RBC or WBC count in the peritoneal lavage fluid may be suggestive of injury. The presence of bile or food fibers in peritoneal lavage effluent is rare. CT scan is not reliable in detecting injuries of the stomach and small bowel unless a large amount of free intraperitoneal air or fluid is present. A negative DPL or CT scan does not rule out the possibility of an injury.

43. What are the indications for surgical intervention in penetrating abdominal trauma?

Gunshot wounds to the abdomen mandate immediate exploration. Patients sustaining abdominal stab wounds may undergo local exploration to determine penetration through the fascia or into the peritoneal cavity. One should suspect gastric or intestinal injury in patients who have sustained stab wounds to the abdomen with peritoneal penetration. Evisceration of omentum or small bowel requires prompt laparotomy.

44. What tetrad of injuries is often caused by lap safety belts?

Lap-only safety belts cause abdominal wall contusions, small bowel rupture, mesenteric tears, and lumbar spine fractures.

DUODENAL INJURIES

45. What mechanism of injury contributes to duodenal trauma?

Duodenal injuries are relatively uncommon (approximately 3% to 5% of all intraabdominal trauma). Three fourths of duodenal injuries result from penetrating trauma. Causes of blunt injury to the duodenum include compression of the epigastric area by the steering wheel or handlebars of bicycles or improperly applied seat belts.

46. Are plain radiograph films of the abdomen indicated in patients with suspected duodenal injury?

Yes. Obliteration of the right psoas shadow, retroperitoneal air bubbles along the right psoas muscle or around the right kidney, or presence of retroperitoneal air is suggestive of duodenal perforation.

47. Is serum amylase sensitive for duodenal injury?

No. A single elevated serum amylase is unreliable for diagnosing duodenal injury; however, a rising or persistently increased serum amylase mandates further evaluation for duodenal injury. Hyperamylasemia also can be seen in patients with facial trauma or recent ethanol ingestion. Duodenal injury frequently occurs without a rise in serum amylase levels.

48. Are all duodenal injuries managed surgically?

No. Duodenal hematomas can be managed nonoperatively, even in the presence of partial duodenal obstruction. Treatment consists of nasogastric suction for decompression and hyperalimentation. Resolution of hematomas occurs in most patients in 1 to 3 weeks. Surgical intervention is recommended for duodenal hematomas with complete occlusions and all other duodenal injuries.

PANCREAS INJURIES

49. What is the incidence of pancreatic injury? What is the mechanism of injury?

Pancreatic trauma is uncommon (7% to 8%), and most injuries are caused by penetrating trauma. Pancreatic injury from blunt trauma most often results from direct impact to the epigastric area (i.e., impact with the steering wheel or bicycle handles).

50. What is the mortality rate for pancreatic injuries?

Although pancreatic injury is relatively uncommon, the mortality rate can be high. Mortality rates are variable and depend on the mechanism of injury, number of associated injuries, time to initial diagnosis, and presence or absence of major ductal injury.

51. **What organs are most frequently injured in association with penetrating wounds of the pancreas?**

Liver and stomach injuries are commonly seen in conjunction with pancreatic injury.

52. **Is serum amylase a sensitive indicator of pancreatic injury?**

No. As with duodenal injury, serum amylase levels are not a reliable indicator of pancreatic injury. Pancreatic isoenzymes, such as lipase, in conjunction with the patient's clinical information may help to determine pancreatic injury.

53. **Is DPL useful in detecting pancreatic injury?**

No. The pancreas is located in the retroperitoneal cavity, and DPL is unreliable in diagnosing injury of the retroperitoneal organs.

54. **What role does CT scan play in the detection of pancreatic injury?**

Abdominal CT scan is currently the diagnostic modality of choice in evaluating pancreatic injury in stable trauma patients. However, the reliability and accuracy of CT scan in detecting pancreatic injury have been questioned. Initial nondiagnostic CT scans do not rule out pancreatic injury, and a repeat CT scan should be done in patients with unexplained or changing abdominal complaints or increasing serum amylase or lipase levels. Many pancreatic injuries that are not initially apparent manifest in 24 to 72 hours after injury; therefore serial lab tests, such as lipase and/or amylase, in conjunction with a repeat CT scan of the abdomen may be useful.

55. **How are pancreatic injuries managed?**

All pancreatic injuries require surgical intervention because there is always leakage of pancreatic enzymes. The required intervention depends on the extent of pancreatic injury, which may range from simple laceration to transection. Surgical intervention may consist of simple external, closed drainage; distal pancreatectomy; or, for major injuries, pancreaticoduodenectomy. The goals of surgery are to control hemorrhage, debride devitalized tissue, and provide adequate drainage.

56. **What are the causes of death in patients with pancreatic injury?**

Most deaths in patients sustaining pancreatic injury are caused by hemorrhage and shock; most of these deaths occur within the first 24 to 48 hours. The causes of late death include intraabdominal and systemic sepsis and pulmonary complications. Deaths specifically related to pancreatic injury are caused by acute severe pancreatitis and/or pancreatic fistula.

RENAL TRAUMA

57. **What is the most common injury to the kidney?**

Blunt contusion.

58. What are some clinical findings suggestive of renal injury?

- Fractures of the posterior lower ribs
- Lumbar fractures
- Grey Turner's sign (Ecchymosis over the flank)
- Gross or microscopic hematuria
- Flank tenderness with palpation

59. How are renal injuries classified?

Kidney injuries have been classified anatomically into five grades based on the size and length of the fracture and the presence of vascular injury by the AAST Organ Injury Scaling Committee. The range is from grade I for a contusion with microscopic or gross hematuria to grade IV for a completely shattered kidney.

60. How are renal injuries diagnosed, and what are some of the advantages and disadvantages of each test?

Comparison of Angiography, CT, and IV Urography for Renal Injuries

Test	Advantages	Disadvantages
Angiography	Delineates vascular injuries.	Invasive.
CT	Delineates grade of injury, shows infarcted segments of the kidney, and identifies other abdominal organ injuries. Shows retroperitoneal structures.	Not appropriate for hemodynamically unstable patients.
IV Urography	90% accurate under the best of conditions. One shot may be helpful to identify contralateral functioning kidney in unstable patient.	Poor study in hypotensive patients; does not evaluate retroperitoneum.

61. Many renal injuries may be handled conservatively; what are some renal injuries that require surgery?

- Vascular injury
- Shattered kidney
- Expanding or pulsatile hematoma
- Persistent extravasation

OPEN BOOK PELVIC FRACTURE

62. What is an open book pelvic fracture?

An open book pelvic fracture occurs when one or both hemipelves rotate externally because of a vertical fracture through the pubic rami or an injury to the symphysis pubis. The mechanism is usually an anteroposterior compression force applied to the pelvis, which splits the symphysis pubis and widens the sacroiliac joint anteriorly. The ipsilateral sacrotuberous and sacrospinous ligaments are often torn while the strong posterior sacroiliac joint remains intact. This gives the appearance of an open book on x-ray.

63. What are some of the complications of open book pelvic fracture?

Patients with open book pelvic fractures usually have multiple high-energy injuries and a high mortality rate. Retroperitoneal hemorrhage and hypovolemic shock may result from tears of the sacral plexus as the fractured pelvic bones move. Neurological injuries may also occur.

64. How is diagnosis of the open book pelvis fracture made?

The diagnosis can be suspected clinically but needs to be confirmed with pelvic x-rays. Additional inlet and outlet views can help identify the full extent of the fracture. Pelvic CT scan may give more details of the injuries.

65. What is pelvic sheeting?

Acute traumatic pelvic ring instability causes severe pain, hemorrhage, and secondary injury with patient movement. Circumferential pelvic sheeting with a bed sheet is a noninvasive resuscitation aid that provides comfort and emergent temporary pelvic stability. Manufactured circumferential Velcro pelvic stabilizers or military antishock trousers (MASTs) with only the pelvic segment inflated may also be used to stabilize the pelvis and may provide better tension for stabilization than sheeting. However, bed sheets are readily available, inexpensive, easily applied, and disposable. For specific details, see Routh, Falicov, Woodhouse, and Schildhauer (2002).

BLADDER TRAUMA

66. How does bladder trauma occur?

Trauma to the bladder is associated with significant trauma to the pelvic and intraabdominal organs. Bladder injuries can be the result of blunt or penetrating trauma. Laceration by pelvic fragments occurs in 5% to 10% of patients with a pelvic fracture. Motor vehicle crashes are a common mechanism of injury.

67. How is bladder trauma classified?

Bladder trauma is classified into five degrees of injury, from partial tears of the mucosa to combined rupture with leakage of both intraperitoneal and extraperitoneal urine.

68. What are some clinical findings suggestive of bladder trauma?

Patients usually have very few symptoms related to bladder injury or even rupture. They do not have a propensity to develop signs and symptoms of peritonitis (rebound tenderness, rigidity, guarding) even with a large amount of uroperitoneum. Some signs suggestive of bladder injury include:
- Gross hematuria (present in 95% of cases)
- Microhematuria (more than 25,000 to 35,000 RBCs per high-power field) present in 5% of cases

- Suprapubic pain
- Pubic rami fracture present
- Pubic symphysis diastasis present
- Lap belt ecchymosis (4% of children with lap belt ecchymosis have bladder rupture)

69. How is diagnosis of bladder injury made, and what is the treatment?

CT cystography or retrograde cystography, performed under urethrography. Usually CT cystography is the study of choice because it can also be used to evaluate other urological organs. Ultrasonography is not sensitive or specific enough to be used for bladder rupture.

Treatment is advanced trauma life-support measures, followed by trauma surgeon and/or urology evaluation and surgical repair.

URETHRAL RUPTURE

70. What is the typical mechanism of injury of a patient with urethral rupture?

Urethral injuries are usually associated with pelvic fractures from high-energy trauma such as motor vehicle crashes or falls from heights. Isolated urethral rupture is usually from straddle-type injuries. Urethral ruptures are rare in women because of the short length and mobility of the urethra. Urethral injuries should be suspected in women with blood at the urinary meatus, urethral hematoma, or urine leaking into the vagina.

71. What is the triad of urethral rupture?

Blood at the urinary meatus, inability to pass urine, and a distended bladder.

72. What are other clinical findings suggestive of urethral rupture?

- Scrotal hematoma
- Butterfly-pattern bruising of the perineum
- High-riding or boggy prostate

73. How is diagnosis of urethral injury made, and what is the treatment?

Diagnosis is made with clinical presentation and a retrograde urethrogram. Treatment is advanced trauma life-support measures followed by urology consultation. If urethral rupture is suspected (see clinical findings discussed previously), do not attempt insertion of a Foley catheter; a urologist will typically place a suprapubic catheter. Additional interventions include IV antibiotics and surgical repair with urethral realignment if necessary.

COLON AND RECTAL INJURIES

74. What mechanism of injury is associated with colon and rectal injuries?

Ninety-six percent of all trauma to the colon and rectum is penetrating. Missile injuries account for approximately 75% of penetrating injuries; the remaining 25% are caused by stab wounds or impalement injuries from falls. Blunt colon trauma has been related to deceleration injuries involving impact with a safety belt or steering wheel. Auto-pedestrian crashes, assaults, and falls also add to the small percentage of blunt colon and rectal injuries. Rectal perforation from foreign bodies is rare.

75. What is the mortality rate for colon and rectal injuries?

The mortality rate for isolated colon and rectal injuries is extremely low (5% to 6%). One of the main factors affecting outcome of colon and rectal injuries is the number and type of associated injuries.

76. What forces or mechanisms produce colonic injury in blunt abdominal trauma?

- **Crush injuries** to the colon are the common type. Most are caused by compression of the colon between the anterior abdominal wall and the lumbar spine. Compression may cause serosal tears, hematomas, or complete laceration. Injuries of this nature most often involve the transverse colon.
- **Deceleration injuries** involve shear stress at points of relative colonic fixation and mobility. Such injuries tend to occur at the hepatic or splenic flexures or in the distal sigmoid colon.
- **Burst injuries** are similar to blunt duodenal and gastric injuries and involve a rapid rise in intraluminal pressure. Burst injuries of the colon most commonly involve the cecum.

77. What safety belt injuries should raise the index of suspicion for colonic injury?

The presence of a Chance fracture and an anterior abdominal wall hematoma should serve as indicators for a potential colon injury.

78. Is the absence of bowel sounds indicative of colon injury?

Yes, but bowel sounds may be present at the time of the initial evaluation. They often disappear after a few hours if bowel perforation has occurred.

79. What physical findings indicate possible peritonitis and colon injury?

Characteristic findings include any change in the abdominal exam suggestive of peritoneal signs, such as guarding and rebound tenderness. Fever, nausea, and vomiting are suggestive of serious pathology. Gross blood from the rectum is also indicative of colonic injury.

80. What is the best method for detecting colon injuries?

Most colon injuries are diagnosed during exploratory laparotomy. The diagnosis of colon injury is often made during laparotomy for associated injuries that have caused peritoneal signs or hypotension.

81. What are the indications for an exploratory laparotomy in patients with colon injuries?

- Hemodynamic instability
- Peritoneal signs or symptoms

- High index of suspicion in blunt trauma
- Patients with anterior penetrating wounds below the fifth intercostal space
- Patients with radiographic evidence of free air or bullets below the diaphragm

82. **Are preoperative antibiotics indicated in patients with suspected colon injuries?**

Patients with suspected colon or rectal injuries should receive preoperative parenteral antibiotics to cover gram-negative aerobes (such as *Escherichia coli*) and anaerobes (such as *Bacteroides fragilis*) so that adequate blood levels can be achieved by the time of laparotomy. A second-generation cephalosporin such as cefotetan or cefoxitin is recommended.

TESTICULAR TRAUMA

83. **What are the three types of testicular trauma and examples of each?**

- **Blunt trauma:** injuries sustained from objects striking the scrotum and testicle with great force, such as a groin kick or a baseball, or falls resulting in a straddle injury.
- **Penetrating trauma:** injuries sustained from sharp objects or gunshot wounds.
- **Degloving trauma:** an uncommon avulsion-type injury in which the scrotal skin is sheared off, such as getting the scrotum caught in farm equipment or heavy machinery.

84. **What is the frequency of testicular trauma?**

Testicular trauma is relatively rare; blunt trauma accounts for close to 85% of cases and penetrating trauma 15%. The most common mechanism of blunt testicular injury is sports, followed by kicks to the groin, motor vehicle crashes, and straddle injuries. The most common cause of penetrating testicular injuries is gunshot wounds. Other causes include stab wounds, self-mutilation, and emasculation.

85. **How is testicular trauma diagnosed?**

- Physical exam
- Scrotal ultrasound imaging with Doppler studies
- CT scan, angiography
- Scrotal exploration for any equivocal testicular trauma

86. **What are some interventions for testicular trauma?**

Conservative treatment for minor trauma includes bed rest for 24 to 48 hours, ice, scrotal support, and nonsteroidal antiinflammatory drugs (NSAIDs).

With the exception of superficial skin injury, all penetrating injuries should undergo surgical exploration. Documented blunt injuries should also undergo surgical exploration because it has proved to improve testicular salvage rates and decrease morbidity.

ABDOMINAL VASCULAR INJURIES

87. Abdominal vasculature includes which blood vessels?

- Midline aorta and inferior vena cava
- Celiac axis, superior mesenteric artery, and superior mesenteric vein
- Renal artery and vein
- Iliac artery and vein
- Hepatic artery, portal veins, and retrohepatic vena cava

88. What mechanism of injury is associated with abdominal vascular injury?

Blunt injury to the blood vessels is caused by deceleration, shear injury, or crushing injury. Rapid deceleration in a motor vehicle crash causes avulsion of the small branches of the major vessels or intimal tears with secondary thrombosis. Direct crush or blow forces cause intimal tears or flaps, with secondary thrombosis or complete disruption of the vessels. Such injuries can occur in pedestrian-vehicle collisions or falls. The majority of severe damage to the vascular system occurs with penetrating trauma. Gunshot wounds account for 25% of all abdominal vascular injuries; stab wounds account for about 10%.

89. What abdominal blood vessels are commonly injured in deceleration-type trauma?

The most commonly injured vessels include the infrarenal abdominal aorta, superior mesenteric artery, and iliac arteries.

90. What are the primary goals of management in patients with abdominal vascular injury?

The goals, listed by priority, include (1) aggressive resuscitation, (2) control of hemorrhage, and (3) early surgical intervention.

91. What CT findings are suggestive of infrarenal vena cava injury?

- Retroperitoneal hematoma around the vena cava
- Irregular vena cava contour and extravasation of contrast-enhanced blood from the cava
- Absence of both renal enhancement and excretion of IV contrast

92. What are the most common abdominal venous injuries?

The inferior vena cava is the most commonly injured. The iliac veins are the second most frequently injured structures.

93. Does a normal pulse distal to the injury rule out vessel injury?

No. Collateral circulation or pressure transmitted through an intimal flap or soft clot may permit normal pulses even with a vessel injury.

94. When should the clinician consider the use of blood during resuscitation?

Patients who require large amounts of crystalloid to maintain blood pressure probably have a severe continuing blood loss. Blood administration should be given after the initial 2 to 3 L of isotonic crystalloid.

95. What is the preferred blood product for replacement during resuscitation?

Type-specific blood should be administered until cross-matched blood is available. Universal donor blood should be administered, if necessary, without waiting for type-specific or cross-matched blood. Men and postmenopausal women may receive type O-Rh-positive blood, whereas girls and women of childbearing age should receive type O-Rh-negative blood to avoid sensitization that may complicate any future pregnancies.

Following coagulopathy protocols and based on laboratory data when possible, consider administering 1 unit of fresh frozen plasma (FFP) and 5 units of platelets for every 5 units of packed RBCs.

96. Hypothermia is a major cause of morbidity and mortality in patients with abdominal vascular injury. What maneuvers can be instituted to prevent hypothermia?

- Warming of all crystalloid and blood infusions
- Warmed humidified oxygen
- Warming blankets and lights
- Covering the patient's head

 Key Points

- If blood is found in any of the sites with the FAST scan, it is presumed the patient has a hemoperitoneum and should undergo abdominal surgical exploration.
- If the first diagnostic exams are negative and a strong clinical suspicion of injury remains, keep looking.
- The spleen is the most commonly injured intraabdominal organ, with mortality rates ranging from 3% to 23%.
- Left lower rib fractures are present in 44% of patients with splenic rupture.
- Massive retroperitoneal hemorrhage may be present without signs of peritonitis (no rebound tenderness, guarding, rigidity).
- Pelvic sheeting is the mechanical compression and securing of the pelvic fragments to prevent movement and additional injury. A bed sheet is applied encircling the pelvis.
- For hemodynamically unstable patients, type-specific blood should be administered until cross-matched blood is available. Men and postmenopausal women may receive type O-Rh-positive blood, whereas girls and women of childbearing age should receive type O-Rh-negative blood.

Internet Resources

Trauma.org:
www.trauma.org

American Association for the Surgery of Trauma:
www.aast.org

American Urological Association:
www.UrologyHealth.com

MedicineNet:
www.MedicineNet.com

eMedicine, *Blunt Abdominal Trauma:*
www.emedicine.com/emerg/topic1.htm

Bibliography

American College of Surgeons, Committee on Trauma: *Advanced trauma life support course for physicians (student manual)*, ed 7, Chicago, 2004, American College of Surgeons.

Cline KJ et al: Penetrating trauma to the male external genitalia, *J Trauma* 44(3):492-494, 1998.

Coley BD et al: Focused abdominal sonography for trauma (FAST) in children with blunt abdominal trauma, *J Trauma* 48(5):902-906, 2000.

Favian TC: What's new in trauma and critical care, *J Am Coll Surg* 192:276-286, 2001.

Greenberg MI et al: *Greenberg's text: Atlas of emergency medicine*, Philadelphia, 2005, Lippincott.

Hoff WS et al: Practice management guidelines for the evaluation of blunt abdominal trauma: The EAST practice management guidelines work group, *J Trauma* 53:602-615, 2002.

Mattox K, Feliciano D, Moore E, editors: *Trauma*, ed 4, New York, 2000, McGraw-Hill.

Moore EE et al: Organ injury scaling: Spleen and liver (1994 revision), *J Trauma* 38:323-324, 1995.

Reiff DA et al: Identifying injuries and motor vehicle collision characteristics that together are suggestive of diaphragmatic rupture, *J Trauma* 53:1139-1145, 2002.

Routh ML Jr et al: Circumferential pelvic antishock sheeting:
A temporary resuscitation, *J Orthop Trauma* 16(1):45-48, 2002.

Rozycki GS et al: Surgeon-performed ultrasound for the assessment of truncal injuries, *Ann Surg* 228:557, 1998.

Sartirekku KH et al: Nonoperative management of hepatic, splenic, and renal injuries in adults with multiple injuries, *J Trauma* 49:56-61, 2000.

Starr AJ et al: Pelvic ring disruptions: Predictions of associated injuries, transfusion requirement, pelvic arteriography, complications, and mortality, *J Orthop Trauma* 16:553-561, 2002.

Udobi KF et al: Role of ultrasonography in penetrating abdominal trauma: A prospective clinical study, *J Trauma* 50(3):475-479, 2001.

Spinal Trauma

Pamela W. Bourg

1. **Why is knowledge about spinal trauma important to emergency nurses?**

   Each year 8000 to 10,000 Americans sustain paralyzing spinal cord injuries. The median age of spinal victims is 25 years; men outnumber women four to one. The cost is estimated at 4 billion dollars per year. Historically, many of those who suffered acute spinal cord injuries died from respiratory complications. Improvements in trauma systems have decreased complications and improved the survival rate. Patient survival and quality of life after acute injury depend on emergency care. Early recognition and care preserve optimal rehabilitative potential.

2. **How many bony vertebrae does the human spine contain?**

   Thirty-three: 7 cervical, 5 sacral, 12 thoracic, 4 coccygeal, and 5 lumbar.

3. **What clinical findings suggest a possible spinal cord injury?**
   - Pain in the neck or spine
   - Point tenderness to palpation along spine
   - Paralysis/abnormal motor exam
   - Paresthesias
   - Priapism
   - Diaphragmatic breathing
   - Neurogenic shock

4. **What level of cervical injury may cause respiratory difficulty?**

   Injuries at the level of C4 or above result in a loss of phrenic nerve (diaphragmatic) and involuntary (intercostal) muscle innervation, which affects respiratory function.

5. **Absence of the biceps reflex and brachioradialis reflexes indicates spinal cord injury at what level?**

   Spinal cord injury at the C5 level, which is vertebral column level C4 to C5. Both reflexes are dependent on innervation from C5 to C6.

6. **What symptoms does a quadriplegic (tetraplegic) patient exhibit?**

   Loss of all motor and sensory function below C4 and loss of bowel or bladder control.

7. What symptoms does a paraplegic patient exhibit?

Loss of all motor and sensory function below the mid-chest, including the trunk muscles, and loss of bowel or bladder function.

8. What is central cord syndrome?

Edema in the central cord exerts pressure on anterior horn cells that results in greater motor deficit in the upper extremities than in the lower extremities. Sensory loss varies but is also more pronounced in upper extremities.

9. What are four movements that may result in spinal cord injury?

Movements That May Cause Spinal Cord Injury

Movement	Mechanism	Likely Cause
Compression (axial loading)	Vertical force to top of the head or buttocks causes longitudinal force on vertebrae and spinal column	Person falls from height and lands on feet or buttocks
		Diving accident
Hyperextension	Head is forced back	Rear-end vehicular collision
	Vertebrae in cervical region are overextended	Commonly seen in elderly as they fall and strike chin
Hyperflexion	Head is forced forward	Seen in head-on collisions and diving accidents
	Vertebrae in cervical region are overflexed	
Rotation	Extreme lateral twisting of head and neck	Motor vehicle crashes
	Ligaments are torn or ruptured so that force causes dislocation and fracture	Falls, sports

10. What are the signs and symptoms of an acute complete transection of the spinal cord?

- Flaccid paralysis of all skeletal muscles below the level of injury
- Loss of all spinal reflexes below the level of injury
- Absence of somatic and visceral sensations below the level of injury
- Bowel and bladder dysfunction

11. What is spinal shock? When is it likely to occur?

Spinal shock results in a state of temporary loss of motor, sensory, and reflex functions below the level of the injury. It usually occurs immediately after the spinal cord is suddenly injured or damaged but may occur several days after the initial injury. Spinal shock usually lasts less than 24 hours. Patients in spinal shock may have an initial increase in blood pressure. Spinal shock is most severe in upper cervical injuries.

12. **Which trauma patients should have spinal immobilization measures implemented?**
   - Patients who sustain trauma and complain of neck or back pain
   - Patients with neurological symptoms characteristic of spinal cord injury
   - Patients with altered mental status or a distracting injury, such as unstable long-bone fracture
   - Patients with a significant mechanism of injury, including falls from a significant height, high-impact motor vehicle crashes, high-impact explosions or blast injuries, and direct or penetrating injuries near the spine

13. **What are the steps of spinal immobilization?**
   - Stabilize the patient's head with in-line stabilization, and instruct the patient *not* to move the neck or head.
   - Assess motor and sensory function.
   - Direct assistants to apply and secure appropriate size rigid cervical collar, logroll patient onto side and place on backboard, and secure backboard strap and head support devices and tape.
   - Reassess motor and sensory function.
   - Maintenance of airway is top priority in all immobilized patients; suction should be readily available. If vomiting occurs, the patient should be logrolled to assist with airway clearance.

   Tip for immobilization of difficult patients (e.g., intoxicated, combative): Use sedation if the airway is intact and no other contraindications are present. Pediatric patients may be comforted by a parent's presence within their line of vision; this can help decrease struggling against immobilization devices.

14. **How should a full-face helmet be removed to avoid further damage to the spinal cord?**
   - Perform a neurological assessment before helmet removal.
   - Using at least one assistant, maintain stabilization of the helmet and mandible and remove the chinstrap and other removable parts of the helmet, including face shield, ear pads, and mouth guards.
   - Direct the assistant to take a position at the patient's side and cup the patient's mandible with the thumb and index finger of one hand and place the other hand on the occipital ride.
   - Ask the assistant to state when he or she is ready and transfer stabilization to the assistant.
   - From the head of the stretcher, spread the sides of the helmet and gently remove it.
   - If a void exists underneath the head, pad under the occiput to maintain neutral head position (external auditory meatus aligned with mid-shoulder).
   - Repeat the neurological assessment and proceed with cervical spine immobilization.

15. An adult patient arrives in the emergency department (ED) with a spinal injury. The physician may order high-dose methylprednisolone. What are the dosages for the initial intravenous (IV) bolus and the maintenance dose for the first 23 hours?

IV bolus: 30 mg/kg over 15 minutes; record the start time. Then there is a 45-minute interval before starting the maintenance infusion at 5.4 mg/kg/hr for 23 hours.

A multicenter study conducted by the National Acute Spinal Cord Injury Study group (Bracken et al, 1997) demonstrated significant improvement for patients treated with high-dose methylprednisolone within 8 hours of injury. Methylprednisolone is used because it crosses nerve cell membrane rapidly and completely. The pediatric dosage is the same, based on weight. See question 27 for discussion of controversy of use.

16. What are the signs and symptoms of a T3 fracture?

Hypotension and bradycardia. Impairment of descending sympathetic pathways results in loss of vasomotor tone and sympathetic innervation to the heart and adrenal glands. Interruption of the pathways leads to vasodilation and maldistribution of blood volume (neurogenic shock).

17. What initial diagnostic radiograph is usually ordered in patients with spinal injuries?

Generally, cross-table lateral radiographs of the cervical spine are ordered first. These films are done without moving the patient. However, many trauma centers are using helical computed tomography (CT) scanning in evaluating unconscious, intubated trauma patients. There is insufficient evidence to suggest cervical spine CT should replace initial screening for less injured patients at low risk for cervical spine injury.

18. How can the visualization of C7 be improved in cross-table lateral films?

Mild traction on the shoulders with the lateral view may help in patients with large shoulders. If the area cannot be seen on plain films, a CT scan may be needed. CT scan is superior for patients at high risk for C-spine injury or in those with depressed mental status.

19. Why is it important to observe respiratory function in a patient with a C7 injury?

Even though the phrenic nerve is intact, the intercostal muscles are not. The patient may develop ascending spinal cord injury, resulting in loss of phrenic nerve function.

20. **Why is it important to prevent secondary injury to the spinal cord?**

Secondary injury results from vascular and neuronal pathological changes and the release of vasoactive agents and cellular enzymes. Hypoxia of gray matter stimulates release of catecholamines, which contributes to hemorrhage, necrosis, and further cord dysfunction.

21. **What are the indications for emergent cervical spine traction?**

It is a physician's decision to reduce and realign fractured and/or dislocated cervical vertebrae. Continuous traction and stabilization with external devices, such as halo or tongs, prevents further damage to the underlying spinal cord and nerves.

Nursing responsibilities include:
- Assembling equipment
- Performing baseline and ongoing neurological assessment
- Shaving and cleansing pin insertion sites
- Assisting with and documenting procedures
- Reassuring the patient as needed

22. **Which radiographic modality is most sensitive for evaluation of spinal injury?**

The CT scan is most sensitive for fractures. CT reconstruction of the spinal canal demonstrates alignment. Magnetic resonance imaging (MRI) is the only modality that visualizes the spinal cord. It can reveal spinal contusions and ligamentous injury.

23. **What are the contraindications for an MRI in patients with suspected spinal injury?**

- Patients with mechanically activated implants (e.g., pacemakers, internal defibrillators, insulin pumps)
- Any other metallic implant (e.g., intrauterine device—IUD, aneurysm clips, sternal wires)
- Pregnant women in the first trimester
- Welders and iron workers require orbital radiographs to exclude metallic fragments in the eye
- Unstable patients who cannot be isolated in the scanner for the length of the exam

24. **Because hypoxia may potentiate spinal cord injury, what actions can maintain tissue oxygenation?**

Ensure stable airway and respiratory status. Maintain oxygen saturation greater than 90% and hematocrit greater than 30%.

25. What are the various types of injury to the spinal cord?

Spinal Cord Injuries

Type of Injury	Description	Mechanism
Concussion	Spinal shock or jarring can cause temporary loss of function for 24-48 hours	Severe shaking of spinal cord or pressure wave within cord
Contusion	Bruising of cord, bleeding into cord, edema, and possible necrosis from compression of edema The extent of neurological deficit depends on severity of contusion and presence of necrosis	Fractures, dislocations, direct trauma
Hemorrhage	Bleeding into or around cord Blood acts as irritant to delicate tissue, resulting in changes in neurochemical components, edema Damage to blood vessels that supply spinal cord (anterior spinal artery or two posterior spinal arteries) may result in ischemia and possible necrosis	The breakdown of RBCs can increase formation of free radicals
Laceration	Actual tear in cord results in permanent injury	Projectile or bone entering spinal cord
Transection	Severing of cord may be complete or incomplete	Physiological transaction resulting from vascular disruption

26. What is a dermatome?

A dermatome refers to an area of skin innervated by the sensory nerves within each segmental nerve (root). Each side of the body has 28 dermatomes (see Figure p. 342).

27. What are the current controversies in management of acute spinal cord injury?

Bracken's (1997) original research on the use of methylprednisolone therapy in acute spinal injury still remains a classic study. Although some studies (National Institute of Neurological Disorders and Stroke, *Spinal Cord Injury: Emerging Concepts)* have argued against methylprednisolone, there is accumulating evidence that it does provide significant benefit in acute spinal cord injury.

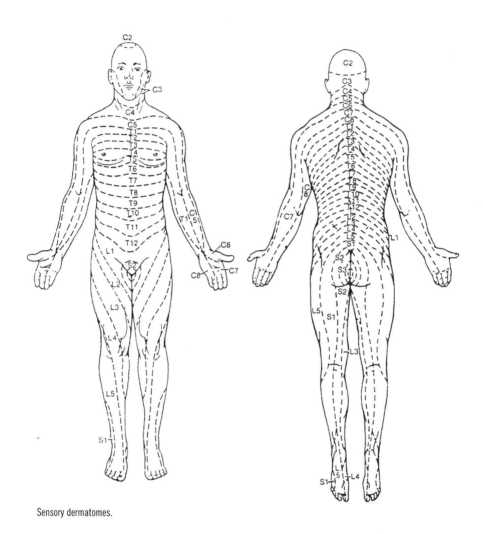

Sensory dermatomes.

28. What does the future hold for treatment of spinal cord injury?

- Researchers in spinal cord injury are now investigating specific changes in cells and molecules that produce the secondary damage. Free radicals are released after spinal cord injury. These and other chemicals attack critical cell structures. Trauma also causes release of excess neurotransmitters, leading to excitotoxicity or secondary damage from overexcited nerve cells. Understanding this cell damage and excitotoxicity may provide answers for reducing damage after spinal cord injuries.
- Damage to axons causes many of the problems associated with spinal cord injury. The newest research findings suggest the axons deteriorate more slowly because the vital transport of molecules and cell components to and from ends of axons is disrupted. The delay provides the opportunity for interventions. Developing therapies are directed toward these causes.

Key Points

- Maintenance of a patent airway should be a top priority with all immobilized patients. Suction should be readily available. If vomiting occurs, logroll the patient to facilitate airway clearance.
- Systemic injuries can be overlooked when vital signs are altered and the assumption is made that the spinal cord injury is the cause. Other systemic injuries must be ruled out.
- Fear and anxiety are primary emotions often seen in the acute phase of spinal cord injury. It is important to provide realistic reassurance. Pharmacological interventions may be necessary.
- Early attention to skin care in the ED can help prevent skin breakdown in spinal cord injured patients.

Internet Resources

National Institute of Neurological Disorders and Stroke, *Spinal Cord Injury: Emerging Concepts:*
www.ninds.nih.gov/news_and_events/proceedings/sci_report.htm

Spinal Cord Injury and Disease Resources:
www.makoa.org/sci.htm

Spinal Cord Injury Information Network:
www.spinalcord.uab.edu

Bibliography

Birchard KR et al: MRI of acute abdominal and pelvic pain in pregnant patients, *Am J Roentgenol* 184: 452-458, 2005.

Bracken MB et al: Administration of methylprednisolone for 24 or 48 hours or tirilazad mesylate for 48 hours in the treatment of acute spinal cord injury. Results of the Third National Acute Spinal Cord Injury Randomized Controlled Trial. National Acute Spinal Cord Injury Study, *JAMA* 277:1597-1604, 1997.

Bracken MB et al: Clinical measurement, statistical analysis, and risk benefit: Controversies from trials of spinal injury, *J Trauma* 48(3):558, 2000.

Brohi K et al: Helical computed tomographic scanning for the evaluation of the cervical spine in unconscious, intubated trauma patient, *J Trauma* 58(5):897, 2005.

Brown C et al: Spinal computed tomography for diagnosis of cervical, thoracic and lumbar spine fractures: Its time has come, *J Trauma* 58(5):890, 2005.

Domeier R et al: Multicenter prospective validation of pre-hospital clinical spinal clearance criteria, *J Trauma* 53(3):744, 2002.

Forstner R et al: Abdominopelvic MR imaging in the non-obstetric evaluation of pregnant patients, *Am J Roentgenol* 166:1139, 1996.

Hockenberger R, Kirshenbaum K: Spine. In Marx JA, Hockenberger RS, Walls RM, editors: *Rosen's emergency medicine concepts and clinical practice*, ed 5, St Louis, 2002, Mosby.

Holmes J, Akkinepalli R: Computed tomography versus plain radiography to screen for cervical spine injury: A meta-analysis, *J Trauma* 58(5):902, 2005.

Lindsey R, Gugala Z: Pneumatic injury to vertebrae and spinal cord. In Feliciano D, Moore EE, Mattox K, editors: *Trauma*, ed 5, New York, 2004, McGraw-Hill.

Meyer P et al: *New spine fracture classification system*, Chicago, 1997, Midwest Regional Spinal Cord Injury Care System. Available at www.northwestern.edu/spine/fxclass.htm.

Russo-McCourt T: Spinal cord injuries. In McQuillan KA et al, editors: *Trauma nursing*, ed 3, Philadelphia, 2002, WB Saunders.

Musculoskeletal Trauma

Sharon Saunderson Cohen

1. What three systems make up the musculoskeletal system?

- Skeletal system (bones)
- Articular system (joints)
- Muscular system (muscles and connective tissue)

2. What are the four developmental areas of a bone?

- Diaphysis: the shaft of the bone
- Epiphysis: the end of the bone that was initially cartilaginous
- Metaphysis: the flared region of the bone at the end of the diaphysis
- Physis: the region of growth cartilage

3. What are the most common fractures in children?

The uniqueness of children is that they tend to fracture where the bones are weakest and ossification is not yet complete. Physeal and metaphyseal fractures are the most common, with buckle (compression) and greenstick (incomplete) also fairly common.

4. What signs and symptoms should be assessed in patients with musculoskeletal injury?

Musculoskeletal Injury Signs and Symptoms

Pain	Swelling	Activity
Location	Location	Continued activity
Onset	Amount/depth	Pain with activity
Intensity	Time occurred	Moves to command
Radiation	Associated with ecchymosis	Moves to pain, unable to bear weight
Quality		No weight bearing
	Pulse	
Sensation	Presence	
Normal	Quality	
Diminished	Loss of pulse (time)	
Burning	Diminished but palpable	
Tingling	With Doppler only	
Numbness		

5. **What complication may follow a crush injury to an extremity?**

Compartment syndrome.

6. **What is compartment syndrome?**

It is an increase in compartmental pressures of an extremity that leads to compromised circulation and nerve function. Untreated compartment syndrome may result in muscle necrosis, partial or complete nerve injury, and vascular compromise that can lead to loss of extremity function or amputation.

7. **What are the signs and symptoms of compartment syndrome?**

Classic signs include pain, especially on passive flexion or extension of the foot; paralysis; paresthesia; and pallor. Pulselessness may be an additional sign, but in most cases, pulses are present because the systolic blood pressure is much higher than the 30-mmHg tissue pressure needed to cause the signs and symptoms of compartment syndrome.

8. **What causes compartment syndrome?**

Internal causes include fractures, vascular compromise (e.g., from a dislocation), reperfusion injury (e.g., crush or prolonged compression), and burns. External causes include constrictive dressings, casts, splints, and in rare cases the use of pneumatic antishock garments (PASGs).

9. **What is the most common site of compartment syndrome?**

The anterior compartment of the lower leg. Tibial fracture is the usual etiology.

10. **How is compartment pressure measured? What level is considered dangerous?**

Compartment pressure is measured directly by inserting a pressure-sensitive device into the affected muscle. Critical values are usually in the range of 30 to 45 mmHg.

11. **How is compartment syndrome treated?**

Treatment includes fasciotomy, within 4 hours if possible. The procedure can be done at the bedside in an emergency or, preferably, in the operating room (OR) under aseptic conditions. Do *not* elevate the extremity before fasciotomy, because elevation further compromises circulation. Instead, place the extremity at the level of the heart to promote arterial inflow.

12. **What is Volkmann's contracture?**

Volkmann's contracture results from prolonged compartment syndrome (with resultant ischemia) of the forearm that has progressed to contracture and paralysis. This description was first documented in 1881 by Richard Volkmann. The clinical presentation includes pain, pallor, pulselessness, paresthesias, and paralysis. Pain is usually the earliest sign. On physical examination, pain worsening by passive stretching seems to be the most reliable finding. Firmness of the tissues may be noted on palpation. Pulselessness and paralysis are late findings.

13. What is the best method to control bleeding of a large wound?

Direct pressure is the best method to control bleeding. A tourniquet should be used as a life-saving measure only if bleeding cannot be controlled by other methods. Topical agents (e.g., powdered thrombin, Gelfoam) may also be used.

14. What is an avulsion?

An avulsion is a full-thickness skin loss in which a segment of skin is torn away.

15. How is an avulsion treated?

A large avulsion can lead to hypovolemic shock. Always begin treatment with assessment and needed interventions for the ABCs (airway, breathing, circulation). In particular, monitor and control bleeding with direct pressure. Gentle irrigation of the flap is often necessary, followed by covering with a moist, sterile, bulky dressing. Definitive treatment may include simple closure or split-thickness skin graft (for a more extensive wound).

16. Should an impaled object ever be removed in the emergency department (ED)?

It depends on the location of the impaled object. Sometimes removal may precipitate further injury or large amounts of bleeding and should be done with surgical support available. However, an object impaled in the cheek, finger, or other less vascular site or in locations without the possibility of underlying organ damage often can be removed without further sequelae.

17. What is the treatment for impalement?

Treatment depends on the location of the impalement. Before definitive treatment, the impaled object should be stabilized, by whatever method works best, to prevent further injury from movement of the object.

18. How is "road rash" (large abrasions) treated?

Most authorities consider road rash to be analogous to a burn. The extent and depth of the road rash dictate the treatments. Simple epithelial road rash may require only irrigation and debridement with an appropriate dressing (maintaining a moist environment speeds reepithelialization), whereas full-thickness injury requires split-thickness skin grafting. Remember to check tetanus status.

19. How are fractures described?

Descriptions of fractures are based on a variety of factors:
- Skin status (open versus closed)
- Bone (proximal, medial, or distal)
- Fracture pattern (spiral, comminuted)
- Degree of angulation or displacement (relation of the distal to the proximal aspects; e.g., lateral, medial, anterior, posterior)

20. What is the best method to immobilize a fractured extremity?

It is best to splint above and below the fracture, including the joints proximally and distally. If definitive treatment of the fracture is to be delayed, a well-padded splint is recommended to help prevent skin breakdown.

21. What should be assessed before and after splinting or casting?

At a minimum, assess circulation and motor and sensory function distal to the fracture.

22. How is extremity circulation assessed?

Assessment should be performed distal to the injury. Circulatory assessment evaluates vascular integrity. Assess for capillary refill distal to the injury. If the refill time is longer than 2 seconds, further evaluation is needed to find the cause and to direct the appropriate intervention. Because capillary refill slows down with age, the 2-second standard may be misleading. It is best to compare the refill in the injured extremity to the uninjured extremity when possible. Assess color of the tissue. Tissue should be pink or normal skin tone, and the skin should be warm. Pulses should be noted for trends in quality and presence.

23. How is neurological assessment of the extremity performed?

Motor and sensory assessments are the focus of the neurological exam. Assess for flexion and extension of the fingers or toes of the affected extremity and determine whether the patient can feel the fingers or toes. Gross sensation is documented, and further examination may be done, if warranted, to discriminate between one and two points and light and sharp/dull touch.

24. What discharge instructions should be given to the patient with crutches, a cast, or another orthopedic appliance?

The most important instruction is the need to monitor neurological and vascular status. Patients need to know whom to call if a problem arises. If the patient is discharged with a cast, cast care instructions need to be given and documented. If the patient is discharged with crutches, proper crutch walking (*not* running) should be demonstrated, and patient performance should be noted. Any orthotic device (e.g., sling, sling and swath, splints) needs to be fully explained to the patient, including why it is needed, proper fitting or use, whether the patient can remove it to bathe, and how to reapply it.

25. What are the goals of fracture treatment?

- Alignment of the bones in both the angular and rotational planes
- Restoration of proper length
- Restoration of apposition of the bone ends
- Adequate immobilization
- Normalization of function

26. What treatments are used for patients with a fracture?

Fracture treatment depends on the location and degree of fracture, as well as the age and premorbid condition of the patient. In general, five treatment methods are used:
- No treatment or at most simple restriction of activity with a sling or crutches
- Closed reduction followed by cast immobilization
- Continuous traction usually followed by cast immobilization
- Open or closed reduction with internal fixation
- Open reduction with external fixation

27. What are the different types of fracture patterns?

- **Angulated fracture:** A fracture with the two bone ends at an angle to each other
- **Avulsion fracture:** A bone chip fracture caused by the tendon being pulled from the bone
- **Buckle fracture:** Seen in children; bending of the cortex of the bone but no disruption
- **Closed fracture:** Intact skin over a fracture site
- **Comminuted fracture:** Fragmentation of bone into more than two parts
- **Displaced fracture:** A fracture that involves *no* angulation—only displacement of the bone ends
- **Greenstick fracture:** Seen in children; an incomplete fracture involving only one side of the cortex of the bone
- **Impaction fracture:** A fracture caused by compression forces in which the ends of the bone are driven into each other without fracture displacement
- **Intraarticular fracture:** A fracture involving the articular surface of the bone
- **Oblique fracture:** A fracture that creates an oblique angle to the long axis of the bone
- **Open fracture:** Fractured bone (compound fracture) communicates with the external environment through the overlying wound; high risk for infection
- **Pathologic fracture:** A fracture through abnormal bone (e.g., bone with tumor, osteoporotic bone, diseased bone)
- **Rotational fracture:** A fracture that has one bone end rotating in relation to the other bone end or the longitudinal axis; most often seen on physical exam, not on radiographs
- **Simple fracture:** "Clean break"; one fracture line divides bone into two parts
- **Spiral fracture:** A severe fracture in which an oblique angle rotates along the long axis of the bone; caused by twisting
- **Stress fracture:** A fracture caused by repetitive forces unloaded onto the bone (as in competitive runners)
- **Transverse fracture:** A fracture that is horizontal to the long axis of the bone

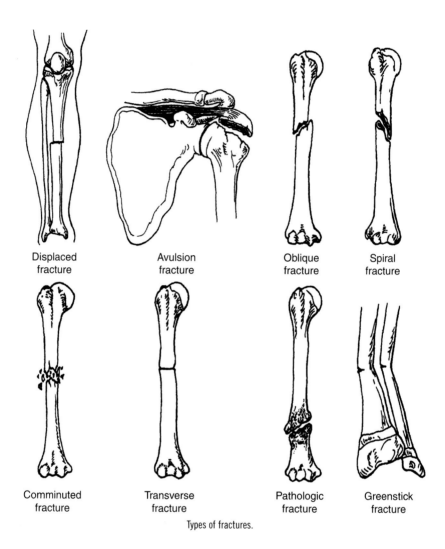

Displaced fracture	Avulsion fracture	Oblique fracture	Spiral fracture
Comminuted fracture	Transverse fracture	Pathologic fracture	Greenstick fracture

Types of fractures.

28. What is the greatest risk with an open fracture?

Infection.

29. What is the initial treatment for an open fracture?

To minimize the risk of infection, treatment should include covering the wound, antibiotic therapy, tetanus prophylaxis, irrigation with possible surgical debridement, and stabilization of the fracture.

30. What is tennis elbow?

Tendonitis of the lateral epicondyle of the humerus.

31. What is osteomyelitis?

Inflammation and infection of the bone marrow and bone. In adults, the most common pathogen is *Staphylococcus aureus.*

32. What is the epiphysis?

It is the growth plate, or the distal ends of the bone involved in bone growth.

33. Why is the growth plate of concern in pediatric fractures?

Injury to the growth plate of the immature or pediatric long bone may compromise the normal bone growth. If there is damage to the entire physis, premature physeal closure occurs with resulting longitudinal growth arrest. Asymmetrical closure leads to angular deformity of the limb.

34. What is fat embolism syndrome (FES)?

A fat embolism occurs when fat enters the vascular system. The syndrome usually develops 24 to 48 hours after injury and most commonly occurs after a long bone injury.

35. What are the most common signs and symptoms of FES?

- Change in level of consciousness
- Dyspnea
- High fever
- Petechial rash (usually over the thorax and upper extremities)
- Hypoxia

36. What is the treatment for FES?

Supportive care with supplemental oxygen and ventilatory support as indicated. Operative stabilization of long bone fractures may help prevent FES.

37. Why is a severe pelvic fracture potentially life threatening?

Major blood loss can occur secondary to disruption of the large and numerous arterial and venous plexuses within the pelvis. In addition, high-energy forces that cause pelvic disruption can result in associated injuries.

38. How is an unstable pelvic fracture stabilized?

There are several methods of pelvic stabilization. External fixation such as the Slatis or Pittsburgh frame or the C-clamp (pelvic stabilizer) may be applied. There are also commercial beltlike devices designed to compress and splint the pelvis (Trauma Pelvic Orthotic Device—T-POD, Sam Sling). These are easily applied in the ED or prehospital setting. Another simple, but not always effective, method is the use of military antishock trousers (MASTs); when inflated over the pelvic region, they provide stabilization, especially in the prehospital setting. In the absence of these devices a sheet wrapped around the pelvis and tied tightly may serve as an interim method.

39. **What is the goal of pelvic stabilization in the emergent setting?**

The goal of pelvic stabilization is to prevent the pelvis from further displacement and to control bleeding by aligning the fractured bones to create a smaller space for blood to accumulate. Pelvic stabilization creates a tamponade effect to help control hemorrhage.

40. **How many liters of blood may be lost in a severe pelvic fracture?**

The retroperitoneal space (a potential space) can accommodate as much as 4 L of blood before tamponade occurs in adults.

41. **What type of anesthesia may be used for suturing a wound in the ED?**

Local anesthesia or blocks are used for proper debridement, exploration, and closure of a wound. A local anesthetic, such as lidocaine with or without epinephrine, often is injected directly into the procedural area. If vasoconstriction is desired, lidocaine with epinephrine is injected. Bupivacaine is an alternative anesthetic often used when longer anesthesia is desirable. Topical preparations containing lidocaine, epinephrine, and tetracaine (LET) are also commonly used in children. In addition, various blocks may be performed, depending on the degree of anesthesia required.
- **Field block:** Anesthetic is injected around the area to be treated
- **Digital block:** Used to anesthetize an entire finger or toe
- **Regional block:** Used to anesthetize a larger area, such as an arm or below the waist

42. **Why should lidocaine with epinephrine be used with caution?**

Lidocaine with epinephrine has vasoconstrictive properties and should never (or very cautiously) be used on the digits, tip of the nose, penis, ears, or any other areas that are distal and may be susceptible to severe vasoconstriction that may lead to tissue ischemia and damage.

43. **What is the difference in the various sutures used in wound closure?**

Sutures Used in Wound Closure

Type	Characteristics
Absorbable	Usually used for layers beneath the skin or mucosal surfaces
Chromic or plain	Absorbs quickly (7-10 days); tensile strength goes quickly
Monofilaments (nylons, propylene, steel wire)	Prolonged tensile strength and low tissue reaction but requires more ties to secure knot
Nonabsorbable	Usually used for skin and subcutaneous pull-out sutures
Silk	Highly tissue-reactive; holds knots well
Synthetic	Causes less inflammatory response; tensile strength lasts longer

44. What are the three types of wound closure?

- **Primary wound closure** is the immediate closure of a wound or laceration with sutures.
- **Delayed primary closure** is suture closure usually 3 to 5 days after incision or injury.
- **Secondary wound closure** is closure *without* sutures; the wound heals by contraction and epithelialization.

45. Is suturing the only form of primary wound closure?

No. Topical skin adhesives (e.g., Dermabond, Indermil) are also used for wound closure. In addition, many types of skin wound tapes (e.g., Steri-Strips, butterfly sutures) approximate wound edges without actual suturing.

46. What precautions should be taken when applying tissue adhesives?

Adhesives are intended for topical application only and should not enter the wound. When used near the eyes, be particularly careful to avoid contact with the eye or lid. Do not apply liquid, ointment medications, or other substances to the wound after closure with adhesive. Such substances can weaken the adhesive and cause wound dehiscence. For the same reason, do not apply adhesive to a wet wound.

47. What is replantation and revascularization?

Replantation is the reattachment of a body part that has been completely severed from the body (amputated). Revascularizaton is the reattachment of a body part that has been partially severed from the body. The terms are sometimes used interchangeably.

48. What is warm ischemia time? When does successful replantation or revascularization become unlikely?

Warm ischemia is the time from loss of perfusion (usually the time of amputation) to reperfusion (usually surgical replantation), not including the time during which the amputated part is cooled. The longer the warm ischemia time, the less successful the replantation. In most cases, 6 hours of warm ischemia time is the limit for successful replantation. Cooled extremity parts, however, may be replanted 10 to 12 hours after injury.

49. Describe the emergency care of the patient with a partial or complete amputation.

Emergency care of all patients begins with stabilization and maintenance of the ACBCs (airway, cervical spine, breathing, circulation). After stabilization of the ACBCs, focus on care of the stump and amputated part.

Care of the stump or wound:
- Generously irrigate the stump or wound with sterile saline to remove gross contamination. Do *not* scrub or use abrasive action. Do *not* use povidone-iodine, hydrogen peroxide, or soaps.

- Apply sterile gauze moistened with saline. If bleeding persists, apply a pressure dressing. Do *not* clamp or tie off any vessels.
- Elevate the stump above the level of the heart.
- If the amputation is not complete, apply a splint. Cool the devascularized portion of the affected extremity with ice packs. Do *not* let any tissue come in direct contact with ice. Elevate above the level of the heart.

Care of the amputated part:

- Generously irrigate the amputated part with sterile saline to remove gross contamination. Do *not* scrub or use abrasive action. Do *not* use povidone-iodine, hydrogen peroxide, or soaps.
- Place the amputated part in sterile gauze moistened with saline and place in a clean, dry, airtight plastic bag or container. Place the container in an ice and water slurry (combination of both). Do *not* allow the amputated part to come in direct contact with ice. Do *not* use salt or dry ice, which is too cold and freezes vessels.

50. What is nursemaid's elbow?

Nursemaid's elbow is a radial head subluxation usually caused by a pull of or fall on an outstretched arm. It occurs in children who have been pulled or swung by the arms.

51. What is the difference between subluxation and dislocation?

Subluxation is an incomplete or partial dislocation.

52. What does RICE mean for the treatment of a sprain or strain?

RICE is the acronym for rest, ice, compression (with an elastic bandage or pneumatic splint), and elevation. This treatment is to be done for 24 to 36 hours after an acute sprain or strain.

53. What is carpal tunnel syndrome?

Compression of the median nerve, resulting in pain along the distribution of the nerve. Common causes of carpal tunnel syndrome are repetitive hand motion, tumor (fibroma, lipoma), ganglion cyst, tenosynovitis secondary to trauma or rheumatoid arthritis, or gout.

54. What is a felon?

Infection of the pulp space of any of the distal phalanges.

55. What is paronychia?

Infection of the lateral nail fold often caused by nail biting, hangnails, or manicures.

56. What are the common presentations of gout?

Middle-age men with complaint of extreme pain in the small joints, especially the first metatarsophalangeal joint. While giving their history, they may admit to alcohol consumption or thiazid diuretic use, which places them at higher risk for gout.

57. What is the most common sports-related injury in the school-age child and adolescent?

The lower extremities are more likely to sustain an injury in this population. Of the lower extremity injuries, the knee and ankle are the most likely to be reinjured, with contusions and sprains the most common type of injury. Fractures and dislocations are less common. Head injuries are the most common cause of sports-related fatality.

58. What is a common cause of medial epicondylitis in the youth playing baseball?

The throwing of curve balls while pitching puts an extra stress on the ulnar collateral ligament of the medial aspect of the elbow, often causing severe strain or partial separation of the apophysis.

59. What musculoskeletal injuries or conditions may constitute an emergent situation?

Open fracture, impending compartment syndrome, dislocation of major joints (e.g., knee, hip, spine), septic arthritis, major arterial injury, FES, and unstable pelvic fracture.

60. What is septic arthritis?

Infection of the joint space, with rheumatoid arthritis and osteoarthritis being a risk factor. Additionally, risky sexual behavior *(Neisseria gonorrhoeae)* and immunocompromised states can lead to septic arthritis.

61. What long-term complications can occur from a dislocated hip or knee?

A dislocated hip can lead to avascular necrosis from injury to the medial and lateral circumflex artery that supplies the femoral head. A dislocated knee, particularly a posterior dislocation, can frequently lead to popliteal artery injury.

 Key Points

- Regardless of the injury or cause of the orthopedic problem, a simple CMS check should be noted and trended.
- Injury to the skin tissues may mean deeper injury to underlying structures (i.e., muscles, ligaments, vasculature, bones). Be sure to assess accordingly.
- Laceration or large avulsions may lead to hypovolemic or hemorrhagic shock. Stop the bleeding as quickly as possible, and monitor the patient closely.
- In caring for patients with orthopedic fractures, assess pulses distal to the injury before and after realignment, casting, or any repositioning or immobilization.

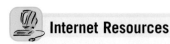
Internet Resources

American Academy of Orthopaedic Surgeons, Advisory Statements:
www.aaos.org/wordhtml/advis.htm

Cochrane Musculoskeletal Group:
www.cochranemsk.org/cmsg

Internet Society of Orthopaedic Surgery and Trauma, Orthogate:
www.orthogate.com

National Association of Orthopaedic Nurses:
www.orthonurse.org

National Institute of Arthritis and Musculoskeletal and Skin Diseases:
www.niams.nih.gov

Nicholas Institute of Sports Medicine and Athletic Trauma, Orthopedic Sports Medicine Corner:
www.nismat.org/orthocor

Bibliography

Bailey J: Getting a fix on orthopedic care, *Nursing* 33(6):58-64, 2003.

Blackbourne LH: *Surgical recall*, ed 3, Baltimore, 2003, Williams & Wilkins.

Brown DE, Neumann RD: *Orthopedic secrets*, ed 3, Philadelphia, 2004, Hanley & Belfus.

Cohen SS: *Trauma nursing secrets*, Philadelphia, 2002, Hanley & Belfus.

Criddle LM: Rhabdomyolysis, pathophysiology, recognition, and management, *Crit Care Nurse* 23(6):
14-28, 2003.

Emergency Nurses Association: *Course in advanced trauma nursing II: A conceptual approach to injury and illness*, Park Ridge, Ill, 2003, Emergency Nurses Association.

Ignatavicius DD: Catching compartment syndrome early, *Nursing* 32(11):10, 2002.

Newberry L, editor: *Sheehy's emergency nursing: Principles and practice*, St Louis, 2003, Mosby.

Chapter **30**

Burn Injury

Elizabeth A. Mann* and Mary Beth Flynn Makic

1. What significant functions of the skin are affected by burns?

As the largest organ of the body, the skin provides a barrier to the external environment, prevents loss of heat and moisture, and inhibits bacteria from entering the body. When burned, the skin loses these vital functions, resulting in hypothermia, vapor losses, and significant potential for infection and sepsis. The skin is also a sensory organ for touch, temperature, and pain. The skin's appearance influences a person's sense of personal identity. Burn injury and resultant wound healing or scars can affect a patient's self-identity based on physical appearance and/or functional limitations.

2. How many layers of skin do humans have?

There are two layers of skin, the epidermis and dermis. The epidermis, the outer layer of skin, is avascular and its primary function is to act as a barrier between the body and the environment. The dermis is vascularized and contains nerves, apocrine sweat glands, sebaceous glands, and hair roots. Connective tissue containing collagen and elastic fibers that provide strength and elasticity are also characteristics of the dermis.

The individual layers of skin are not visible to the naked eye; so, when determining depth of burn injury it is helpful to remember that the dermis is the layer that will bleed. Superficial and full-thickness burns do not bleed because the epidermis and subcutaneous layers are avascular.

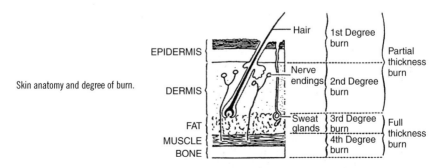

Skin anatomy and degree of burn.

---

*The views expressed in this chapter are those of the authors and do not reflect the official policy of the Department of the Army, the Department of Defense, or the U.S. Government.

357

3. Does the skin vary in thickness?

Yes, the skin varies in thickness anatomically as well as by gender and age. In general males have thicker skin than females, whereas infants and the elderly have thinner, more fragile skin. The skin is most thick on the soles of the feet and palms of hands. Burns in these areas are difficult to heal because of the thickness of the epidermis. The thinnest skin is on the face, especially the eyelids. In patients with facial burns, the very thin skin of the eyelid predisposes injury to the globe of the eye.

4. What are the five possible types of burn injury?

Traumatic burn injury is defined by the mechanism or agent that results in tissue damage. Burns may be caused by thermal, chemical, electrical, and radiation sources of heat. Inhalation injury is also a category of burn injury that typically occurs with thermal heat sources.

- **Thermal:** Flame, contact, scald, and steam are types of thermal burns. Thermal burns may be attenuated by removing the source of heat and cooling the affected area.
- **Chemical:** Alkalis, acids, and organic compounds are classes of chemicals that may cause burn injury. Burning properties of chemicals persist until all remnants of the compound are removed from the skin.
- **Electrical:** Alternating current (AC), direct current (DC), lightning, and arc burns are types of electrical injury. Low-voltage AC electrical injuries usually occur from contact with common household wires. High-voltage AC and DC injuries happen with exposure to electrical transformers, power lines, buried wires, and lightning strikes.
- **Radiation:** Ionizing radiation injury may result from small-scale laboratory or treatment accidents, large industrial accidents such as nuclear reactor leaks or explosions, and nuclear weapon detonation. Contaminated clothing should be removed and the skin flushed with copious amounts of normal saline or water. Ionizing radiation is not immediately life threatening; however, acute radiation syndrome usually begins within hours of exposure.
- **Inhalation injury:** This type of burn injury results from the inhalation of superheated gases and should be considered when burn victims are injured in a closed-space fire or are found unconscious at the scene.

5. What recommendations does the American Burn Association (ABA) make for referral to one of the country's approximately 130 burn centers?

Patients with the following burn injuries should be transferred to the nearest burn center for treatment. Referral criteria include:

- Partial-thickness burns covering more than 10% total body surface area (TBSA)
- Burns that involve the face, hands, feet, genitalia, perineum, or major joints
- Full-thickness burns in any age group
- Electrical burns, including lightning injury
- Chemical burns
- Inhalation injury
- Burn injury in patients with preexisting medical disorders that could complicate management, prolong recovery, or affect mortality

- Any patients with burns and concomitant trauma (such as fractures) in which the burn injury poses the greatest risk of morbidity or mortality
- Burned children in hospitals without qualified personnel or equipment for the care of children
- Burn injury in patients who will require special social, emotional, or long-term rehabilitative intervention

Other injuries that benefit from treatment in specialized burn centers include cold injuries (e.g., frostbite) and necrotizing diseases (e.g., toxic epidermal necrolysis—TEN, necrotizing fasciitis).

6. **What populations are most vulnerable to thermal burns?**

Age groups at highest risk for thermal burn injury include infants, young children, older adults, and persons with disabilities. Individuals in these groups may not be able to escape a fire. When burned, the thin skin of very young and older individuals predisposes them to potentially deeper burn injury. Scalds are the most common burn injury. Abuse or neglect should be considered and reported to the appropriate authorities when children, elderly, or disabled patients present with suspicious burn injury patterns. Additional risk factors for thermal injury include occupational hazards, patient history of substance abuse, physical disability, mental illness, and smoking.

7. **What factors influence the depth of a burn wound?**

Factors that influence the extent of the burn injury include duration of contact with the burning agent, temperature or concentration of the agent, and amount of body surface area affected by burn trauma. Lack of perfusion to the burn wound bed also influences the depth of tissue loss. Initial treatment priorities focus on maintaining thermoregulation, fluid resuscitation, and hemodynamic stability to minimize dermal tissue injury loss from lack of perfusion.

8. **What are the various classifications of burn injury?**

Burn Injury Classifications

Depth	Degree	Appearance	Wound Closure
Superficial	First	Epidermal injury only; dry, reddened, painful	Heals within 7-10 days
Superficial partial-thickness	Second	Some dermis involved; moist; blisters may be present; painful; may bleed	May progress to deep dermal or full-thickness injury; usually heals within 21 days; grafting may be required
Deep partial-thickness	Second	Significant amount of dermis is lost; tissue is dark red to yellowish in color; only slightly moist; inconsistent sensation; may bleed	May progress to full-thickness; usually heals within 21 days; grafting may be required for more rapid closure of wound

Continued

Burn Injury Classifications—cont'd

Depth	Degree	Appearance	Wound Closure
Full-thickness	Third	Nonblanching; tight; insensate; dry; does not bleed; eschar present; skin color may range from dark brown (leathery) to pearly white	Autologous grafting required for wound closure; areas surrounding full-thickness burn are painful
Full-thickness	Fourth	Bone, muscle, subcutaneous tissues involved	Autologous grafting required for wound closure

9. **What is the significance of zones of burn injury?**

The center of the burn (zone of coagulation) is the area of most significant tissue injury or tissue death. The surrounding area (zone of stasis) is the most vulnerable area of the burn wound. Tissue in this area is viable; however, lack of perfusion to this zone can convert the wound to a deeper burn injury. The outermost area of injury is called the zone of hyperemia and is viable tissue showing signs of the inflammatory response. The goal of early burn care is to provide maximal perfusion to burn wounds so that the zone of coagulation (tissue death) is minimized and tissues surrounding the worst part of burn wounds (zone of stasis) remain well perfused and do not convert to deeper burn injury (tissue loss).

10. **What specific information should the emergency department (ED) nurse obtain from family or rescue personnel about the burn-injured patient?**

The nurse should determine the mechanism of burn injury (including what materials were burning), time elapsed between burn injury and arrival of emergency services, patient's neurological status at the scene of injury, extraction time, patient confinement in a burning space, significant past medical history, history of substance abuse, and preburn weight. Tetanus prophylaxis is recommended if the burn covers more than 10% TBSA.

11. **How is the percentage of TBSA burned calculated?**

Three methods can be used to estimate TBSA. The rule of nines is the most expeditious method for use in the ED. Using this method, each major body part is calculated as a multiple of 9%. The percents of the rule of nines are slightly different for children younger than 9 years of age because of differing body proportions in this population.

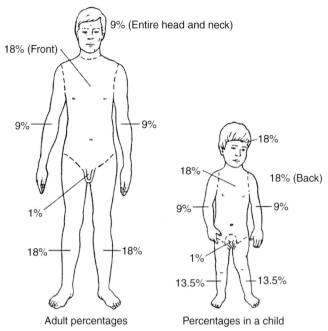

9% (Entire head and neck)

18% (Front)

9% — — 9%

1%

18% — — 18%

Adult percentages

18%

18% — 18% (Back)

9% — — 9%

1%

13.5% — — 13.5%

Percentages in a child

Rule of nines for children and adults.

An alternative method that is much more precise for estimating TBSA burned is to use the Lund-Browder Chart. This chart estimates TBSA in all age groups and is more appropriate for use in the burn center.

Finally, the "palm method" uses the size of the patient's palm to estimate approximately 1% TBSA. There is no consensus if the fingers should be included as part of the palm. This method is useful with smaller, localized burns. Keep in mind that women and obese patients have differing proportions from men and this should be taken into consideration when estimating extent of burn injury. In addition to the percent of burn, an estimation of the depth of burn is also made. However, the true depth of the burn is not usually declared for 24 hours.

Serial TBSA burn injury estimates are completed in the prehospital setting, ED, and upon admission to the burn unit. Often ongoing TBSA assessments continue for several days after injury because tissue damage may extend deeper during the first few hours to days after injury because of lack of adequate tissue perfusion. The importance of calculating the TBSA burned is to help determine fluid resuscitation needs and to determine whether the patient should be transported to a burn center.

Lastly, superficial burn injuries are not calculated into the TBSA of a burn injury assessment. Superficial burn injuries do not produce systemic effects nor require aggressive fluid resuscitation. The TBSA of partial-thickness and full-thickness burns are estimated using the rule of nines or the Lund-Browder Chart.

12. **How is burn shock different from other types of shock?**

Burn shock occurs in patients with burns over more than 20% TBSA. It is a staged shock that results in relative hypovolemia and distribution abnormalities because of massive fluid shifts out of the vascular space into the interstitial space. Chemical mediators are released, causing profound systemic effects on vascular permeability, myocardial depression, and hypoperfusion that impair organ function. Therapeutic goals in treating burn shock focus on aggressive fluid resuscitation. In conjunction with adequate fluid resuscitation, vasopressors such as norepinephrine or dopamine, or an inotrope such as dobutamine, may be added to maintain adequate tissue perfusion during resuscitation. Systemic inflammatory response syndrome (SIRS) and multiple organ dysfunction syndrome (MODS) may result as a complication of burn shock.

13. **What are the initial priorities in burn resuscitation?**

For any traumatic injury, initial priority should be given to management of the patient's ABCDs (airway, breathing, circulation, determination of disability—neurological status). The cervical spine should be stabilized for mechanisms of injury when concomitant trauma may have occurred, as with electrical or lightning injury or associated trauma from blasts. The cause of the burn injury should be determined and the agent removed from the body to stop the burning process (e.g., chemicals, clothes, metals, leather belts).

Partial-thickness burn wounds do not bleed enough to alter hematocrit concentrations. So if significant bleeding is present or the patient's hematocrit is dropping, a secondary survey to assess for an underlying source of traumatic bleeding is indicated.

When a burned patient presents to the ED unconscious, carbon monoxide (CO) poisoning and head trauma should be considered. Lastly, all rings, bracelets, and necklaces should be removed early because generalized edema occurs during fluid resuscitation.

14. **How are fluid resuscitation requirements calculated for the burn patient?**

Two formulas are commonly used to calculate fluid resuscitation requirements for burn-injured patients. The Parkland Formula (also known as the Consensus Formula) is recommended by the ABA. Fluid requirements are calculated as follows:

Adults: 2 to 4ml of lactated Ringer's solution × weight in kg × % TBSA injury

Children younger than 3 years of age: 3 to 4 ml of lactated Ringer's solution × weight in kg × % TBSA injury (a maintenance infusion with a solution containing dextrose is also administered)

Half of the calculated total volume is administered in the first 8 hours after the burn injury, with the remaining volume administered over the following 16 hours.

The Modified Brooke Resuscitation Formula is also widely used in the United States. This formula is similar to the Parkland Formula for the initial 24 hours; however, it includes infusion of colloids (5% albumin in lactated Ringer's solution) at a rate based on % TBSA injury. Typically, lactated Ringer's solution is the fluid of choice for fluid resuscitation; however, some burn centers use various hypertonic solutions with good patient outcomes.

Fluid received before arrival in the ED is considered in the total amount of fluid needed for burn resuscitation. Timing the first 8 hours begins with the estimated time of injury. Rate of administration may require adjustment to ensure the initial 8-hour calculated volume is delivered or "caught up." Optimizing perfusion to the wound with adequate fluid resuscitation is a central principle in treating burn-injured patients.

Fluid requirements may vary among patients; thus it is vital to titrate fluid resuscitation to measurable endpoints to avoid over or under resuscitation. Possible complications during fluid resuscitation are abdominal compartment syndrome or pulmonary edema. Ongoing assessment of the burn-injured extremity and cardiopulmonary, hepatic, and renal systems is essential in evaluating effectiveness and complications of fluid resuscitation. Children will require dextrose-containing fluids because of their higher metabolic rate. Patients with superficial partial-thickness burns covering less than 15% to 20% TBSA (without inhalation injury) may not require fluid resuscitation.

15. **How is the calculated resuscitation fluid administered to the burn patient?**

The nurse should avoid bolusing resuscitation fluid in the burn victim. Capillary pressures are already elevated and vascular permeability results from burn injury, so the increased hydrostatic pressures resulting from fluid boluses could potentiate further vascular fluid loss. The required resuscitation fluid should be administered via infusion pump, with infusion rate calculated according to amount of fluid required for that particular 8- or 16-hour period.

16. **When will a burn injury require additional fluid administration?**

Inhalation injuries, electrical injuries, and large full-thickness burns generally require a significantly greater amount of fluid resuscitation than the consensus formula recommends, often as much as or exceeding 5 ml/kg/TBSA. In these cases, fluid resuscitation should be titrated for urine output of 0.5 to 1 ml/kg/hr, and as much as 2 ml/kg/hr for significant electrical burns, in addition to the appropriate endpoints discussed later.

17. **What are the primary endpoints of adequate fluid resuscitation?**

The easiest method in the ED for monitoring fluid resuscitation is urine output. For burns covering less than 30% TBSA, a urine output of 0.5 to 1 ml/kg/hr is usually adequate. For burns covering more than 30% TBSA, urine output is not as reliable an indicator of adequate fluid resuscitation. For seriously injured burn patients, the arterial base deficit (target range of ±3 mmol/L) is a more reliable measurement of adequate tissue perfusion. Elevated serum lactate levels correlate with inadequate resuscitation and can serve as a method for monitoring patient response to fluid administration. Central venous oxygen saturation ($ScvO_2$) measurements obtained via oximetric central venous catheters correlate well with true mixed venous oxygen content. The clinician must take time to evaluate the accuracy of the $ScvO_2$ during rapid resuscitation; stopping or slowing the fluid infusion for 30 seconds allows stabilization of the $ScvO_2$ reading. These methods reflect true oxygen availability and extraction at the tissue level, which is often diminished in the presence of normal vital signs and adequate urine output in the patient experiencing shock. In electrical injury or severe burn injury muscle may be damaged, causing the release of myoglobin. Fluid resuscitation should be titrated to achieve a urine output of 75 to 100 ml/hr, or 1 to 2 ml/kg/hr to minimize myoglobinurea and renal tubular damage.

18. **If urine output is less than 0.5 ml/kg/hr during fluid resuscitation, should diuretics be administered?**

No. The nature of fluid shifting from the vascular space to the interstitial space in the burn-injured patient requires increased fluid administration to achieve adequate tissue perfusion. Diuretics will mask the effectiveness of resuscitation and result in loss of vascular fluid and subsequently decrease tissue perfusion. An exception to this is in the presence of myoglobinurea with diminished urine output. Osmotic diuretics (such as mannitol) may be required to ensure clearance of cellular wastes in patients with myoglobinurea.

19. **What are signs and symptoms of inhalation injury? What should be included in the initial treatment of these patients?**

Inhalation injury is always suspected if the burn injury occurred in a closed space (e.g., house fire, under the hood of a car). The presence of singed nasal or facial hair, soot around the mouth or nose, carbonaceous sputum, deep-sounding cough, hoarseness, dyspnea, wheezing, stridor, oral pharynx or upper airway edema, disorientation, obtundation, and unexplained hypoxia are highly suspect for inhalation injury. Unconscious patients or patients who experienced exposure to toxic fumes or smoke in an enclosed space should be suspect for inhalation injury. Early radiographic changes are rarely present in the patient with inhalation injury; fiberoptic bronchoscopy is the diagnostic method routinely used to determine extent of pulmonary injury. Early management of the airway is crucial. Early intubation before significant airway edema occurs is a priority treatment in patients with suspected inhalation injury. CO toxicity should also be ruled out for all suspected inhalation injury patients.

20. **What is the best method for determining arterial CO levels?**

Serum carboxyhemoglobin (COHb) is the best method for assessing CO toxicity. Pulse oximetry (SpO_2) is an unreliable indicator of CO toxicity and may display normal SpO_2 levels in the presence of elevated serum CO. CO has a stronger affinity than oxygen on the hemoglobin molecule. Thus CO will bind to hemoglobin over oxygen, creating a hypoxemic state for the patient. Pulse oximetry monitoring assesses the saturation of hemoglobin, not what the hemoglobin molecule is saturated with (e.g., CO, oxygen). Thus the pulse oximeter is unreliable in patients with CO toxicity.

21. **What are the signs and symptoms associated with CO toxicity?**

Carbon Monoxide Toxicity Signs and Symptoms

CO Level	Signs and Symptoms
Less than 5%	Asymptomatic
5%-10%	Impaired visual acuity
11%-20%	Flushing, headache
21%-30%	Nausea, impaired dexterity
31%-40%	Vomiting, dizziness, syncope
41%-50%	Tachypnea, altered mental status
More than 50%	Coma, death

22. **What is the optimal method for treating a patient with elevated CO levels?**

Fortunately, elevated CO is easily treated by applying 100% oxygen administered via face mask. Oxygen should be delivered until serum levels of CO fall below 5% and signs and symptoms of toxicity are resolved. Hyperbaric oxygen therapy has not been shown to be a superior intervention. The half-life of COHb is approximately 4½ hours on room air and 1½ hours with 100% oxygen via face mask. The duration of treatment with 100% oxygen should be approximately 4 to 6 hours with COHb levels less than 20%. CO toxicity decreases tissue oxygen delivery, causing myocardial depression and poor organ perfusion. In addition to monitoring vital signs, assessment of the patient is important to evaluate improved neurological status that occurs as the CO is replaced with oxygen on the hemoglobin. Concomitant cyanide poisoning is rare but should be considered in patients with inhalation injury associated with textile materials.

23. **What is eschar, and when is an escharotomy performed?**

Eschar is dead tissue. Eschar is essentially an open wound that lacks all protective properties of normal skin and is a medium for bacterial growth. Eschar needs to be removed from the wound bed for wound depth to be assessed. It should be excised surgically or enzymatically to allow for wound healing. In patients with full-thickness burns, the eschar is dry and noncompliant. If the eschar extends circumferentially around a limb or the trunk, compartment syndrome will likely result. To reverse vascular or respiratory compromise, an escharotomy is needed to release the pressure and restore perfusion or ventilation within the compartment. The escharotomy is frequently performed at the bedside by a surgeon. Intravenous (IV) analgesia should be administered before the procedure because the entire area requiring decompression may not be insensate.

24. **How is vascular compromise assessed in a burned extremity?**

Early signs of vascular compromise include paresthesia, deep tissue pain, and cold sensation of the extremity. However, these symptoms may be masked in a severely burned extremity because of extensive nerve damage. Late signs include pallor, cyanosis, decreased capillary refill, and ultimately diminished or absent pulse. If pulses are not palpable, Doppler ultrasound and direct tissue pressures are reliable methods to assess for adequate perfusion in the burned extremity. Continued neurovascular assessment of limbs affected by circumferential burns or high-voltage electrical injury is essential to prevent compartment syndrome and permanent damage.

25. How should pain be treated in the patient with a severe burn injury?

Analgesia should be administered via IV to the burn-injured patient. Morphine or fentanyl administered via IV in small, regular doses is the most commonly used analgesic for acute burn injuries. In addition, benzodiazepines may be administered to decrease anxiety and act synergistically with narcotics, decreasing pain during the acute injury phase. If respiratory drive is threatened because the patient requires increasing amounts of narcotics to maintain pain control, intubation should be considered. Pain management is the ultimate responsibility of the nurse; burn patients tend to require large amounts of narcotic analgesics for comfort and thus require close monitoring.

26. What is the best initial treatment of burn wounds in the ED?

After the burn patient is stabilized and secondary trauma is ruled out, burn wound care can be addressed by the emergency nurse. Minor superficial burns can be cleaned with mild antibacterial soap, treated with topical ointments, and loosely covered with dry gauze. Deeper partial-thickness, deep dermal, and full-thickness burn wounds should be covered with a dry sheet and the patient covered in blankets. Cool saline should not be applied to burn wounds after the initial management because of the risk of causing hypothermia. Wound debridement or application of topical agents to deep burns before transport to a burn center is not necessary. Simply cover the wounds with dry dressings and ensure tissue perfusion (fluid resuscitation) is maximized to prevent conversion of partial-thickness wounds into full-thickness wounds.

Intact blisters should not be disturbed; ruptured blisters may be debrided and dressed with dry gauze before the patient is transported to the local burn center. Burned extremities should be elevated at or above the level of the heart to reduce peripheral edema and compartment syndrome. The head of the bed should be elevated to more than 30 degrees for facial or trunk burns to decrease edema and protect the airway. Avoid use of pillows for head, neck, or ear burns.

27. How are tar and asphalt burns treated?

The initial treatment priority is to cool the burning substance with cool saline or water poured over the affected area. Body temperature should be monitored to ensure the patient does not become hypothermic. After the tar is cooled, the burning process has stopped so the tar does not need to be removed immediately from the skin. Petroleum jelly, mineral oil, or even mayonnaise is effective for removal of tar. Apply the ointment, allow it to soak in, then gently remove the tar with gauze. Avoid peeling tar from skin without first softening with a solvent. When all the tar is removed from the skin, the depth and TBSA burned are assessed.

28. **When is insertion of a nasogastric tube (NGT) indicated?**

Placement of an NGT is indicated in presence of nausea, vomiting, or gastric distention, or for deep burns covering more than 20% TBSA. In severely burned or hemodynamically unstable patients, the NGT can be used to facilitate early gastric feedings. In addition, placement of the NGT in the ED may prevent associated complications (e.g., ileus).

29. **What are some common topical agents that may be used in the ED to treat small partial-thickness burn wounds?**

First, before applying a topical agent or dressing, clean the burn wound with mild antibacterial soap and water and gently remove debris from the wound. Topical agents and dressings are applied based on the wound depth and wound drainage (absorptive) needs.

Bacitracin is the most common petroleum-based antibacterial ointment used for minor burns. It is applied in a thin coat over superficial and partial-thickness burns. The wound may be left open or covered loosely with gauze to absorb wound drainage.

Silver sulfadiazine cream (Silvadene) is a broad-spectrum antimicrobial ointment, applied in a $\frac{1}{4}$-inch to $\frac{1}{2}$-inch layer over partial-thickness burns. The use of silver sulfadiazine in patients with allergy to sulfa may be contraindicated. Long-term use of silver sulfadiazine may cause leukopenia in patients with larger TBSA burns. The wound is typically covered with a secondary gauze dressing to absorb wound drainage.

Other dressings such as hydrocolloids (DuoDERM) and silver-based antimicrobial dressings (Acticoat, SilverSorb, AQUACEL Ag) can also be applied to burn wounds.

30. **Should antibiotics be administered to burn victims?**

No. Unless a patient has a preexisting infection, antibiotics are not recommended as prophylaxis for the burned patient.

ELECTRICAL INJURIES

31. **What types of electrical current cause burn injury?**

There are two types of electrical current: AC and DC. AC is found at low voltage (110 to 220 volts) in households; intermediate voltage (220 to 1000 volts) to high voltage (more than 1000 volts) is found in industrial use or in high-tension wires. DC is found in car batteries and lightning. Contact with electrical current causes deep tissue damage, as well as localized and flash burns. The higher the voltage encountered by the patient, the more severe the tissue damage and associated mortality.

32. **Why are high-voltage electrical injuries difficult to assess?**

Electrical injuries may have a disproportional small contact point relative to the extent of internal damage. Electricity follows the path of least resistance in the body, traveling along nerve pathways deeper in tissues and along muscles.

The energy travels throughout the body and damages a great deal of tissue despite external appearance of entrance or exit wounds. The exit wound may be overwhelming in nature but the main focus is on internal tissue damage caused by the path of electrical energy through the body. Priorities for care of patients with electrical burns are to ensure adequate fluid resuscitation (frequently more than fluid resuscitation formulas estimate), cardiac monitoring, assessment and treatment of myoglobinurea, and neurovascular assessment for compartment syndrome.

33. In the patient with electrical trauma, what are the most commonly associated injuries?

Low- and intermediate-voltage injuries are generally localized without incidence of compartment syndrome, loss of consciousness, or rhabdomyolysis. Tissue burns will be noted at the points of contact with the electrical source. In toddlers, the most common injury is biting or chewing of a household electrical cord. Oral burns and extensive edema are associated with this type of injury, and delayed hemorrhage from the labial artery may occur when the eschar sloughs off.

High-voltage injuries pose significant risk for concomitant trauma from a fall at the time of contact with the energy source. Muscle contractions stimulated by the electrical energy can cause long bone or spinal fractures. Cardiac arrhythmias, compartment syndrome, and rhabdomyolysis with associated renal compromise are also significant concerns for focused assessment in patients with high-voltage electrical injuries. Lastly, ongoing neurological assessment is indicated because permanent neurological impairment may ensue.

External thermal injury, arc or flash burns, or burns from ignited clothing may accompany electrical burn injury. It is important to obtain a careful history of the incident to ascertain potential trauma associated with the electrical injury. If these patients survive the initial injury and do not experience cardiac arrest, the chance of recovery is good.

34. Is cardiac monitoring necessary for patients with electrical burn injury?

Yes. Cardiac monitoring is recommended for a minimum of 24 hours and as long as 72 hours after the patient experiences an electrical injury to evaluate cardiac insult. Electrical current travels randomly through the body following nerve pathways, so electrical impulses can interfere with normal cardiac contraction cycles and cause arrhythmias. If arrhythmias occur, they are generally noted within the first few hours after injury. A complete cardiac assessment to include laboratory analysis (e.g., creatine kinase MB isoenzyme—CK-MB, cardiac troponin) and function tests (e.g., echocardiogram) may be indicated.

The most common cause of death in lightning strike victims is cardiac arrest caused by massive counter shock to the myocardium. If the patient survives the lightning strike, cardiac monitoring and serial serum enzymes to assess myocardial damage are indicated.

35. What is the appropriate treatment for myoglobinurea associated with electrical burns?

High-voltage electrical injury causes an extensive breakdown of muscle tissue and release of large amounts of cellular debris. Fluid resuscitation should be titrated to maintain a urine output of 75 to 100 ml/hr or 1 to 2 ml/kg/hr. Osmotic diuretics such as mannitol may be used to enhance urine output, and sodium bicarbonate may be administered via IV to alkalinize the urine and protect the renal tubules in patients with myoglobinurea.

CHEMICAL BURNS

36. What are some examples of the common agents that may cause chemical trauma?

Agents That Cause Chemical Trauma

Class	Compound	Common Uses
Acids	Hydrochloric acid, hydrofluoric acid, oxalic acid, sulfuric acid	Bathroom cleaners, acidifiers for swimming pools (hydrochloric acid), rust removers (oxalic acid), industrial drain cleaners (sulfuric acid)
Alkalis	Hydroxides; carbonates; caustic sodas of sodium, potassium, ammonium, lithium, barium, and calcium	Oven cleaners, drain cleaners, fertilizers, heavy industrial cleaners, cement or concrete
Organic compounds	Phenols, creosote, petroleum products	Chemical disinfectants (phenols), gasoline (petroleum)

37. What factors influence the extent of a chemical injury?

The extent of injury depends on concentration of the chemical, extent and depth of exposure, and systemic absorption of the chemical. The true extent of the injury may not be apparent for several days after the injury. Daily assessment of the burn, laboratory values, and organ function are needed to fully evaluate the extent of chemical burn injury.

38. How can the nurse reduce the severity of chemical burns?

Care should be taken when treating the chemical burn to avoid spreading the agent to unaffected areas or contaminating members of the healthcare team. All contaminated clothing, shoes, and jewelry should be immediately removed from the patient. Determination of the causative agent should be made. Chemical agents in powder form should be carefully brushed off, with a mask on the patient and caregivers to protect the airway, before initiating irrigation of the area.

Thorough removal of liquid agents and copious irrigation with water should continue for 30 minutes or longer until the "soapy" feel of alkalis is gone. Tissue injury will occur until all traces of chemical substance are removed. The patient should be protected from hypothermia if large areas require irrigation.

39. How is treatment of chemical burns different from thermal burns?

The only difference in treating a chemical burn versus a thermal injury is the necessary evaluation of systemic toxicity, electrolyte imbalances, or organ dysfunction caused by exposure to the chemical. Otherwise, after the causative agent is thoroughly removed from the skin, assessment and treatment of the wound is similar to that of thermal injuries. Determination of the TBSA affected and wound depth is made, and appropriate referral to the local burn center is initiated. The burned areas should be covered with gauze or a clean dry sheet, and the patient should be kept warm. Evaluating the patient for systemic toxicity or electrolyte imbalances is necessary; appropriate labs should be drawn and renal function assessed.

Key Points

- Monitor the ABCDs first, then treat the burn injuries.
- Approach all severely burned patients as having the potential for multiple traumas.
- The rule of nines is the best method for determining the extent of burns in the ED.
- Consider potential for abuse or neglect with suspicious burns in patients of all age groups.
- Patients with less than 15% TBSA burned may not require fluid resuscitation.
- Administer fluids via continuous infusion; avoid bolusing fluid.
- Fluid administration formulas are only a guide; administer fluid to achieve physiological endpoints of adequate perfusion (i.e., urine output).
- In children, electrical and inhalation injuries require significantly more fluid resuscitation. Children need dextrose-containing maintenance fluids in addition to resuscitative fluids.
- Diuretics are not recommended during resuscitation of the burned patient.
- Prompt intubation for facial burns and suspected inhalation injury is necessary to protect the airway.
- Treat CO exposure with 100% oxygen via face mask.
- Cover major burns in the ED with a clean dry sheet or gauze, apply no topical ointments, and prepare for transport to a regional burn center.
- Electrical injuries are generally more extensive than they appear.

Internet Resources

American Burn Association:
www.ameriburn.org

Burn Survivors Online:
www.burnsurvivorsonline.com

BurnSurgery.org:
www.burnsurgery.org

Children's Burn Foundation:
www.childburn.org

International Society for Burn Injuries:
www.worldburn.org

National Center for the Dissemination of Disability Research, An Easy Guide to Outpatient Burn Rehabilitation:
www.ncddr.org/rr/burn/burnguide.html

Radiation Emergency Assistance Center/Training Site (REAC/TS), Managing Radiation Emergencies:
www.orau.gov/reacts/emergency.htm#Triage

Bibliography

Ahrns KS: Trends in burn resuscitation: Shifting the focus from fluids to adequate endpoint monitoring, edema control, and adjuvant therapies, *Crit Care Nurs Clin North Am* 16:75-98, 2004.

American Burn Association: *Burn unit referral criteria*, 1999. Available at www.ameriburn.org/BurnUnitReferral.pdf.

Beale RJ et al: Vasopressor and inotropic support in septic shock: An evidence-based review, *Crit Care Med* 32:455-465, 2004.

Cancio LC et al: Predicting increased fluid requirements during the resuscitation of thermally injured patients, *J Trauma* 56:404-414, 2004.

Cartotto RC et al: How well does the Parkland Formula estimate actual fluid resuscitation volumes? *J Burn Care Rehabil* 23:258-265, 2002.

Dellinger RP et al: Surviving sepsis campaign guidelines for management of severe sepsis and septic shock, *Crit Care Med* 32:858-872, 2004.

Flynn MB: Nutritional support for the burn-injured patient, *Crit Care Nurs Clin North Am* 16:139-144, 2004.

LaBorde P: Burn epidemiology: The patient, the nation, the statistics, and the data resources, *Crit Care Nurs Clin North Am* 16:13-25, 2004.

Merz J et al: Wound care of the pediatric burn patient, *AACN Clin Issues* 14:429-441, 2003.

Montonye J: Burns. In Oman K, Koziol-McLain J, Scheetz L, editors: *Emergency nursing secrets*, Philadelphia, 2001, Hanley & Belfus.

Papp A et al: Myocardial function and haemodynamics in extensive burn trauma: Evaluation by clinical signs, invasive monitoring, echocardiography and cytokine concentrations. A prospective clinical study, *Acta Anaesthesiol Scand* 47:1257-1263, 2003.

Radiation Emergency Assistance Center/Training Site (REAC/TS): *Guidance for radiation accident management*, 2002. Available at www.orau.gov/reacts/emergency.htm#Triage.

Rhodes A, Bennett ED: Early goal-directed therapy: An evidence-based review, *Crit Care Med* 32:448-450, 2004.

Richards MS, Johnson RM: Managing superficial burn wounds, *Adv Skin Wound Care* 15:246-247, 2002.

Rivers EP, Ander DS, Powell D: Central venous oxygen saturation monitoring in the critically ill patient, *Curr Opin Crit Care* 7:204-211, 2001.

Sheridan RL: Burns, *Crit Care Med* 30:S500-S514, 2002.

Sheridan RL: Burns. In Fink MP et al, editors: *Textbook of critical care,* ed 5, Philadelphia, 2005, Elsevier Saunders.

Stübgen JP, Plum F: Coma. In Fink MP et al, editors: *Textbook of critical care,* ed 5, Philadelphia, 2005, Elsevier Saunders.

Supple KG: Physiologic response to burn injury, *Crit Care Nurs Clin North Am* 16:119-126, 2004.

White SR: Carbon monoxide poisoning. In Kruse JA, Fink MP, Carlson RW, editors: *Saunders manual of critical care*, Philadelphia, 2003, Saunders.

Trauma During Pregnancy

Connie J. Mattera

1. How often do pregnant women experience trauma?

The true incidence of trauma in pregnancy is unknown. About 8 million women become pregnant annually in the United States. Maull (2001) note that the peak age for pregnancy coincides with the peak age for trauma. It is estimated that 6% to 8% of pregnant women will suffer some form of injury. Fewer than 1 in 14 seek medical assistance for injury, and less than 5% are hospitalized as a result of trauma.

2. Are pregnant women more susceptible to injury?

Yes. Many more injuries are seen in pregnant women today because they are more active and often work and travel throughout all stages of pregnancy. In addition, there is a significant incidence of violence and battering of pregnant women.

Factors that predispose a woman to accidental injury in early pregnancy are syncopal episodes, hyperventilation, and easy fatigability. Factors that cause gait unsteadiness and a predisposition to falls during the last trimester include a protuberant abdomen that changes the woman's center of gravity; loosening of pelvic ligaments and joints; and pelvic pressure, which causes pain and neuromuscular dysfunction of the lower extremities.

The enlarging abdomen increases susceptibility to blunt and penetrating trauma after the first trimester when the uterus rises to become an abdominal organ. Motor vehicle crashes in which the seat belt is not used or is used in an improper position are common causes of trauma, as is violence.

3. What effect does trauma have on pregnancy?

- Minor trauma usually is not a risk to maternal or fetal well-being.
- Major trauma may lead to fetal injury or interruption of the pregnancy.
- Physiological changes of pregnancy may mimic pathological conditions (e.g., shock).
- Pregnancy may alter the pattern and severity of injury.
- Trauma management must be modified to accommodate and preserve the physiological changes in pregnancy.

4. What are the possible outcomes or complications of trauma in pregnancy?

- Maternal or fetal injury or distress
- Maternal or fetal death

- Fetomaternal hemorrhage (placental abruption)
- Preterm labor and delivery
- Uterine rupture

5. **What factors contribute to maternal and fetal morbidity and mortality from trauma?**

Trauma is the leading cause of nonobstetrical maternal death during pregnancy. Pregnancy does not increase mortality or morbidity after trauma but it does influence the pattern of injury (see question 2).

The leading cause of fetal death is placental abruption; the second leading cause is maternal death. Maternal and fetal death are highest in patients with internal injuries to the thorax, abdomen, and pelvis. Gestational age is the most significant predictor of fetal, neonatal, and infant mortality. Rogers et al reported in 1999 that fetal deaths are higher in the maternal population with higher injury severity scores (ISSs) (above 25), lower Glasgow Coma Scale scores, lower admitting pH levels, shock, or fetal heart rates lower than 110 beats/min at some time during hospitalization. Fetal fatality rates above 50% have been reported in mothers whose ISSs are 12 or higher, although lower scores have still been associated with significantly elevated adverse outcomes.

6. **What normal physiological changes in pregnant patients alter assessment and treatment of the pulmonary system?**

As a result of an increased blood volume the upper respiratory passages become engorged by swollen capillaries, making the pregnant patient more susceptible to nosebleeds and upper airway obstruction. Intubate with caution. Avoid nasal intubation. If it must be performed, select a smaller, well-lubricated tube and insert very gently.

As pregnancy progresses, the diaphragm is pushed upward 4 cm, causing the lungs to shorten by 4 cm and decreasing oxygen reserve. Chest circumference increases by 6 cm and transverse diameter by 2 cm to compensate for the diminished lung length. Residual volume decreases to 800 ml, and functional residual capacity (volume of gas that remains in the lungs at the end of normal expiration) decreases by 20% to 1350 ml. Ligamentous relaxation and outward flaring of the rib margins compensate for this decreased capacity. Vital capacity is essentially unchanged. These changes predispose the patient to hypoxia and a feeling of shortness of breath. As the diaphragm elevates, lower lobes of the lungs become more difficult to expand, predisposing the patient to atelectasis. Dyspnea occurs in 60% of pregnant women. Therefore, it is especially important to avoid placing a pregnant patient in Trendelenburg's position because she may not be able to breathe adequately.

Oxygen requirements can increase 10% to 20% above the nonpregnant state in response to fetal growth and increased maternal metabolism. Tidal volume increases to 600 ml and respiratory rate may increase by 15%, thereby increasing the minute volume by as much as 26% to 50%. These changes result in a chronic state of hyperventilation and compensated respiratory alkalosis.

Arterial blood gas (ABG) changes include increased partial pressure of oxygen (100 to 104 mmHg) and oxygen saturation (at or above 96%) and decreased partial pressure of carbon dioxide ($PaCO_2$ 25 to 32 mmHg) and bicarbonate (18 to 22 mEq/L). Such changes provide a gradient for the exchange of oxygen and carbon dioxide favoring the fetus. A $PaCO_2$ in arterial blood of 35 to 40 mmHg may indicate respiratory acidosis for pregnant women. The pH compensates via excretion of bicarbonate from the kidneys, which leaves the pregnant patient with decreased buffering capacity after trauma.

7. **What normal physiological changes of pregnancy alter assessment and treatment of the cardiovascular system?**

Pregnancy simulates a stress test for the cardiovascular system. Changes start at 4 to 6 weeks and continue to approximately 34 weeks. All of these alterations are designed to protect both mother and fetus and to provide increased oxygen and nutrient delivery to the fetus.

Anatomical changes to the heart: As the uterus enlarges and elevates the diaphragm, the heart is pushed upward and rotated forward and toward the left, causing a leftward shift of the electrical axis by 15 degrees, producing Q waves in leads II and aV_F. Cardiac hypertrophy is caused by increased blood volume. Systolic ejection murmurs are present in 90% of pregnant women. There is increased loudness of the first and third heart sounds with an exaggerated split between mitral and tricuspid closure. There are no significant electrocardiogram (ECG) changes, although premature atrial and ventricular contractions are common. Flattened or inverted T waves (lead III) also may be present.

Cardiac output (CO): Pregnant women experience a high-output, low-resistance state. CO increases 20% to 30% or by 1.5 L/min during the first trimester and peaks at 6 to 7 L/min (40% to 50% increase) at the end of the second trimester because of catecholamine release or as a response to the functional 20% to 30% arteriovenous shunt produced by the low-resistance placental circuit. CO remains increased to term when measured in the lateral recumbent position.

Heart rate: Increases 10 to 20 beats/min over prepregnant levels by the third trimester because of increased blood volume and oxygen demand. Pulses of 80 to 95 beats/min are considered normal in both awake and sleeping states. Sustained heart rates of more than 100 beats/min may indicate hypovolemia.

Arterial blood pressure: Little change in the first trimester. During the second and third trimesters vessels dilate because of the release of progesterone, resulting in a relative resistance to the vasopressor effects of renin and angiotensin II. Systolic blood pressure decreases by 5 to 15 mmHg and diastolic blood pressure by 5 to 10 mmHg in the second trimester (nadir at 28 weeks gestation) to an average of 102/55 mmHg. The pulse pressure also widens. Blood pressure then rebounds during the third trimester to an average of 108/67 mmHg because of an increase in blood volume and venous congestion.

It is never normal to have a blood pressure higher than the prepregnant level. Pregnant women with preeclampsia have lost resistance to angiotensin and have become hyperreactive to renin and angiotensin in the supine position to counter-regulate the perceived decrease in blood return. A diastolic blood pressure higher than 90 mmHg may indicate hypertension of pregnancy and is cause to alert a physician.

Venous pressure: Central venous pressure drops to half of nonpregnant levels by the third trimester because of venous pooling and stasis. Vena caval compression from the uterus results in increased pelvic and peripheral venous pressures and congestion in the lower extremities, which may cause increased bleeding from soft tissue injuries, pelvic fractures, and even minor wounds to the lower extremities. This compression may also cause varicose veins and leg cramps.

Peripheral blood flow: In the first and second trimesters, decreased peripheral resistance is associated with increased peripheral circulation. Thus, the pregnant patient in shock may be warm and dry, rather than cool and moist.

8. What normal physiological changes of pregnancy alter the hematological assessment?

Plasma volume: Begins to increase by the tenth week to fill the uteroplacental vasculature. By the thirty-second week, volume increases 35% to 50% or 40 to 70 ml/kg (1200 to 1600 ml) to a total of 7 to 8 L at term. This hypervolemia can mask a 30% (1500 to 2000 ml) gradual loss of maternal blood volume or a 25% acute blood loss before measurable changes in vital signs appear. The average pregnant patient can tolerate a 1500-ml (30% to 35%) volume loss before becoming extremely hypotensive. When blood loss occurs, maternal vital signs may be maintained at the expense of perfusion to the uterus, placing the fetus at early risk for hypoxia. Maternal shock is associated with an 80% fetal mortality rate.

Total red blood cell (RBC) mass: Increases by 20% to 35% (25 to 30 ml/kg) as a result of placental erythropoietin secretion to meet the fetal need for oxygen. Given that plasma volume increases over RBC mass, the pregnant patient becomes physiologically anemic and is easily fatigued. A normal prepregnancy hematocrit of 40% to 45% may drop 10 to 12 g/dl, to 32% to 34% by week 30 as a result of hemodilution caused by the increase in plasma volume.

Leukocytosis: Occurs during the last half of pregnancy and labor, producing a white blood cell (WBC) count of 12,000 to 18,000/m³. Levels may rise as high as 25,000 in response to stress. There is no change in the differential or in platelets.

Coagulation factors: The sedimentation rate increases as a result of increased fibrinogen (from 80 to 180 mg/dl to 350 to 450 mg/dl). Pregnancy produces a hypercoagulable state with increased risk of thromboembolic disease. Estrogen-mediated increases in hepatic production of fibrinogen (1.5 times normal) and factors VII, VIII, IX, X, and XII and decreased plasminogen activator (fibrinolytic activity) may result in spontaneous thrombus formation and impaired clot lysis, especially if the woman is immobilized. This pattern becomes a potential benefit if hemorrhage occurs.

Both the uterus and the placenta contain large amounts of thromboplastin. If released, it can precipitate disseminated intravascular coagulation (DIC). Abruptio placenta with DIC is frequently accompanied by a drop in fibrinogen levels. The harbingers of disaster may be missed if the clinician is unaware of normal fibrinogen increases in pregnancy. Prothrombin time (PT) and partial thromboplastin time (PTT) are both mildly reduced as pregnancy progresses. If anticoagulants are needed, physicians are more likely to order heparin because warfarin crosses the placenta.

9. **What normal physiological changes of pregnancy alter assessment and treatment of the gastrointestinal (GI) system?**

Abdominal wall: The peritoneum has decreased sensitivity. General laxity and stretching of the abdominal wall often masks typical findings of guarding, rigidity, and rebound tenderness, suggesting intraperitoneal injury and making an abdominal assessment by palpation unreliable in trauma.

Abdominal contents: Compartmentalization of the abdominal organs displaces the small bowel and other organs laterally and cephalad by the enlarging uterus and changes pain referral patterns. The uterine mass interferes with attempts to palpate abdominal viscera or masses and thus impairs the ability to detect intraperitoneal bleeding clinically.

Stomach and GI tract: Loss of gastroesophageal sphincter control coupled with a progesterone-induced suppression in gastric motility causes delayed gastric emptying, prolonged intestinal transit times, and an increase in gastric secretions. Such changes generally lead to heartburn and constipation but also may make the patient more prone to vomiting and aspiration during trauma and intubation; they may also mimic a silent abdomen. The bowel is compressed, increasing the likelihood of significant injury. The appendix is in the right *upper* quadrant during the third trimester.

Liver and spleen: These organs become mildly distended, compressed, or displaced, making them more vulnerable to injury or rupture. Aspartate aminotransferase (AST) and alanine aminotransferase (ALT) are normal; alkaline phosphatase (ALP) is elevated (placental origin).

10. **What normal physiological changes of pregnancy alter assessment and treatment of the genitourinary system?**

The bladder is attached to the lower uterine segment and usually is compressed between the uterus and abdominal wall because it is displaced upward and anteriorly as a result of uterine growth, beyond the protection of the pelvic ring (twelfth week). It is especially vulnerable to rupture with direct trauma to the suprapubic area. Hypertrophy of the kidneys and dilation of the calyces and ureters (mild physiological hydronephrosis of pregnancy) should be considered when urograms are interpreted.

Urinary frequency during the first and third trimesters is caused by increased renal filtration (30% increase in renal blood flow) and compression of the bladder. This increase in renal vascular supply may lead to augmented blood loss in trauma in comparison with similar injuries in nonpregnant women. The glomerular filtration rate is increased, creatinine clearance is increased, and serum creatinine and blood urea nitrogen (BUN) are decreased. Although glycosuria is common, hematuria and albuminuria are abnormal.

11. **What characteristics of the reproductive and obstetrical organs become significant in assessing a pregnant trauma patient?**

The uterus grows from 60 to 80 g to 900 to 1200 g at term. It enlarges 10 to 20 times its nonpregnant size, remaining an intrapelvic organ until week 12 when it rises to become an abdominal organ. At 20 weeks, the fundus is level with the umbilicus and reaches the costal margin at 36 weeks. The uterus is a passive pressure organ with no autoregulation. Although the uterus usually exists in a state of maximal vasodilation, uterine vessels constrict in response to compensatory catecholamines released in early shock. This constriction markedly diminishes blood flow to the fetus by 20% to 30% before any blood pressure changes in the mother are detectable.

Uterine blood flow is markedly increased (500%) from 2% of the CO to approximately 20% or 500 to 700 ml/min at term. As a result, injuries can produce rapid and profound blood loss. The entire blood volume circulates through the uterus every 8 to 11 minutes.

The mature placenta is discoid and flattened, measuring 20 cm in diameter and 2.5 cm in thickness at the center and weighing approximately 500 g at birth. Interposed between the fetal and maternal circulations, it serves as a source of hormones and provides transfer of nutrients, wastes, antibodies, hormones, and electrolytes. Drugs and infectious organisms may cross the placental barrier. The fetal surface is smooth and glistening because of the amnion and chorion, which are continuous with the edges of the placenta and form the amniotic sac. The maternal surface is rough and raised into 10 to 38 cotyledons that attach to the uterine wall. Premature separation of one or more cotyledons results in fetal distress and hypoxia (abruptio placenta).

The umbilical cord has two arteries and one large vein. The arteries carry unoxygenated blood from the fetus to the placenta, and the umbilical vein returns oxygenated blood to the fetus. The vessels are surrounded by connective tissue called Wharton's jelly. At birth, the cord is about 50 cm in length and 12 mm in diameter. It remains stiff during development because of the blood flowing through it. When blood flow is interrupted by trauma or compression, the fetus experiences hypoxia and distress.

The amniotic sac or bag of waters provides a sterile environment, maintains a constant temperature for fetal development, prevents the amnion from adhering to the developing embryo, permits symmetrical growth and free movements of the fetus, serves as a cushion, and decreases the force of insult to the fetus. Risk for fetal injury is highest in the third trimester when the fetal head is engaged, the torso is exposed, and the ratio between fetal size and amniotic fluid volume diminishes.

The amniotic sac initially contains fluid produced by its cellular walls, but the majority comes from maternal blood. At week 37, approximately 1000 ml of fluid is exchanged every 3 hours via placental membranes. The fetus swallows and absorbs about 400 ml/day and in late pregnancy excretes 500 ml of fetal urine per day into the fluid. A distressed fetus may also excrete meconium into the fluid, tingeing it brownish-black or green and giving it a "pea soup" appearance.

12. **What factors should be assessed when examining the uterus and its contents?**

Palpate for uterine irritability and fetal movement. The gravid uterus is highly vulnerable to irritation by physical stimuli. Therefore, injury to the abdomen may initiate active labor. Prolonged periods without movement may suggest fetal demise.

Measure fundal height. The distance from the symphysis pubis to the top of the uterus (fundus), measured in centimeters, is an approximate indicator of gestational age. From weeks 16 to 36 from the last menstrual period (LMP), each centimeter approximates 1 week of gestation.

Ask the patient about the status of the membranes. A sudden gush of fluid from the vagina after an abdominal impact suggests rupture of the membranes. The pH of amniotic fluid is 7 to 7.5, whereas the pH of urine is 4.8 to 6. Check for leakage of amniotic fluid and meconium staining. Nitrazine pH paper turns black in the presence of amniotic fluid.

Auscultate fetal heart tones (FHTs). Normal FHTs range between 120 and 160 beats/min. They are the best indicator of fetal condition because FHTs change before maternal vital signs. Fetal bradycardia is a grave sign, suggesting fetal anoxia, and requires immediate action for fetal survival. If FHTs are present, they should be monitored sonographically until there is good presumptive evidence that the fetus has tolerated the traumatic episode well. If FHTs are not present, it is essential to confirm fetal death. Doppler ultrasonography should confirm the presence of fetal heart activity if it exists. If fetal death is presumed to have occurred after injury, maternal injuries should be treated. The mother should be observed until her condition is stable. Labor can then be induced for a vaginal delivery.

13. **What factors should be included in the abdominal exam?**

- Note the shape and contour of the abdomen. Inspect for deformity, contusions, abrasions, punctures, and wounds.
- Assess the onset (abrupt or gradual), provocation, quality, location, radiation, severity, and duration of abdominal pain.
- Auscultate bowel sounds superiorly and laterally.
- Palpate for tenderness, guarding, and rigidity; note whether pain is generalized or localized to the uterus.
- Percuss for shifting dullness (if skilled in the procedure).

14. **What is supine hypotensive syndrome? How can it be avoided in trauma patients?**

In the supine position, vena caval and aortic compression by the uterus and its contents may decrease venous return (reduce preload) and CO by 30% to 40% after 20 weeks, resulting in 30% less effective circulating blood volume and diminished uteroplacental perfusion. These changes make it difficult to evaluate the effects of acute blood loss producing shock. A supine position also increases pelvic venous pressures and may worsen placental separation. Tachycardia and hypotension assessed in a supine pregnant trauma patient may represent shock or be caused by position. All blood pressure measurements taken on patients in their second and third trimesters should be done when the patient is in the left or right lateral recumbent position. Displacing the uterus from the inferior vena cava can increase CO up to 25%. The uterus can be displaced off the vena cava by manual manipulation, by tilting the spine board or patient to the side, or by using a hip wedge to tilt the uterus.

15. What are the major mechanisms of injury in pregnancy?

Blunt trauma caused by motor vehicle crashes, falls, and interpersonal violence are the most frequent causes of maternal and fetal injury.

16. What types of injuries are sustained from blunt trauma?

- Most common: fractures, dislocations, sprains, and strains
- Shock
- Head injury with skull fracture, cerebral contusion, or intracranial hemorrhage
- Vertebral fracture
- Spinal cord injury
- Chest injury requiring thoracostomy
- Abdominal injury: hepatic, spleen, and retroperitoneal injuries and hematomas caused by increased vascularity
- Genitourinary injury requiring surgery
- Pelvic fractures

17. What is the primary cause of significant blunt trauma and death during pregnancy?

Motor vehicle crashes result in 1300 to 3900 fetal losses per year. Deceleration and shearing forces during impact cause placental abruption, uterine damage, and rupture. Head injury is the leading cause of maternal death, followed by chest trauma. However, intraabdominal injury is nearly as frequent a cause of maternal death.

18. What determines the severity of injury in a motor vehicle crash?

- Speed of vehicle at impact
- Damage to the vehicle
- Position of the victim at time of impact
- Type of collision (head-on, rear-end, side impact, rollover)
- Side of the vehicle on which the impact occurred in relation to the patient's position
- Weight and size of the vehicle
- Use of occupant restraints

Seats belts, used properly (shoulder harness across chest, lap belt under pregnant abdomen), and air bags usually limit the severity of injury. However, an isolated case has been reported of extensive brain injury in a premature infant with minimal maternal trauma associated with deployment of an air bag. Lap belts alone allow significant forward flexion and, if worn too high, result in direct compression to the abdomen. Either wearing a lap belt alone or wearing a lap belt too high can result in pressures sufficient to rupture the uterus or amniotic sac. Deceleration forces are transmitted directly to the uterus. Lap belts with shoulder harnesses are essential to provide equal distribution of forces and to prevent forward flexion of the mother. Proper use of restraints improves fetal survival. Without the shoulder harness, the protuberant uterus not only receives the impact of the steering wheel or dashboard but also may suffer the effects of the inertial forces of mass versus momentum.

Intrauterine impact pressures can rise to 550 mmHg because of flexion of the mother's torso and deceleration forces (10 times the pressure of normal labor). Such pressures can result in lacerations, rupture, and complete avulsion of the uterus, as well as severe placental and fetal injuries (50% fetal death).

19. **What is the risk of falls in pregnant women?**

Falls are a significant cause of blunt trauma in pregnant women. Kady et al (2004) found them to be the leading mechanism with the severest injuries and worst outcomes. Contributing factors include fatigue; relaxed pelvic ligaments, which cause pelvic tilt and increase lordosis; joint laxity caused by the effects of progesterone; altered gait and balance; and assaults. The severity of injury is proportional to the force of impact and the specific body part sustaining the impact. More serious injuries include pelvic fractures, lower extremity fractures, and head and spinal cord trauma.

Obtain the following history: events preceding the fall; height from which the patient fell; the patient's ability to break the fall by grasping onto something, which can decrease velocity; and the surface onto which the patient fell (energy-absorbing capabilities; e.g., wood chips versus concrete). Pregnant women usually land on the buttocks, not the abdomen; therefore injuries are more likely to be sustained by the mother than by the fetus.

20. **What is the significance of penetrating trauma in pregnancy?**

Penetrating trauma is almost always intentional. It occurs less frequently than blunt trauma, and the prognosis depends on the type of missile involved and the number of organs injured. The usual pattern of injury is altered during the late second and third trimesters because the gravid uterus occupies such a large portion of the abdomen that other organs are protected. This results in a lower maternal mortality rate.

Gunshot wounds are the most common type of penetrating trauma. The incidence of fetal injury is 60% to 90%. Maternal mortality is rare because bullets are likely to strike the uterus because of its large size. Much of the projectile's energy is dissipated in penetrating the thick, muscular uterus. However, injury to the fetus, cord, placenta, and amniotic membranes is generally severe with a fetal mortality rate of 40% to 80% if the fetus is wounded, depending on gestational age. If the bullet does not strike the uterus, vascular wounds are likely and multiple entry and exit wounds may occur in the bowel because of crowding and reduplication.

The incidence of severe injury is lower in stab wounds than gunshot wounds because abdominal organs can slide away from the less rapidly advancing weapon. Stab wounds to the upper abdomen often carry a high incidence of visceral injury, especially to the small bowel. Fetal mortality is directly related to maternal mortality.

21. **What factors should be considered in resuscitating a pregnant woman with burn and/or inhalation trauma?**

The greatest dangers to the fetus are from stress, maternal shock, catecholamine release, and sepsis. Fluid resuscitation needs are greater to maintain adequate uterine blood flow. Fetal mortality increases when maternal burns involve more than 20% of the total body surface area (TBSA). Carbon monoxide (CO) exposure should be considered in all smoke-inhalation cases, and 100% oxygen should be administered because nonlethal maternal CO levels can be lethal to the fetus, in which carboxyhemoglobin levels are 10% to 15% higher. Fetal complications include cerebral palsy.

Burn Mortality Rates

Maternal Burn Area (TBSA)	Maternal Mortality Rate	Fetal Mortality Rate
20%-40%	3%	17%-27%
50%	25%	53%
100%	100%	100%

22. **Is a pregnant patient at risk with even a minor electrical burn?**

No matter how minor the shock appears, fetal monitoring is essential. The low resistance of the vascular uterus and its amniotic fluid may funnel much of the electrical energy through the fetus, resulting in a high fetal mortality rate.

23. **When an injured pregnant woman is seen, should physical abuse be suspected?**

Yes. Up to 33% of women report abuse or battery. Maintain a high index of suspicion and gently probe for details surrounding the injury. Use an abuse assessment screen on all pregnant trauma victims regardless of trauma type and mechanism of injury.

24. **Why is abruptio placenta the leading cause of fetal death associated with trauma?**

Abruptio placenta is premature separation of the placenta from the uterine wall. It occurs in 5% of major motor vehicle crashes after acute deceleration and in up to 40% of those with severe blunt abdominal trauma. On impact, the uterus flattens against the abdominal wall. Resulting waves in the amniotic fluid cause the relatively elastic uterus to elongate rapidly and to shorten along its vertical axis. The nonelastic placenta is unable to undergo such elongation and shortening and is torn from its uterine attachments. Disruption of maternal-fetal circulation causes hemorrhage in the mother and hypoxia in the infant. The maternal mortality rate is generally less than 1%, whereas the fetal mortality rate may reach 100%. The degree of fetal danger depends on the extent of separation. Up to 25% placental separation may be well tolerated, but fetal demise is universal with 50% or more. Premature labor is a frequent complication. Thirty percent of abruptions occur within 48 hours; observe at least overnight.

25. What clinical presentation suggests abruptio placenta?

Initial signs and symptoms can be vague, depending on the extent of separation and amount of bleeding. Assess the patient for the following:
- Sudden onset of sharp, constant abdominal pain
- Local uterine rigidity with tetanic contractions (boardlike)
- Expanding fundal height
- Asymmetry of uterine shape
- Dark red vaginal bleeding (present in 80% of cases)
- Evidence of volume deficit and shock
- Premature labor
- Fetal distress; alteration in FHTs (normal 120 to 160 beats/min)
- DIC

26. What are the priorities of management for patients with suspected or known abruptio placenta?

- Monitor maternal vital signs every 15 minutes while the mother is unstable.
- Continuously monitor FHTs; use sonograms and obstetrical nurses if possible.
- Monitor fundal height and abdominal girth every 30 minutes.
- Maintain continuous cardiotocographic monitoring (fetal heart rate and uterine contractions) in patients at 20 weeks gestation if possible. Note uterine contraction patterns, FHT deceleration patterns, and beat-to-beat variability. Consultation with an obstetrical nurse, nurse midwife, or obstetrician is advised in the interpretation of fetal monitoring.
- Observe for signs and symptoms of DIC: uncontrolled bleeding from intravenous (IV) line sites, mucous membranes, and traumatic wounds; petechiae, ecchymosis, and development of hematomas; thrombosis of extremities evidenced by cyanosis and mottling; decreased urine output; and impaired oxygenation.
- Monitor serial lab tests for decreased fibrinogen levels; decreased platelet counts; and prolonged PT, PTT, and clotting times.
- The Kleihauer-Betke (KB) test is frequently drawn as part of the routine labs profile of pregnant trauma patients, but its use remains controversial. To date, no study has shown its efficacy as a predictor of fetal or maternal morbidity or mortality or as a confirmatory test for abruption. Muench et al (2004) concluded that a negative KB test excludes preterm labor and positively suggests close fetal surveillance, including electronic monitoring and serial KB testing every 6 to 12 hours to determine the fetal effects of placental injury. KB testing may provide a false-positive result in patients with sickle cell disease because of the presence of hemoglobin F and thalassemia. In these cases the maternal erythrocytes may look like fetal RBCs. Flow cytometry or using monoclonal antibodies against fetal hemoglobin and fluorescent microscopy is an equivalent or superior substitute for the KB testing to measure transplacental hemorrhage volume.

27. What type of direct trauma can be sustained by the placenta?

Laceration. Although rare in blunt injuries, placental lacerations may be mediated by either direct forces or contrecoup mechanisms. With an anteriorly placed placenta, initial decelerating forces applied to the anterior uterine wall propel the fetus forward. The amniotic fluid is noncompressible and allows the fetus to move forward with sufficient force applied to the placenta to cause a bursting or irregular laceration of the fetal surface. After disruption of placental circulation, the fetus bleeds to death in utero.

28. **Under what circumstances should uterine rupture be suspected?**

Uterine rupture occurs in less than 1% of pregnant trauma patients. In early pregnancy, the uterus is behind the bony pelvis and the uterine wall is thicker, providing more protection. As the uterus enlarges it thins out and moves out of the pelvis and therefore has less protection. The rupture may be complete or incomplete when the visceral peritoneum remains intact. Women who have had a previous cesarean section have an increased risk for rupture, as do those with direct, severe abdominal impact. Maintain a high index of suspicion if any of the following are present:
- Sudden onset of sharp abdominal or suprapubic pain
- Diaphragmatic irritation; tachypnea and shallow respirations
- Hypotension/shock
- Slowing or absent FHTs
- Asymmetry of the uterus (palpation of fetal body parts in the abdomen)
- Contractions that may be associated with increased fetal activity (distress) or cessation of fetal activity

29. **What complication should be anticipated with premature rupture of membranes (PROM)?**

Possible prolapsed cord caused by excessive uterine activity and increased intra-amniotic pressures associated with severe blunt trauma. Inspect the perineum for evidence of prolapsed cord. If absent, monitor the patient's temperature and prepare for cervical culture. The patient will have labor induced if amnionitis develops. If amnionitis is present, prepare for emergent cesarean section.

30. **What are the risks and guidelines for treating a pregnant patient in traumatic arrest?**

- If a pregnant woman has been critically injured during the second half of pregnancy, there are two lives to be saved. It may not be possible to save both, but sometimes the fetus can be saved even if the mother cannot.
- All efforts to resuscitate the mother should be initiated in the field and continued during transport until medical evaluation at the hospital is complete. Good cardiopulmonary resuscitation (CPR) and ventilation with 100% oxygen may keep the fetus alive, even after the mother is biologically dead.
- The principles of resuscitation (airway, breathing, circulation—ABCs) are the same as those for nonpregnant patients except for the need to implement methods to reduce the effects of aortocaval compression caused by supine positioning.
- Prepare for an emergency cesarean section and attempt to deliver the fetus alive. CPR and maternal ventilation must continue until the fetus is delivered.

Physicians usually consider the gestational age of the fetus and the amount of time the mother has been in arrest before performing an emergency cesarean section.

- Neonatal resuscitation must be immediately available in the emergency department (ED). Maternal brain death may require ventilatory and hemodynamic support of the mother until the fetus is mature enough to survive after cesarean delivery.

31. What are the most common types of fetal injuries?

Direct injury to the fetus from blunt trauma is rare (less than 1 in 10,000 births) because amniotic fluid serves as a natural buffer. Skull fracture and intracranial hemorrhage are most common in vertex presentations associated with pelvic fractures in the mother. Nonfatal injuries to the fetus may heal before delivery, and residual damage (especially neurological) caused by remote trauma can rarely be proved to be the causative agent. Isolated fractures of the mandible, clavicle, vertebrae, and all the long bones, which heal slowly in utero, have been reported.

32. Is there a correlation between trauma and miscarriage?

It is difficult to pinpoint the causal relationship between trauma and miscarriage because 20% of all pregnancies terminate in a spontaneous abortion. Loss of pregnancy that occurs within days of trauma already may have been in progress. Injury to the embryo or fetus may not result in a miscarriage for weeks to months after the trauma.

33. What is the significance of vaginal bleeding after trauma?

Vaginal bleeding may be the earliest symptom of placental separation, spontaneous abortion, or preterm labor. It may also be associated with traumatic injuries to the genital tract. Note the presence, amount, color, and consistency of vaginal bleeding.

34. In addition to uterine trauma, what other injuries may the mother sustain?

- Perimetric hemorrhage (surrounding the uterus)
- Splenic or hepatic rupture
- Rupture of an epigastric vessel, which may simulate an acute abdomen or concealed placental abruption
- Intestinal perforation caused by penetrating trauma
- Retroperitoneal hematoma leading to shock
- Rupture of abdominal viscera

35. What are the priorities of emergency management in obstetrical trauma?

Management of the pregnant trauma patient requires a team approach involving emergency, trauma, and obstetrical professionals. Specific assessments and outcomes will be influenced by the type of injury, gestational age, and associated complications.

ABCs:
- Immediate resuscitative priorities are the same regardless of the patient's pregnant state. Initial management is directed at resuscitation and stabilization of the mother because the fetus's life is dependent on the mother's. Early aggressive resuscitative efforts should be directed at the mother, because the fetus is dependent on maternal stability and the mother may be compensating at the expense of the fetus.

Potential for impaired airway or impaired gas exchange:
- Obtain, secure, and maintain a patent airway. If emergent intubation is required, prepare the patient and equipment for rapid sequence and/or drug-assisted intubation, rescue airways, and cricothyrotomy. Use the Sellick maneuver during tube placement to minimize aspiration.
- In a patient who has adequate spontaneous ventilations, administer oxygen at 12 to 15 L by tight-fitting, nonrebreather mask, even in the absence of maternal respiratory distress, to reduce or prevent hypoxia. It is important to remember that fetal blood is usually unsaturated with a different oxyhemoglobin dissociation curve. Even small amounts of supplemental oxygen can be beneficial to the fetus.
- Bag-valve-mask ventilation carries an increased risk of aspiration because of delayed gastric emptying. Early passage of an orogastric or nasogastric tube (NGT) is advised to evacuate the stomach and protect the airway when ventilatory assistance is necessary.
- Take vomiting precautions and keep a suction source readily available.

Potential for maternal hemorrhage, vascular volume deficit, and cellular hypoxia related to shock:
- If more than 24 weeks gestation, position the patient to avoid supine hypotensive syndrome. Displace the uterus off the vena cava.
- Maintain adequate circulatory volumes with warmed normal saline or lactated Ringer's solution infused through large-bore (14 to 16 g) IV catheters. Permissive hypotension may be catastrophic for the pregnant trauma patient and fetus. Patients may be prone to pulmonary edema with over-vigorous fluid replacement because of decreased colloid osmotic pressure and a tendency to leak plasma from the vascular compartment. Anticipate the need for blood or blood products (packed RBCs) if the patient has a critical oxygen-carrying capacity deficit.
- Obtain trauma lab profile: complete blood count (CBC), coagulation panel, urinalysis, type and screen or cross match, and DIC screen.
- Physicians order drugs cautiously in pregnant patients because of the potentially toxic effects to the fetus or the propensity to shunt blood away from the uterus. However, pressors or inotropes may be necessary to save the mother's life when volume replacement has been adequate, hemorrhage is controlled, and hypotension continues.

Chest trauma:
- Modified placement of the chest tube 1 to 2 interspaces higher than normal is necessary because of an elevated diaphragm.

Adjuncts to the primary survey:
- If not contraindicated, place an indwelling urinary catheter if injuries are moderate to severe to monitor urinary output and to keep the bladder decompressed.
- Place an NGT or orogastric tube as needed to decrease incidence of aspiration and to keep the stomach decompressed.

Secondary survey:
- Review systems; complete a head to toe assessment.
- Monitor fundal height, uterine tone, fetal position, vaginal discharge, FHTs, and fetal activity. If contractions are present, assess cervical effacement and dilation if not contraindicated. Continuous fetal monitoring should be started as soon as possible.
- If no vaginal bleeding is present, prepare for vaginal speculum exam.
- Test vaginal fluid for pH and ferning to determine whether membranes have ruptured. A pH of 7 suggests amniotic fluid. Vaginal pH is generally 5.
- Examine for vaginal lacerations or bone fragments in the vagina that may suggest a pelvic fracture.
- Perform a FAST (Focused Assessment with Sonography for Trauma) scan on the uterus and abdomen.

36. What factors should be considered when determining the need for an emergency cesarean section?

- Gestational age
- Fetal monitoring findings (heart tone decelerations)
- Risk of prematurity
- Maternal and fetal prognosis if undelivered
- Presence of procedure indications, such as placental separation, uterine rupture, unstable pelvic fractures, inadequate exposure to repair injuries found during abdominal exploration, and DIC

37. What factors should be considered before performing a postmortem cesarean section?

- Fetal viability or near-term status: Better outcome if gestational age is 28 weeks or greater
- Cause of maternal death
- Resuscitative efforts applied to mother and fetal status
- Interval between maternal death and delivery or life support of mother
  Emergent delivery by cesarean section should be started within 4 minutes after initiation of CPR during the third trimester for both maternal and fetal benefits.

Fetal Prognosis after Maternal Arrest

Length of Arrest	Prognosis
Less than 5 min	Excellent
5-10 min	Good
10-15 min	Fair
15-20 min	Poor
20-25 min	Unlikely

38. Does pregnancy contraindicate radiographic studies?

Not usually. Although fetal organs are most sensitive to radiation when less than 8 weeks gestation, growth impairment and possible malignant changes can be seen at later gestational ages. A radiation dose under 5 to 10 rads should carry no significant fetal risk. For example, the pelvic radiation dose of a chest film is 3 mrads; a cervical spine film is less than 1 mrad; and a computed tomography (CT) scan of the head is less than 1 rad. However, a pelvic CT may carry a radiation dose as high as 9 rads. Radiographic studies should be completed after physicians consider the risks versus benefits and should be done with appropriate fetal shielding. Although ultrasound can detect fetal distress, use of screening CT allows a concurrent evaluation of multiple areas in the pregnant trauma patient, including the uterus. A limitation of CT screening is that the normal gravid uterus and physiological changes of pregnancy can confound interpretation. Clinically indicated studies should be performed if nonradiographic alternatives are not an option.

39. What are the nonradiographic diagnostic options?

Real-time ultrasound can be used to assess fetal size, gestational age, status of the amniotic fluid, cardiac movements, and placental location. It may not detect placental abruption until at least 200 ml of blood is evident. Tocodynamometry (measuring the force of contractions) is more sensitive for diagnosis of abruptio placenta. The presence of contractions more frequent than one every 10 minutes may suggest a 20% risk of placental disruption. Diagnostic peritoneal lavage (DPL) is safe if performed using an open, supraumbilical approach.

Key Points

- The challenge of major trauma to the pregnant woman is to resuscitate two lives. The best predictor of fetal survival is maternal survival.
- A successful outcome for both patients depends on a team approach involving emergency nurses, physicians, trauma surgeons, OR personnel, and perinatology.
- The leading cause of fetal death is placental abruption, followed by maternal death.
- Because of the vasodilatory effects of hormones, the pregnant patient in shock may be warm and dry, rather than cool and moist.
- The average pregnant patient can tolerate a 1500-ml volume loss before becoming extremely hypotensive. When blood loss occurs, maternal vital signs may be maintained at the expense of perfusion to the uterus, placing the fetus at early risk for hypoxia. Treat shock before it is severe. Do not wait for classic signs and symptoms.
- Uterine constriction in early shock diminishes blood flow to the fetus by 20% to 30% before any blood pressure changes in the mother are detectable.
- FHTs are the best indicator of fetal condition because they change before maternal vital signs; fetal bradycardia is a grave sign and requires immediate action for fetal survival.
- Patients in the second and third trimester should be placed in a left or right lateral recumbent position to displace the uterus from the inferior vena cava. The uterus can be displaced by tilting the patient on her side using a hip wedge or spine board, or by manual manipulation.
- Even small amounts of supplemental oxygen to the mother can be beneficial to the fetus.

 Internet Resource

eMedicine, Pregnancy and Reproduction Resource Center:
www.emedicine.com/rc/rc/i18/pregnancy.htm

Bibliography

Bradley W: Trauma in pregnancy. In Campbell JE, editor: *Basic trauma life support*, ed 5, Upper Saddle River, NJ, 2004, Pearson Prentice Hall.

Chang AK: *Pregnancy, trauma*, eMedicine, 2004. Available at www.emedicine.com/emerg/topic484.htm.

D'Amico C: Trauma in pregnancy, *Top Emerg Med* 24:26-39, 2002.

Desjardins G: *Management of the injured pregnant patient*, Trauma.org. Available at www.trauma.org/resus/pregnancytrauma.html.

Dhanraj D, Lambers D: The incidence of positive Kleihauer-Betke test in low-risk pregnancies and maternal trauma patients, *Am J Obstet Gynecol* 190:1461-1463, 2004.

DiLeo G: *Trauma in pregnancy*, Virtual OB-GYN Office, 1999. Available at www.gynob.com/traumiup.htm.

Grossman NB: Blunt trauma in pregnancy, *Am Fam Physician* 70(7):1303-1310, 2004.

Kady DE et al: Trauma during pregnancy: An analysis of maternal and fetal outcomes in a large population, *Am J Obstet Gynecol* 190:1661-1668, 2004.

Karimi P et al: Extensive brain injury in a premature infant following a relatively minor maternal motor vehicle accident with airbag deployment, *J Perinatol* 24(7):454-457, 2004.

Martel MJ et al: Hemorrhagic shock, *J Obstet Gynaecol Can* 24(6):521-524, 2002.

Mattera CJ: Trauma during pregnancy. In Oman K, Koziol-McLain J, Scheetz L, editors: *Emergency nursing secrets*, Philadelphia, 2001, Hanley & Belfus.

Maull K: Maternal-fetal trauma, *Semin Pediatr Surg* 10(1):32-34, 2001.

Muench MV et al: Kleihauer-Betke testing is important in all cases of maternal hemorrhage, *J Trauma* 57:1094-1098, 2004.

Newton ER: *Trauma and pregnancy*, eMedicine, 2003. Available at www.emedicine.com/med/topic3268.htm.

Rogers FB et al: A multi-institutional study of factors associated with fetal death in injured pregnant patients, *Arch Surg* 134:274-1277, 1999.

Sugrue ME, O'Connor MC, D'Amours SK: Trauma during pregnancy, *ADF Health* 5(1):24-28, 2004. Available at www.defence.gov.au/dpe/dhs/infocentre/publications/journals/NoIDs/ adfhealth_apr04/ADFHealth_5_1_24-28.pdf.

Van Hook JW: Trauma in pregnancy, *Clin Obstet Gynecol* 45:414-424, 2002.

Warner MW et al: Management of trauma during pregnancy, *ANZ J Surg* 74:125-128, 2004.

Wright G: *Blunt abdominal trauma during pregnancy*, Emerald Health Care, 2004. Available at www.statdoc.com/Emerald/pubs/Wright_pubs/pregtrau.htm.

Pediatric Trauma

Donna Ojanen Thomas and Nancy L. Mecham

1. What are the most common mechanisms of injury in the pediatric trauma patient?

The most common mechanism of injury in the pediatric patient is blunt trauma. The most common types of fatal childhood injuries amenable to prevention strategies are motor vehicle passenger injuries, pedestrian injuries, bicycle injuries, submersion, burns, and firearm injuries. Unlike adults, a large proportion of children injured by automobiles are pedestrians. Although falls account for a large number of emergency department (ED) visits, they are infrequently the cause of fatalities. Death from unintentional injury accounts for 50% of all deaths in children younger than 19 years of age and is the most common cause of death in people age 1 to 24 years. Homicide and suicide rank second and third as causes of mortality from trauma in the first 19 years of life.

Although the injury death rate dropped from the year 2000 to 2001, the rate of decrease in deaths from medical causes has consistently dropped more than trauma mortality. Twenty percent of all pediatric hospitalizations result from trauma. About 30,000 children who are injured experience permanent disabilities annually, and the economic cost of trauma in childhood is $5 billion to $8 billion annually in the United States.

2. What exactly is a pediatric trauma center?

The American College of Surgeons' Committee on Trauma has stated that injured children have special needs that can be optimally met in a children's hospital with a demonstrated commitment to trauma care. In most states, trauma center accreditation follows the strict guidelines set forth by the American College of Surgeons to verify hospitals on levels of I to IV, pediatric, adult, or pediatric and adult. Level I pediatric trauma centers provide the highest level of care for children. This criterion includes availability of pediatric specialists both in-house and on-call, equipment, training and education, and research. As a result, pediatric trauma centers evolved to improve the care of injured children in the United States. As of April 2005, there were 13 published pediatric level I trauma centers within children's hospitals. Another 9 adult hospitals have both a level I adult and pediatric trauma center designation. Because of the high number of pediatric injuries and the relatively few pediatric trauma centers, most children continue to be treated at adult trauma centers. Hospital EDs are required by law to assess and stabilize all patients who present for treatment. Therefore, all EDs must be prepared to care for pediatric trauma patients properly and to arrange for transfer and transport to a qualified institution if indicated. Recent studies have shown that children with severe head, liver, or spleen injuries that are treated at a pediatric trauma center have significantly better outcomes than those treated at adult trauma centers.

3. **What are the most common pediatric injuries?**

Head injury is the most common type of pediatric injury. Sixty-eighty percent of children with multiple injuries sustain head injuries. Reasons for this are discussed in question 4. Abdominal injuries can be a result of a lap belt in a motor vehicle crash or bicycle handlebars. Laceration of the liver is a major cause of morbidity and mortality in children. Abdominal trauma is the most commonly unrecognized fatal injury. Musculoskeletal trauma is common in children with multiple injuries but can also be a single-system injury resulting from sports or recreational activities.

4. **Why do children sustain head injuries so frequently?**

The head of the infant and young child is large and heavy in proportion to the rest of the body. A large head, high center of gravity, and less-developed neck muscles predispose infants and children to an increased chance for head injuries. The malleable skull provides less protection to the underlying brain structures, making them vulnerable to blunt and penetrating injury forces. In infants and toddlers, the open fontanels allow for skull expansion, which helps prevent increased intracranial pressure (ICP); however, they also allow transmission of injury forces to the brain.

5. **Are long-term sequelae common after pediatric head injury?**

No. The central nervous system is in a process of rapid development and change from early in gestation until several years postnatal. So although pediatric patients may be more susceptible to sustain injury, they are often protected from long-term neurological sequelae from the injury because of this central nervous system immaturity.

6. **Are spinal cord injuries common?**

No. Children 16 years of age and younger account for only 1% to 14% of all spinal cord injuries per year, but when they do occur, they are devastating to the child and family. Anatomical factors that place children at risk for spinal cord injuries include underdeveloped cervical musculature and vertebral joints and lax spinal ligaments. The most common causes of spinal cord injuries in children are high-speed motor vehicle crashes, auto-pedestrian crashes, and falls from a significant height. Although the vertebrae are not likely to fracture, the spinal cord can be injured by flexion/extension and acceleration/deceleration forces. A child may present with signs and symptoms of spinal cord injury, but the radiographic images are normal (no vertebral fractures or dislocations). This phenomenon is called spinal cord injury without radiographic abnormality (SCIWORA) and occurs when ligaments allow significant movement of bony structures resulting in injury to the cord even though no spinal fracture is present. This injury occurs most commonly in children 8 years of age or younger. The signs and symptoms from this injury may last for minutes to days.

7. How can the nurse effectively assess a scared child who wants to get out of the immobilization devices?

Preverbal children can be challenging during C-spine immobilization and clearance. First, consider the mechanism of injury. If a head injury is suspected, pay close attention when assessing the child's level of consciousness. Also determine whether the movements are purposeful; for example, is the child kicking to avoid clothing removal and grabbing and pinching to avoid blood pressure measurement or venous cannulation? If the movements are purposeful, try to calm the child. Be reassured that a vigorously crying child has an open airway, excellent respiratory capacity, and adequate circulatory and neurological perfusion. To calm the child, assign one nurse as the support person, who stands at the child's chest level to maintain eye contact. Speak slowly and calmly and explain what is happening in words that the child can understand. Consider having the parent(s) present in the trauma room, in the child's line of sight if possible, to provide verbal and tactile comfort to the child. Surprisingly, infants and young children often calm down and actually feel comforted by being placed in a spinal immobilization. The swaddling effect appears to give comfort and security in an insecure situation to this age group. Even toddlers, who dislike being held down, often respond to distraction techniques such as toys, stories, or music to comfort them while immobilized.

8. What is recommended to clear a child's cervical spine?

Cervical spine radiographs are taken early in the treatment to check for vertebral alignment. The child is assessed for signs of neurological deficit (numbness, tingling, paralysis, or weakness). Careful palpation of the spine allows detection of tenderness and deformities. If the child denies pain, is awake and alert, and is neurologically intact, the devices may be removed after the complete neurological examination and radiographs are completed and read. The devices are not removed if the child is unconscious or has an altered level of consciousness, when a complete examination is not possible, or if the child has symptoms suggestive of spinal cord injury.

9. When should an abdominal injury be suspected?

Suspicion of abdominal injuries should be based on the mechanism of injury and physical assessment findings. Because the organs within the abdominal cavity are in close proximity to each other, externally applied blunt forces are easily transmitted to all abdominal organs. The spleen is the most commonly injured organ, followed by the liver. Abdominal trauma is the most common cause of unrecognized fatal injury in children. Note any bruising to the abdomen, which indicates where the forces were applied; for example, a lap belt leaves a bruise pattern around the middle to lower abdominal area. Also observe for distention and complaints of pain or guarding. Auscultate for bowel sounds. Perform gentle palpation. If severe pain or guarding is elicited, surgical consultation should be obtained and deep palpation deferred. Finally, because the liver and spleen are highly vascular, carefully monitor the patient for signs of shock.

10. How are fractures in children different?

Children's bones are still growing, and the periosteum is strong and vascular. Consequently, blunt forces applied to a bone can result in a bending of the bone instead of a fracture. These injuries are often called greenstick or buckle fractures. Young bones also heal quickly because they are growing (osteogenic). The growth plate (epiphysis) is the source of longitudinal bone growth; the closure of these growth plates varies with each long bone. Generally, all long bones have completed growth by the end of adolescence. A fracture to the growth plate (often called a Salter-Harris fracture) can result in growth arrest of the affected bone. Care in the ED should be directed to prevent loss of function, abnormal growth, or deformity.

11. How is a pediatric trauma patient assessed?

The principles and priorities of trauma management (primary and secondary assessments) are the same for children as for adults. Unique anatomical and physiological differences must be considered in both the assessments and interventions. The step-by-step process for the initial assessment of a pediatric trauma patient is outlined in the following table.

Initial Assessment of the Pediatric Trauma Patient

Assessment Area	Interventions	Considerations
Primary Assessment		
A: Airway/simultaneous cervical spine stabilization	Assess for airway patency Observe for loose teeth, emesis, or other obstructions, including tongue obstruction in the unresponsive patient Suction airway to remove any obstructions such as teeth, emesis, or other foreign body Reposition head to open airway using jaw thrust only to avoid movement of cervical spine Maintain neutral cervical spine alignment Evaluate correct size and placement of cervical collar, cervical immobilization device, or other immobilization equipment Open cervical collar to observe for tracheal deviation and jugular vein distention	Remind children to answer questions verbally and not to nod or shake their heads as a response to questioning Cervical collar is properly fitted when child's chin rests in chin holder, bottom of collar rests on sternum, and collar does not cover ears Ensure that for children younger than 3 years of age there is a layer of padding under the torso to maintain neutral alignment of spine

Adapted from Hawkins HS et al, editors: *Emergency nursing pediatric course,* ed 3, Des Plains, Ill, 2004, Emergency Nurses Association.

Initial Assessment of the Pediatric Trauma Patient—cont'd

Assessment Area	Interventions	Considerations
B: Breathing	Auscultate breath sounds in anterior chest and axillae for presence and equality Observe rate and quality of respirations; look and listen for signs of respiratory distress or increased work of breathing Apply high-flow oxygen via a nonrebreather mask Prepare for intubation depending on patient condition Assess chest for contusions, penetrating wounds, abrasions, or paradoxical movements	Breath sounds are easily transmitted across entire chest, especially in crying children; listen carefully Flail chest is rare in young children
C: Circulation	Assess apical pulse for rate, rhythm, and quality; compare apical and peripheral pulses for quality and equality Evaluate capillary refill (should be less than 2 seconds) Evaluate skin color, temperature, and moisture Note open wounds or uncontrolled bleeding; apply direct pressure and appropriate dressings to control any bleeding Obtain vascular access; site and type of access is dependent on clinical status of patient	Congenital heart disease may be present, as well as innocent or pathological murmurs Observe for chest scars from previous surgeries Ask the parent for clarification about any heart problems Intraosseous access should be attempted during CPR or severe shock or if venous access cannot be rapidly achieved
D: Disability	Assess level of consciousness, by assessing response to verbal and/or painful stimuli A: Awake and alert V: Responsive only to verbal stimulation P: Responsive only to painful stimulation U: Completely unresponsive For infants, assess alertness and response to familiar faces and objects Measure pupil size, reactivity to light, and equality	Mild anisocoria (unequal pupil size) and strabismus may be normal findings but warrant further evaluation or questioning of parent

Continued

Initial Assessment of the Pediatric Trauma Patient—cont'd

Assessment Area	Interventions	Considerations
E: Exposure and environmental control to prevent heat loss	Remove clothing to allow visual inspection of entire body Obtain temperature measurement	Initiate methods to keep patient warm: Increased ambient room temperature Warm blankets Warm IV solutions Overhead warming lights
Secondary Assessment		
F: Full set of vital signs	Obtain full set of vital signs if not done during primary assessment: Respirations Heart rate Blood pressure Temperature Weight in kilograms Apply continuous cardiorespiratory and oximetry monitors	Obtain an apical heart rate as a baseline; compare central and peripheral pulses Hypotension is defined by age and can occur with blood loss, sepsis, or medications; it is a late sign of shock in pediatrics Obtain oral, rectal, or axillary temperature depending on patient's age and condition Weight is for calculating medication doses and fluid amounts
G: Give comfort measures	Evaluate presence and level of pain: Self-report Behavioral observation Physiological measures	Administer analgesics as prescribed Stabilize suspected fractures Dress open wounds Consider nonpharmacological developmentally appropriate techniques to reduce pain
H: Head to toe assessment (general appearance) Head/face/neck	Assess activity level: interaction with environment, outward appearance, and reactions to caregivers Assess scalp for lacerations, step-off defects, depressions, and open wounds; palpate for hematomas and pain Palpate forehead, orbits, maxilla, and mandible for crepitus, deformities, step-off defects, pain, and stability; evaluate for malocclusion; note any open wounds Evaluate facial symmetry by having child smile, grimace, and open/close mouth	Body position, alignment, protective movements, and unusual odors Assess anterior fontanels in infants for fullness, bulging, or depression Orthodontia may be damaged and should be assessed for intactness or loose parts The trachea is very soft in young children; even low-force trauma can result in edema of airway and vocal cords

Initial Assessment of the Pediatric Trauma Patient—cont'd

Assessment Area	Interventions	Considerations
	Assess anterior neck for jugular vein distention and tracheal deviation; note any bruising, edema, open wounds, pain, or crepitus	
Eyes/ears/nose	Listen for hoarseness or changes in child's voice	Observe for raccoon eyes (periorbital ecchymosis) and Battle's sign (postauricular ecchymosis)
	Assess pupils for equality and reactivity; assess eyes for extraocular movements; inquire about child's visual acuity	
	Assess for eye and eyelid position, drainage, bleeding, or lacerations	
	Assess for ecchymosis and bruising	
	Assess ears and nose for rhinorrhea and otorrhea	
Chest	Observe inspiration and expiration for symmetry or paradoxical movement, as well as use of accessory muscles	The chest wall of a young child is softer and more pliable than an adult's and provides less protection for underlying structures
	Check for lacerations, abrasions, contusions, or impaled objects	
	Palpate chest wall and sternum for pain, tenderness, and crepitus	
Abdomen	Observe abdomen for bruising, lacerations, and distention	A physician usually performs rectal tone assessment; note any injury or bleeding; stool sample may be tested for blood
	Auscultate bowel sounds briefly in all four quadrants	
	Consider gastric decompression using a nasogastric or orogastric tube	
Pelvis and genitalia	Assess pelvis for tenderness and stability	Measure urine output when and if Foley catheter is ordered; observe for gross hematuria
	Palpate bladder for distention and tenderness	
	Assess urinary meatus and vagina for blood	
	Observe for signs of priapism, scrotal bleeding or edema, and any other genital trauma	
Extremities	Observe extremities for deformities, swelling, lacerations, or other injuries	Ask child to wiggle toes and fingers
	Observe for abnormal movement	Patterned injuries or injuries in different stages of healing may be suggestive of child maltreatment
	Assess for strength	

Continued

Initial Assessment of the Pediatric Trauma Patient—cont'd

Assessment Area	Interventions	Considerations
	Palpate distal pulses for equality, rate, and rhythm; compare with central pulses	
Posterior surfaces	Logroll child as unit to inspect back Maintain spinal alignment; Palpate each vertebral body for tenderness, pain, deformity, and stability Assess flank area for bruising and tenderness	Observe for bruising and open wounds

12. What ED equipment is necessary for the care of pediatric trauma patients?

The amount of equipment varies based on pediatric patient volumes and trauma level designation. All facilities should have supplies available to treat and stabilize a pediatric patient for transfer. This includes equipment for airway and C-spine management, oxygen delivery and resuscitation bags and masks, airway adjuncts, endotracheal tubes (ETTs), pediatric sized blood pressure cuffs, pediatric intravenous (IV) catheters and interosseous needles, and devices to keep the child warm. In addition to equipment and supplies, medications used in pediatric advanced life support should be stocked in EDs caring for children. Pediatric supplies are also discussed in Chapter 36.

The National Emergency Medical Services for Children Resource Alliance has published equipment and supply guidelines. The American College of Surgeons also provides guidelines for equipment requirements for verified trauma centers. Many other publications, such as the American Heart Association's (AHA's) *Pediatric Advanced Life Support* (PALS) manual, suggest additional optional equipment. Equally important is having staff trained to use the equipment. EDs can collaborate with a pediatric trauma center for equipment suggestions and training support.

13. What are the most common errors in caring for a pediatric trauma patient?

The four most common errors in pediatric trauma resuscitation according to PALS are:
- Failure to open and maintain an airway along with spinal immobilization
- Failure to provide appropriate oxygenation and ventilation
- Failure to provide appropriate fluid resuscitation
- Failure to recognize and treat hemorrhage

14. What leads to the errors related to oxygenation and ventilation?

The child's upper and lower airway diameters are relatively narrow, allowing for easy obstruction with mucus and edema. The young child's ribs are pliable and do not provide protection to underlying chest structures. Kinetic forces striking the chest during blunt force injury can result in pulmonary and cardiac contusions. Rib fractures are rare in young children; their presence should raise a high index of suspicion for child maltreatment or violence because a great amount of direct force is necessary to cause such fractures. Children have a baseline higher metabolic rate and oxygen requirement compared with adults; thus, providing high-flow oxygen to all pediatric trauma patients is of high priority. Tachycardia is the body's first response to decreased oxygenation. When this compensatory mechanism fails to improve oxygenation, tissue hypoxia, hypercapnia, and brady-cardia result. Bradycardia is a late sign of hypoxia and cardiac decompensation in the injured child.

15. What leads to the errors related to circulation?

The estimated blood volume in children is 80 ml/kg. Although this amount is low, it is a higher relative volume than in adults. Therefore, small amounts of blood loss can result in decreased perfusion and decreased circulating blood volume. Children also have large cardiac reserves, allowing them to maintain a relatively high or normal blood pressure in the presence of blood loss. Therefore, hypotension is a late sign of hypovolemia in the pediatric trauma patient. A child can lose 20% to 25% of circulating blood volume before the onset of hypotension. Frequent serial assessment of circulation status (pulses, capillary refill time, and blood pressure) is vital to recognize shock early. Rapid intervention with fluid resuscitation is also important in the pediatric trauma patient. Adequate and rapid fluid resuscitation will prevent the trauma patient from developing a potentially life-threatening metabolic acidosis.

16. Is body temperature an issue for the pediatric trauma patient?

Yes. Hypothermia is a serious problem in pediatric trauma because children have a high body surface area to weight ratio; they are at increased risk for heat loss through convection, conduction, and radiation. Hypothermia results in decreased release of oxygen from hemoglobin to the tissues and can also contribute to life-threatening coagulation problems. Infants younger than 6 months of age, as well as children who are pharmacologically paralyzed, sedated, and intubated, cannot shiver to keep warm and must have external heat sources to prevent hypothermia. Steps should be taken quickly to ensure that all pediatric trauma patients remain normothermic. Continuous temperature monitoring should be instituted on all multiple trauma patients. Bladder, rectal, or esophageal probes are the least invasive and easiest to insert. External devices such as convective warming covers (e.g., Bair Hugger), warm blankets, or over-head lights should be used as soon as the patient arrives in the trauma bay. Administering warm fluids and warmed blood products during resuscitation can also help reduce heat loss.

17. When is the best time to teach a child and family about injury prevention?

A recent study showed that caregivers who received counseling during a primary care visit were more likely to provide a safe home environment for their children. Targeted injury prevention counseling during a non–injury-related ED visit has also been shown to have a positive impact on injury prevention behaviors after discharge. Targeted counseling makes a positive impact on behavior after discharge when caregivers report unsafe practices during an unrelated ED encounter. Discuss injury prevention during ED visits even if it is difficult to do so. Gear injury prevention efforts to the types of childhood injuries that are common in the area. Having safety information, posters, videos, and other media in the ED may stimulate discussion among children and families presenting for care. Many computerized discharge instructions include injury prevention tips such as seat belt and helmet use that can be included on every discharge instruction. Some hospitals give away bicycle helmets or have literature on obtaining and properly using infant seats.

18. **What discharge instructions should parents be given after a child suffers a mild head injury?**

Parents should be taught to observe the child's level of awareness. The child should know where he or she is and who the parents are. Parents should be told to contact their healthcare provider or ED if the child seems confused or sleepy, has severe headaches, or has projectile vomiting or persistent vomiting (more than three times in 24 hours). Changes in the child's gait or balance should be cause for concern and a call to the healthcare provider. Parents should be encouraged to provide quiet activities for the child, such as board games, and to give acetaminophen for head pain. Generally, the child should feel better in a few days. Parents should be told about the possibility of postconcussive syndrome, which usually lasts 4 to 6 weeks and includes symptoms such as memory loss, headaches, fatigue, mood changes, sleep changes, and difficulty in remembering directions and activities.

 Key Points

- The mechanism of injury in the pediatric patient is primarily blunt trauma.
- Head injury is the most common type of pediatric injury.
- Abdominal trauma is the most commonly unrecognized cause of fatal injuries.
- The principles of trauma management (primary and secondary assessments) are the same for children as for adults. The unique anatomical and physiological differences must be considered in both the assessments and interventions.
- Do not remove C-spine immobilization devices if the child is unconscious or has an altered level of consciousness, when a complete neurological examination is not possible, or if symptoms are suggestive of spinal cord injury.
- Steps should be taken quickly to ensure that all pediatric trauma patients remain normothermic because children have a high body surface area to weight ratio and are at risk for heat loss that can lead to hypothermia.
- It is important to discuss injury prevention during ED visits, even though doing so is often difficult in a busy ED.

Internet Resources

American Academy of Pediatrics:
www.aap.org

American College of Surgeons:
www.facs.org

American College of Surgeons, *National Trauma Data Bank Pediatric Report 2004* (pdf document, Adobe Acrobat Reader software required):
www.facs.org/trauma/ntdbpediatric2004.pdf

American College of Surgeons, Verified Trauma Centers:
www.facs.org/trauma/verified.html

Centers for Disease Control and Prevention, National Center for Injury Prevention and Control:
www.cdc.gov/ncipc

Emergency Medical Services for Children:
www.ems-c.org

National Association of Children's Hospitals and Related Institutions:
www.childrenshospitals.net

National Guideline Clearinghouse:
www.guidelines.gov

Pediatric Emergency Care Applied Research Network:
www.pecarn.org

Bibliography

American College of Emergency Physicians, American Academy of Pediatrics: Care of children in the emergency department: Guidelines for preparedness, *Ann Emerg Med* 37(4):389-391, 2001.

Campbell L, Thomas D: Musculoskeletal trauma. In Thomas D, Bernardo L, Herman B, editors: *Core curriculum for pediatric emergency nursing,* Boston, 2003, Jones & Bartlett.

Claudius I, Nager A: The utility of safety counseling in a pediatric emergency department, *Pediatrics* 115(4):423-427, 2005.

Eddy V, Morris J, Cullinane D: Hypothermia, coagulopathy, and acidosis. Critical care of the trauma patient, *Surg Clin North Am* 80(3):845-853, 2000.

Greenes D: Neurotrauma. In Fleisher G, Ludwig G, Henretig F, editors: *Textbook of pediatric emergency medicine,* Philadelphia, 2006, Lippincott Williams & Wilkins.

Haley K, Mecham N: Abdominal trauma. In Thomas D, Bernardo L, Herman B: *Core curriculum for pediatric emergency nursing,* Boston, 2003, Jones & Bartlett.

Haley K, Mecham N: Mechanisms of injury. In Thomas D, Bernardo L, Herman B: *Core curriculum for pediatric emergency nursing,* Boston, 2003, Jones & Bartlett.

Hawkins HS et al, editors: *Emergency nursing pediatric course,* ed 3, Des Plains, Ill, 2004, Emergency Nurses Association.

Hazinski M, editor: *Textbook of pediatric advanced life support,* Chicago, 2002, American Academy of Pediatrics and American Heart Association.

Muir R, Town D: Spinal cord injury. In Moloney-Harmon P, Czerwinski S: *Nursing care of the pediatric trauma patient,* St Louis, 2003, Mosby.

Potoka D et al: Impact of pediatric trauma centers on mortality in a statewide system, *J Trauma* 49(2): 237-245, 2000.

Ruddy R, Fleisher G: An approach to the injured child. In Fleisher G, Ludwig S, Henretig F, editors: *Textbook of pediatric emergency medicine,* Philadelphia, 2006, Lippincott Williams & Wilkins.

Rupp L, Day M: Children are different: Pediatric differences and the impact on trauma. In Maloney-Harmon P, Czerwinski S, editors: *Nursing care of the pediatric trauma patient,* St Louis, 2003, Mosby.

Simone S: Abdominal/genitourinary injury. In Moloney-Harmon P, Czerwinski S, editors: *Nursing care of the pediatric trauma patient,* St Louis, 2003, Mosby.

Vernon-Levett P: Traumatic brain injury in children. In Moloney-Harmon P, Czerwinski S, editors: *Nursing care of the pediatric trauma patient,* St Louis, 2003, Mosby.

Psychosocial Aspects of Trauma

Catherine T. Kelly

1. What are the most common psychosocial reactions to trauma?

No matter what causes a specific traumatic event, the common reaction is complete disorganization. The person's view of the normal world has suddenly changed, thought patterns are disrupted, and he or she may feel unsure of self and others.

2. What does the trauma patient experience?

Each situation is different, but there are some common concerns. Many patients fear that they are going to die or be permanently disabled. It is important to tell them the truth about their injuries and expected course of treatment. By evading a patient's question or lying, healthcare providers can lose the patient's trust. An inability to trust caretakers may complicate the recovery period and cause additional stress.

3. How should a nurse intervene with a person or family responding to a traumatic event?

The most important point is to provide information. Because traumatic events happen suddenly, many questions need to be answered. Explaining the event and all activities that take place helps patients and families to process information and adapt to the situation.

4. What can the nurse do to help a patient or family experiencing an anxiety attack?

After introducing yourself, explain to the patient or family that you are there to help. Their whole life has suddenly changed, and they need to know that someone will help them; they need to feel a sense of safety. Tell anxious persons that they need to breathe more slowly; show them how it is done. Take the opportunity to explain what has happened and what will be done. It may be helpful to use the sequential notification technique described in Chapter 4.

5. How often should information be repeated to the patient and/or family?

Information may need to be repeated several times before the patient or family actually processes the message. The higher the stress level, the more times you may need to explain what is happening. Repeat all of the basic information as additional friends and family arrive. Repeating the information will help everyone to understand the situation better. New arrivals can then ask the healthcare provider clarifying questions. This access to direct information from the healthcare provider will reduce the need for other family or friends to answer difficult questions, removing an additional stressor.

6. Families and patients often tell the same story about the event over and over again. Is this something to worry about?

No. In fact, retelling the story may be helpful for the patient and family. This "reliving" of the event helps the people involved to understand what has happened and begins the process of incorporating the traumatic event into their lives. Healthcare personnel can help the recovery process by filling in gaps of missing or incorrect information or identifying people who can be contacted (e.g., police) to complete the story.

7. What is the first step in working with a patient or family in crisis?

First, reassure the patient and family that they are in a safe place and that appropriate steps are being taken to care for them and their loved ones. Then ask the patient or family what is most important for them at this time. Healthcare providers sometimes make assumptions about what is best for the patient or family based on past experiences. However, each patient and family is unique to some degree. It is okay to ask what they need first, then to prioritize from there. Help them to focus on short-term goals instead of trying to deal with everything at once.

8. Considering that there are so many different types of trauma, how can a nurse help patients and families?

Be prepared when the next trauma patient arrives in the emergency department (ED). Most EDs have protocols in place to address patients' physical needs. But protocols to address patients' psychological needs and the needs of the family are often lacking. Therefore, consider developing a collaborative trauma care response protocol that can meet the many needs of patients and their families. A comprehensive response protocol provides a valuable system of support for patients and families. Addressing the family's immediate needs for information as well as physical and psychological comfort should be part of the protocol. The protocol also should deal with bereavement to address the many needs of the patient's survivors, from admission to the ED through death. Chaplaincy and social work may be included as members of the trauma response team so that intervention with the family can begin immediately.

During trauma resuscitation, one nurse should be assigned to communicate with the patient, informing him or her of what is being done and providing psychological support. Stay within the patient's line of vision, if possible, and accompany the patient to any other areas for diagnostic studies.

It is a good idea to have a designated "family room," either in the ED or nearby, where family members can gather as the patient is cared for. In addition to providing privacy, the family room should provide telephone access. Other basic needs, such as food, fluids, and bathroom facilities, should be available. One nurse should be responsible for providing regular updates to the family and answering questions. Allow the family to see the patient, even if only briefly, as soon as possible. Sometimes this is the family's last opportunity to see their loved one alive.

Community resources and support services should be identified for patients and families. Some EDs have established a follow-up service for trauma patients and families, contacting them a few weeks after the event by telephone or a written note to answer questions and iterate available community support services.

9. **When multiple people are injured or killed, what should the survivors be told?**

Honesty is usually the best policy, even though the acute pain and grief reaction may be intensified. Try to identify friends or family who can provide support to the survivor(s), discuss the situation with them first, and then have them go with you to tell the survivors. This method helps to support the survivor even if he or she is discharged. Telling the support person the details about the situation enables him or her to review the event with survivors as they ask questions or need clarification.

10. **Do certain traumatic events cause more distress than others?**

Everyone's story and response can be different. However, a few situations may cause more distress than others. Suicide may create feelings of blame and guilt among survivors. Social stigma associated with suicide frequently makes it difficult for family members and friends to grieve openly. The inability to grieve openly can lead to disenfranchised grief that is difficult to resolve. Homicide may create an increased sense of personal vulnerability for the people involved. Trauma deaths, especially those of children, often result in "could have" or "should have" statements and internal feelings of self-blame. End-of-life decisions can be traumatic for friends and families.

11. **What is posttraumatic stress disorder (PTSD)?**

PTSD is a type of stress disorder that may occur in people who have experienced a situation that they perceive to be violent and life threatening. Events that may trigger PTSD include vehicle crashes, personal assaults, sudden infant death syndrome (SIDS), hostage situations, and natural disasters.

PTSD can develop at any age and is more common in women. The most common signs and symptoms are sleep disturbances (a physiological hyperarousal); constantly thinking about the situation (often described as replaying a video of the event, intrusive memories); depression; inability to focus on work, school, or family; and fatigue (signifying avoidance behavior or an emotional numbing). After a mass casualty, people with PTSD may also feel "survival guilt" and wonder why they weren't injured or killed as others were. Alcohol use and substance abuse may increase in people with PTSD.

12. **Can friends and family of the trauma patient experience PTSD?**

Yes. PTSD can occur in anyone who is involved in a traumatic situation. Most people know that PTSD can affect the patient but are unprepared for PTSD in themselves, other members of the healthcare team, family, and friends.

EDs should have referral mechanisms for those who are closely involved in traumatic incidents.

13. **What risk factors predict acute stress disorder (ASD) or PTSD?**

Determining whether a person is "at risk" in the acute phase of an event is difficult. ASD is diagnosed when the stress-related symptoms, including a cluster of dissociative symptoms, appear from 2 days to 4 weeks of the event. If symptoms last more than 1 month, the diagnosis is PTSD. PTSD may develop any time after the traumatic event, even after 30 years. Up to 8% of people will experience PTSD in their lifetime. Recurrent traumatic events can also lead to reliving earlier experiences. People experiencing ASD and PTSD should be referred to healthcare providers with special training in trauma-focused care.

14. **How does treating trauma victims affect healthcare providers?**

Cumulative stress and grief can develop in healthcare providers who are exposed to multiple traumas and deaths. Critical incident stress debriefing (CISD), a group intervention tool provided after exposure to a significant traumatic event, is often part of a wider program of critical incident stress management (CISM). Although *compulsory* debriefing (CISD) is currently not recommended because it may prolong the recovery process for some people, it should remain a choice available to staff. Appropriate referral services for healthcare provider trauma-focused care (individual and group) should be available within 24 hours of major traumatic events, as well as months (and even years) later.

 Key Points

- The most common psychological reaction to trauma is disorganization.
- Tell patients the truth about injuries and expected outcomes to foster a trusting relationship.
- Repeat information as necessary. "Fill in" information as soon as possible.
- Assign one team member to be the family liaison.
- Suicide, homicide, child deaths, and involvement in end-of-life decisions often cause survivors to blame themselves and require special intervention.
- PTSD can occur in family and friends of trauma patients.

Internet Resources

Association for Death Education and Counseling:
www.adec.org

At Health, Effects of Traumatic Experiences:
www.athealth.com/Consumer/disorders/traumaeffects.html

Gift From Within: An International Nonprofit Organization for Survivors of Trauma and Victimization:
www.giftfromwithin.org

National Association of Social Workers, Bereavement/End of Life Care:
www.socialworkers.org/practice/bereavement

U.S. Department of Veterans Affairs, National Center for Post Traumatic Stress Disorder, Casualty and Death Notification:
www.ncptsd.va.gov/facts/disasters/fs_death_notification.html

U.S. Department of Veterans Affairs, National Center for Post Traumatic Stress Disorder, Helping Survivors in the Wake of Disaster:
www.ncptsd.va.gov/facts/disasters/fs_helping_survivors.html

Bibliography

Azoulay E et al: Risk of post-traumatic symptoms in family members of intensive care unit patients, *Am J Respir Crit Care Med* 171(9):987-994, 2005.

Doka KJ: *Living with grief after sudden loss: Suicide, homicide, accidents, heart attack, stroke*, Bristol, Pa, 1996, Taylor & Francis.

Figley CR: *Treating compassion fatigue*, New York, 2002, Brunner-Routledge.

Harms L: After the accident: Survivors' perceptions of recovery following road trauma, *Aust Soc Work* 57(2):161-174, 2004.

Lantz MS, Buchalter EN: Post-traumatic stress disorder: When current events cause relapse, *Clin Geriatr* 13(2):20-23, 2005.

Larson DG: *The helper's journey*, Champaign, Ill, 1993, Research Press.

Leasch RM: *Death notification*, Hinesburg, Vt, 1994, Upper Access.

Ritchie EC: *Trauma, war and violence. Public health in socio-cultural context*, New York, 2002, Kluwer Academic/Plenum Publishers.

Spates CR et al: Behavioral aspects of trauma in children and youth, *Pediatr Clin North Am* 50(4):901-918, 2003.

Special Populations

Chapter 34

Pregnant Women

Virginia M. Koziel

1. What history should be elicited when triaging a pregnant patient?

Women suspected of being pregnant should be asked the following about their past medical history:
- Medication allergies
- Daily medications
- Date of last menstrual period (LMP), duration, and amount of flow
- Contraceptive usage
- Previous pregnancies, abortions (differentiate spontaneous from therapeutic), and ectopic pregnancies
- Past dysmenorrhea, dysfunctional uterine bleeding, or dyspareunia (pain during intercourse)
- Current bleeding (duration, presence of tissue or clots, length of time for pad or tampon saturation)
- Current pain
- Trauma from intercourse, domestic violence, or sexual assault (ask in private)
- Gynecological surgeries

Women known to be pregnant should also be asked about the following:
- Complications with current or previous pregnancies
- Social history (drug, alcohol, or tobacco use)
- Anticipated multiple birth
- Current contractions
- Presence of fetal movement

Be cautious with assumptions related to the following:
- The patient's sexual orientation
- Whether the person accompanying the patient is the father of the child

2. How can pregnancy be diagnosed in the emergency department (ED)?

All currently used qualitative pregnancy tests rely on the presence of human chorionic gonadotropin (HCG) hormone in the serum or urine. Current technology allows detection of HCG within 2 or 3 days after implantation. A qualitative HCG blood or urine test will give a positive or negative result, whereas a quantitative blood test measures the exact units of HCG present. The earliest visual confirmation of heart activity is about 6 weeks with sonographic devices. Detection of fetal heart tones (FHTs) by fetoscope or Doppler ultrasound is also indicative of pregnancy.

3. When and where can FHTs be detected?

FHTs are audible by Doppler ultrasound device at about 9 to 12 weeks of gestation and by fetoscope at 18 to 20 weeks. Differentiate between the FHTs and maternal heart rate by feeling the pulse of the mother while auscultating FHTs. A "whooshing" sound indicates placental circulation.

To know where to start looking, first ask the patient where the heart tones were heard the last time they were checked. If this is the first episode of assessing FHTs, palpate the abdomen to confirm fetal position. Use warm conductive gel on the abdomen. Start at the suprapubic hairline, and move the Doppler device slowly until FHTs are heard. This task is most successful if the direction of the angle of the probe is changed while the Doppler device head is moved slowly. Count the FHTs for 1 full minute, noting any increases or decreases in heart rate. If unable to auscultate FHTs, reassure the patient that it is not unusual to have some difficulty in locating the heart tones. Then promptly consult with an obstetrical nurse or physician.

4. What is the normal fetal heart rate? What causes an increase or decrease?

Normal baseline FHTs range from 120 to 160 beats/min. Fetal activity may cause a brief increase in baseline heart rate above 160 beats/min. Maternal fever, intraamniotic infection, maternal thyrotoxicosis, fetal anemia, or hypoxia may cause prolonged fetal tachycardia. Certain drugs that increase maternal heart rate, such as parasympatholytic drugs, also may result in fetal tachycardia.

Fetal bradycardia, a heart rate below 120 beats/min, may be related to fetal hypoxia and require emergent surgical delivery. Fetal head compression, cord compression, maternal hypothermia, prolonged hypoglycemia, or use of maternal beta blockers may cause fetal bradycardia.

5. When should continuous fetal monitoring be done in the ED?

If a pregnant patient is admitted to the ED with trauma, especially to the abdomen, FHTs and uterine contractions should be monitored continuously. Not until a pregnant patient is "medically cleared" should she be transferred to the labor and delivery unit for further monitoring. Whether the patient is in the ED or in labor and delivery, a nurse who has been verified as competent in fetal monitoring should watch the monitor. Fetal monitoring is also recommended for unstable medical conditions such as preeclampsia.

6. What pain medications are safe to administer in pregnancy?

Category A or B drugs (presumed safe for use in pregnancy) include acetaminophen, meperidine, morphine, and hydrocodone. Category C drugs (use with caution) include fentanyl, codeine, ibuprofen, salicylates, and indomethacin. Aspirin and ibuprofen should be avoided in the third trimester, unless specifically prescribed by a physician.

7. **What causes vaginal bleeding in the first trimester of pregnancy?**

Bleeding in the first trimester is not uncommon; 20% to 25% of all pregnant women spot or bleed lightly in the first trimester. Causes of bleeding include the following:

- **Implantation bleeding** is common and consists of minimal bleeding around the time of the first missed menstrual period. After pelvic examination, a brownish-tinged mucus may be noted. Prolonged bleeding does not occur, and bleeding in excess of the normal menstrual flow is rare.
- **Threatened abortion** is defined as any bleeding in the first 20 weeks of pregnancy without passage of tissue or cervical dilation. Abdominal cramping usually accompanies the bleeding. Approximately 62% of spontaneous miscarriages (abortions) are associated with abnormal embryonic development. Fifty percent of threatened abortions result in complete or incomplete abortions within a few hours.
- **Inevitable abortion** occurs when the cervix dilates and products of conception pass through the internal os or when bleeding is profuse.
- **Complete abortion** is passage of all fetal tissue before 20 weeks of gestation, closure of the internal os, and a decrease in bleeding and cramping.
- **Incomplete abortion** occurs when only a part of the products of conception has been expelled; it is likely to occur between 6 and 14 weeks of gestation.
- **Missed abortion** is defined as a fetal death at less than 20 weeks gestation without passage of any fetal tissue. There may be minimal dark red or brown vaginal bleeding, and pregnancy tests may remain positive for quite some time.
- **Ectopic pregnancy** results when implantation occurs outside the uterine cavity. Most commonly, ectopic pregnancies are located in the fallopian tubes and cause symptoms within the first 12 weeks of pregnancy. This condition can be life threatening if rupture occurs.

8. **How is first-trimester vaginal bleeding treated?**

- Initial assessment with complete vital signs and serial vital signs as needed. Document the amount of blood loss. The rule of thumb is that a saturated pad or tampon equals approximately 20 to 30 ml of blood. Rh-negative patients should receive Rh-immune globulin (RhoGAM).
- Intravenous (IV) hydration, using a minimum of an 18-gauge angiocatheter, with normal saline or lactated Ringer's solution.
- Laboratory tests include baseline hematocrit, blood type (ABO) and Rh factor, and serum pregnancy test. If hematocrit is less than 30% or it is likely that the patient may be admitted to the operating room (OR), type and screen for 2 to 4 units of whole blood.
- Prepare the patient for a pelvic examination; her bladder should be emptied before examination.
- Prepare the patient for diagnostic ultrasound.
- Provide for patient privacy.
- Be supportive of expressions of fear or guilt, and allow interaction with family members or friends as the patient desires.
- Obtain additional support for the patient as appropriate, such as clergy.
- If the patient is discharged from the ED, provide written discharge instructions, medication instructions, and follow-up information.

9. **What is the treatment for various types of abortions?**

Manual vacuum aspiration syringes are used for first-trimester incomplete abortions. Equipment consists of a single- or double-valve syringe and sterile, flexible cannulae of various sizes.

Surgical abortion through the cervix is performed by first dilating the cervix and then evacuating the pregnancy by mechanically scraping out the contents (sharp curettage), by electric vacuum aspiration (suction curettage), or both. This procedure is usually performed in an outpatient surgery suite or the OR. The procedure should be performed before 14 weeks.

Laminaria is often used to dilate the cervix before surgical abortion (dilation and curettage—D&C). Laminaria is the dried stalks of seaweed that swell to about six times their volume and are used for abortion induction. Another option for abortion is vaginal insertion of misoprostol, which also dilates the cervix and is classified as a prostaglandin. Both laminaria and misoprostol are used in early second-trimester abortions (13 to 20 weeks).

10. **What are the signs and symptoms of an ectopic pregnancy? How is it diagnosed?**

Pelvic pain and vaginal bleeding or spotting in a woman of childbearing age should be treated as an ectopic pregnancy until this critical condition is ruled out. Predisposing factors for ectopic pregnancy are previous ectopic pregnancies, adhesions, surgeries, pelvic infections, and presence of an intrauterine device (IUD). Common signs and symptoms are vaginal bleeding and abdominal tenderness. If the ectopic pregnancy is leaking or ruptured, the diaphragm becomes irritated from blood in the peritoneum, which causes referred pain to the shoulder. This is known as Kehr's sign. Tachycardia and hypotension may be signs of a ruptured ectopic pregnancy, along with a hematocrit less than 30%. Bimanual exam reveals adnexal tenderness and a palpable adnexal mass in 50% of women with ectopic pregnancy.

Prepare the patient for IV access, pelvic exam, and ultrasound. If diagnostic ultrasound is not available, culdocentesis may be used to diagnose ectopic pregnancy. Culdocentesis is the aspiration of fluid from the cul-de-sac of Douglas. Culdocentesis is negative if serous fluid is aspirated and positive if nonclotting blood is aspirated.

11. **What are the treatment options after an ectopic pregnancy is diagnosed?**

For hemodynamically stable patients, there are two treatment options: operative laparoscopy and systemic methotrexate.
  · If operative laparoscopy is to be done, start a large-bore infusion, send laboratory tests as ordered, and prepare the patient for the OR according to hospital protocol. Reassure the patient and significant others.
  · Methotrexate is an option for stable patients up to 8 weeks gestation with unruptured ectopic pregnancy measuring less than 4 cm in diameter. Methotrexate interferes with folic acid synthesis, thereby halting continued growth of the pregnancy. Follow hospital protocol for administration of methotrexate, and provide written discharge information. The patient should understand ectopic precautions (see question 12), as well as the side effects of

methotrexate (mild abdominal pain, nausea, vomiting, indigestion, and fatigue) and what to avoid (alcohol, aspirin, nonsteroidal antiinflammatory drugs— NSAIDs, and vitamins with folic acid).

For hemodynamically unstable patients, treatment includes oxygen, fluid administration with a large-bore angiocatheter, type-specific blood as needed, and immediate gynecological consultation for surgical management.

12. Many women are discharged home with "ectopic precautions." What does this mean?

A serial quantitative HCG should be done 48 hours after discharge from the ED. In normal intrauterine pregnancies, the HCG level doubles approximately every 2 days from 4 to 6 weeks since the LMP. This fact has led to the frequent clinical use of serial quantitative HCG in stable patients to assess whether there is an appropriate increase in 2 days. Ectopic gestations have a slower increase in HCG titer. Therefore, women are instructed to return to the ED or their healthcare provider in 2 days for serial quantitative HCG. Warning signs that require immediate return to the ED are acute onset of lower abdominal pain, dizziness or syncope, shortness of breath, or extreme fatigue.

Patients discharged home for either "rule-out" ectopic pregnancy or threatened abortion should be instructed to return to the ED if bleeding increases, large clots or tissue is passed, or cramping increases. Women usually are told to save and bring to the ED anything that is passed from the vagina. In addition, women are instructed to refrain from intercourse and tampon usage.

13. What is the treatment for hyperemesis gravidarum?

When a pregnant patient presents to the ED with intractable vomiting, dehydration, and weight loss and laboratory studies that reveal either hypokalemia or ketonuria, the criteria are met for the diagnosis of hyperemesis gravidarum. Nursing care should include the following:
- Withhold all forms of oral ingestion.
- Start an infusion of 5% dextrose (D5) and normal saline or D5 and lactated Ringer's solution, infusing 30 to 40 ml/kg (usually 2 to 5 L).
- Assess urine ketones and specific gravity until the patient is rehydrated.
- Administer antiemetics as ordered. The following antiemetics are presumed safe in pregnancy: dimenhydrinate (Dramamine), promethazine (Phenergan), prochlorperazine (Compazine), diphenhydramine (Benadryl), and ondansetron (Zofran).
- Before discharge, the patient should be able to retain oral fluids or crackers.

14. What discharge instructions are indicated for women with hyperemesis gravidarum?

- Avoid triggers for nausea or vomiting (e.g., strong odors such as cigarette smoke and cooking odors or fumes).
- Decrease the size and increase the frequency of meals.
- Discontinue prenatal vitamins and iron supplements.
- Avoid mixing solids and liquids.
- Avoid fatty or spicy foods.

- Maintain oral hydration with electrolyte-rich drinks such as Gatorade or bouillon; avoid sweet drinks.
- Start oral intake with clear liquids or soups; follow with complex starches such as noodles, pasta, potatoes, and rice; then add protein such as chicken, turkey, or beef.

15. What can cause bleeding in the third trimester?

Placenta previa, placental abruption, "bloody show," local trauma, or cervical lesions.

16. How can placenta previa be differentiated from placental abruption? What is the role of the emergency nurse?

Placenta previa occurs when the placenta implants on or near the cervical os. Ultrasound studies are accurate in locating the placenta. Placenta previa causes *painless* vaginal bleeding with bright red discharge. There are three types of placenta previa that are defined by how much of the cervical os is covered:
- Total: The placenta completely covers the os.
- Partial: The placenta partially covers the os.
- Marginal or low implantation: The placenta is adjacent but does not extend beyond the margin of the os.

Hemorrhage is the first, most commonly seen sign in placenta previa. If placenta previa is suspected, a manual or speculum exam should be avoided because it could precipitate hemorrhage.

Placental abruption occurs spontaneously or after trauma. Predisposing factors include maternal hypertension, cocaine use, and sudden uterine decompression. Hypertonic uterine contractions and fetal distress may be present. The patient usually reports severe pain, although in early stages or with a small abruption the pain may not be severe. Vaginal bleeding may not be present. If vaginal bleeding is present, the blood is usually dark red in color.

Nursing care for both placenta previa and placental abruption includes a large-bore infusion, oxygen, fetal heart monitoring, maternal vital sign monitoring, laboratory studies, and an immediate ultrasound. Also, position the patient on the left side to facilitate venous return. Unstable patients should be taken directly to the OR or delivery suite.

17. What should a clinician look for in a pregnant woman with hypertension?

- **Preeclampsia:** Also called pregnancy-induced hypertension; the patient develops edema, protein in the urine, and hypertension greater than 140/90 mmHg. Preeclampsia almost always occurs after 20 weeks of gestation.
- **Eclampsia:** Occurs with the onset of seizures in a patient with preeclampsia and can occur as long as 1 week after delivery. Warning signs for eclampsia include hyperreflexia, visual disturbances, right upper quadrant pain, and severe headache. The treatment of choice is magnesium sulfate. A loading dose of 4 to 6 g in a 10% solution should be infused slowly over 15 to 30 minutes. The maintenance dose is 1 to 3 g/hr via IV. Risks of magnesium therapy are loss of reflexes, hypotension, hypocalcemia, and respiratory arrest. The antidote for magnesium sulfate toxicity is calcium gluconate, 1 g, given slowly via IV.

18. **What is hemolysis, elevated liver enzymes, low platelet count (HELLP) syndrome?**

HELLP syndrome is either a variant of severe preeclampsia or a separate complication of pregnancy. In addition to hypertension, the pregnant patient usually presents with complaints of epigastric or right upper quadrant pain, nausea or vomiting, and nonspecific viral-like symptoms. Malaise for a few days before presentation may be reported. Liver enzymes (aspartate aminotransferase—AST and alanine aminotransferase—ALT) are elevated. Thrombocytopenia, with a platelet count of less than 150,000/mm^3, also may be present. Proteinuria may be absent or minimal. HELLP syndrome is more common among multigravida women. Treatment for HELLP syndrome usually follows the same pathway as treatment for severe preeclampsia, including correction of coagulopathies. Ultimately, delivery is necessary after maternal condition is stabilized.

19. **A woman presents to the ED saying, "My bag broke." How can ruptured membranes be confirmed?**

When a pregnant patient presents with possible ruptured membranes, vaginal secretions with a pH of 7 to 7.5 are indicative of leaking amniotic fluid. Nitrazine pH paper is frequently used; it turns black in the presence of amniotic fluid.

20. **What are common signs and symptoms of an imminent delivery?**
  - Bloody show
  - Bulging perineum or perianal flattening
  - Crowning
  - Uncontrollable desire to push. Some women request to go to the bathroom.

21. **What equipment should be prepared for a precipitous delivery?**

Many EDs have a "precip" pack with the following equipment:
  - Sterile gloves
  - Baby blanket
  - Bulb syringe
  - Dry towels
  - Two sterile cord clamps or Kelly clamps
  - Basin for placenta
  - Sterile scissors

22. **What is the best way to handle a precipitous delivery?**

It is important to remain calm and in control to help reassure the mother. After it is determined that delivery is imminent, do the following:
  - Obtain important information related to the pregnancy. This information should include the estimated date of confinement (EDC), rupture of membranes and color of fluid, complications during the pregnancy, known multiple gestation, and presence of fetal movement.
  - Explain to the mother what to expect during the delivery.

- Assist the mother in using breathing techniques so that she can control and slow the delivery. Instruct her in deep abdominal breathing. She should inhale through her mouth and exhale slowly through pursed lips. Breathe with her if necessary.
- After the head is delivered, support the baby's head and have the mother "pant like a puppy" to control expulsion.
- Suction the infant's mouth, then nose, using a bulb syringe. Avoid traumatization of the infant's nose and mouth. At this point, check for the umbilical cord around the neck. If the cord is loose, carefully slip it over the infant's neck. If it is tight, clamp in two places and cut the cord. Lower the infant's head to facilitate delivery of the anterior shoulder.
- After the shoulders are delivered, the infant slips out quickly and is quite slippery. Note the time of delivery.
- Suction the mouth and nose again.
- Dry the infant as quickly as possible, and place the infant skin-to-skin on the mother's abdomen; cover both with a dry blanket. Be sure to cover the infant's head.
- Clamp the umbilical cord in two places at least 6 inches from the umbilicus. Use sterile scissors to cut the cord between the two clamps. The cord can be cut as soon as it is convenient, usually when it has stopped pulsating.
- Using gentle pressure on the cord, ask the mother to bear down to facilitate delivery of the placenta in a sterile basin. Save the placenta.
- Assess the condition of the fundus by placing the open palm of one hand just above the symphysis pubis and the other open palm at the umbilicus. Gently exert pressure with the hand at the umbilicus so that the fundus is between both hands. If the fundus feels about the size and firmness of a grapefruit, massage is not necessary. If the fundus is soft or "boggy," gently massage your hands together until it firms up.
- Check for firmness every 5 minutes to ensure that the fundus remains firm. Place a sterile sanitary napkin on the mother after washing off any blood. Obtain vital signs of the mother, and continue to assess the infant until transportation to the labor and delivery unit.

23. What should be done if the umbilical cord is prolapsed?

A prolapsed cord is an obstetrical emergency. This occurs when the umbilical cord precedes the fetus through the birth canal and obstructs the fetal circulation. Intervention is aimed at relieving pressure on the cord and minimizing fetal anoxia. This is accomplished by placing the mother on her left side to relieve pressure from the uterus on the abdominal aorta. The exposed cord will dry out and should be covered with saline-moistened sterile gauze.

24. What are the Apgar scoring criteria?

The Apgar scoring system has been used as an indicator to assess the need for resuscitation at birth. Apgar scores are noted at 1 and 5 minutes after birth. Apgar scores and criteria are listed in the following box and table.

Apgar Scores

7-10: Infant is stable at this time
4-6: Moderate distress
0-3: Severe distress requiring resuscitative measures

Apgar Scoring*

Criteria	0	1	2
Heart rate	Absent	Fewer than 100 beats/min	More than 100 beats/min
Respiratory effort	Absent	Slow or irregular	Normal
Muscle tone	Flaccid	Some extremity flexion	Active movement
Reflect irritability	No response	Grimace	Cry
Color	Pale or blue	Body pink; extremities blue	Completely pink

*Apgar scores should be taken at 1 and 5 minutes after delivery.

If breathing is absent or heart rate is below 60 beats/min despite 30 seconds of assisted ventilation, begin neonatal resuscitation. A useful mnemonic for newborn resuscitation is TABS:

T	Temperature
A	Airway
B	Beats (heart rate)
S	Sugar

25. What are some causes of cardiac arrest in the pregnant woman?

Cardiac arrest is generally related to changes and events at the time of delivery, including amniotic fluid embolus, eclampsia, and drug toxicity. Other physiological changes associated with pregnancy that may cause arrest are pulmonary embolism (PE), hemorrhage caused by pregnancy-related pathology (placenta previa or placental abruption), trauma-related problems, and aortic dissection.

26. Are there modifications for basic life support (BLS) and advanced cardiac life support (ACLS) algorithms for the pregnant woman?

BLS: Do not straddle the pregnant patient. Place the heel of the lower hand on the center of the breastbone at the nipple line. Start chest compressions after the woman is placed on her left side with back angled 30 degrees. Foam wedges work best because they provide a wide surface that will support the tilted body during compressions. The pregnant woman's uterus may press down on the inferior vena cava, reducing blood flow. This lack of venous return can produce hypotension and possible shock.

ACLS: There are no modifications to the ACLS algorithms for the pregnant individual other than those listed under BLS. Emergent cesarean section is accepted as part of the resuscitation of a pregnant woman who has no evidence of peripheral pulses. When ACLS is not successful, a perimortem cesarean section should be considered. The goal is to deliver the fetus or infant within 4 to 5 minutes after onset of arrest. When a pregnant patient needs resuscitation, the gestational age of the fetus should be considered. Most references list a range of viability from 23 to 28 weeks gestation. Positive outcomes are dependent on the availability of institutional resources, availability of skilled personnel, and viable gestation of the fetus (23 to 28 weeks).

27. Unfortunately, infant death sometimes occurs. How can an ED nurse facilitate the patient grieving a miscarriage or stillbirth loss?

Parents begin forming attachments to an expected child early in pregnancy; most experience shock, emotional numbing, and an unreal sense of "This can't be happening" when they are first aware of the infant's death. Be aware that such reactions are not limited to parents who planned a pregnancy. Expect a grief reaction whenever an unexpected loss occurs, even if the woman did not know that she was pregnant before coming to the ED or reports that the pregnancy was not wanted.

Mothers should be supported if they wish to see the products of conception or stillborn child. They should be encouraged to see and hold the stillborn after delivery; this is the only time that they will have with their child. The emergency nurse can facilitate grieving by allowing the parents time to realize the loss. Photographs of the infant can be taken if the family wishes. Parents and family members should be assured of privacy in a quiet area. Either pastoral care or other support service (e.g., perinatal loss coordinator, mental health services, social services) can provide additional emotional support.

Most cities have support groups for perinatal loss, and the parents should be given a written list of such groups before discharge from the ED. Women who have been treated in an ED for a miscarriage find a follow-up telephone call very helpful. Women will often have the following questions:

· What happened to me in the ED?
· Was the miscarriage my fault?
· Can I have a normal pregnancy?
· How do I deal with the loss?

If a pregnancy is lost, it is often considered a death within the family. Supporting a family through the grieving process can be an emotionally rewarding experience for the emergency nurse.

Key Points

- Normal FHTs are 120 to 160 beats/min and are audible with Doppler ultrasound at about 9 to 12 weeks gestation.
- Most abortions happen in the first trimester of pregnancy. Half of all threatened abortions result in complete or incomplete abortions within a few hours.
- Rh-negative pregnant patients with vaginal bleeding should receive RhoGAM.
- After an ectopic pregnancy is diagnosed, hemodynamically unstable patients should have immediate gynecological consultation for surgical management.
- Placenta previa causes painless bright red vaginal bleeding with bright red discharge.
- Placental abruption causes severe pain with no bleeding or blood that is usually dark red.
- An Apgar score should be taken at 1 and 5 minutes after delivery. A score of 7 to 10 indicates the infant is stable at this time.
- The treatment of choice for eclampsia is magnesium sulfate, 4 to 6 g infused slowly over 15 to 30 minutes.

 Internet Resources

Early Path Medical Consultation Services:
www.earlypath.com

FertilityPlus:
www.fertilityplus.org

Ipas, Protecting Women's Health, Advancing Women's Reproductive Rights:
www.ipas.org

Perinatology.com:
perinatology.com

SafeFetus.com, Drugs in Pregnancy and Lactation:
www.safefetus.com

Bibliography

Abbrescia K, Sheridan B: Complications of second and third trimester pregnancies, *Emerg Med Clin North Am* 21:695-710, 2003.

Benrubi G: *Handbook of obstetric and gynecologic emergencies*, ed 2, Philadelphia, 2001, Lippincott Williams & Wilkins.

Berg T, Smith C: Pharmacologic therapy for peripartum emergencies, *Clin Obstet Gynecol* 45:125-135, 2002.

Budassi-Sheehy S: *Sheehy's emergency nursing principles and practice*, St Louis, 2003, Mosby.

Cancienne G: Pregnant women. In Oman K, Koziel-McLain J, Scheetz, L, editors: *Emergency nursing secrets*, Philadelphia, 2001, Hanley & Belfus.

Cummins R: *ACLS provider manual*, Dallas, 2002, American Heart Association.

Cunningham F et al, editors: *Williams obstetrics*, ed 21, New York, 2000, McGraw-Hill.

Emergency Nurses Association: Obstetrical and gynecological emergencies. In *Orientation to emergency nursing: Concepts, competencies and critical thinking*, Des Plaines, Ill, 2000, ENA.

Gilbert SE, Harmon JS: *Manual of high risk pregnancy and delivery*, ed 3, St Louis, 2003, Mosby.

Stallard T, Burns B: Emergency delivery and perimortem C-section, *Emerg Med Clin North Am* 21: 679-693, 2003.

Thompson S et al: Clinical risk management in obstetrics: Eclampsia drills, *BMJ* 328:269-271, 2004.

Chapter 35

Seniors

Karen Hayes

1. Are seniors a substantial part of the emergency department (ED) population?

Yes. Adults older than age 65 account for up to 19% of the ED patient population, higher than the 13% they represent in the general population. By 2030, 20% of the U.S. population will be over age 65 with almost 5% over age 85. Seniors account for 36% of ambulance transports, 43% of all hospital admissions, and 48% of admissions to ICUs. With the aging of society, seniors will continue to be a significant portion of the ED patient population.

2. Are seniors significantly different than younger adults with similar problems?

Seniors tend to be more ill at presentation, stay longer in the ED, are more often admitted to the hospital, and have higher ED charges than younger adults. They are more likely to have preexisting conditions and take medications that impair their ability to compensate for the effects of illness or injury and make them more likely to experience complications of injury or illness. Geriatric emergencies are multifocal events requiring a high level of skill in an emergency nurse.

3. What is the most challenging aspect of care for the senior person in the ED?

Seniors living independently have an average of three chronic medical problems. This number increases to 10 for those living in care facilities. These chronic problems complicate the evaluation of the acute problem. A frequent pitfall is to focus too closely on the patient's presenting problem without looking for underlying medical and social conditions that may have caused the acute problem.

4. What is the effect of normal physiological changes of aging on health and functional status? Does aging change the assessment process?

Assessment of seniors is more complex and requires an understanding of the difference between normal age-related physiological changes and pathology. For example, after age 75, cardiac output decreases up to 50%, and there is a 30% loss in pulmonary function. The normal physiological changes of aging and their relationship to nursing assessment outcomes are outlined in the following table.

Physiological Changes of Aging

Changes	Assessment Implications
Cardiovascular System	
Loss of myocardial elasticity and strength	Decreased cardiac output and blood flow to brain, heart, kidney, liver; slower adaptation to change in activity
Fibrosis of blood vessel lumen; calcification of arteries	Increased systolic blood pressure (155/90 mmHg), hypertension, pulse pressure
Thickening of vessel membranes; decreased elasticity	Edema, increased diastolic blood pressure, decreased baroreceptor sensitivity
Increased perivascular fibrosis	Increased peripheral resistance to blood flow; edema; coolness of extremities
Thickened and more rigid valves	Decreased cardiac output; 65% of elderly have diastolic murmurs, especially of mitral or aortic valve
Respiratory System	
Increase in residual lung volume	Distressed breathing; fear, anxiety; shallow breathing; carbon dioxide retention
Muscle atrophy and rigidity	Impaired ventilation, decreased vital capacity, reduced ability to cough and deep breathe
Thickened membranes, alveoli, and capillaries	Increased anteroposterior diameter, impaired diffusion of oxygen, tissue hypoxia, impaired pulmonary circulation
Skin and Cutaneous Tissue	
Atrophy of sweat glands, sebaceous glands, subcutaneous tissues	Decreased perspiration; dry, thin skin; increased susceptibility to trauma and abrasions; inability to regulate body temperature
Uneven deposits of melanin	Lentigines, keratoses, spotty pigmentation
Loss of elasticity of tissues	Skin wrinkles, more fragile, subcutaneous and muscle tissue becomes flabby
Sensory System	
Decreased sense of smell	Loss of appetite; decrease in salivary flow; safety hazards of gas leaks, fires
Decreased tactile sensation and sense of body position	Tendency to drop items, sustain injuries, and fall more readily
Increase in amount and thickness of cerumen	Plugging of ear canal, decreased hearing
Decrease in rods and cones; thickening of lens	Decrease in visual acuity, loss in peripheral vision, presbyopia, decrease in adaptation to dark
Atrophy and sclerosis of tympanic membrane	Decreased acuity of hearing, especially loss of high tones and consonants
Reticuloendothelial System	
Decreased production of cellular components of blood	Slight anemia, slight leukopenia, increased bleeding time

Physiological Changes of Aging—cont'd

Changes	Assessment Implications
Decreased immune system functions	Decreased resistance to disease, infection, and slowed response to inflammation
Gastrointestinal System	
Atrophy of mucosal linings; diminished production of hydrochloric acid and other digestive enzymes	Delayed gastric emptying, slowed digestion, impaired absorption, increased gas formation
Smooth muscle weakness; muscle atrophy	Decreased excretory efficiency, incontinence, constipation, diminished peristalsis, tendency toward hiatal hernia
Increased tendency to choke when swallowing	Risk of aspiration
Musculoskeletal System	
Calcification of vertebral ligaments	Postural change: kyphosis, scoliosis, kyphoscoliosis
Fibrocartilaginous atrophy; muscle atrophy	Loss of muscle power; flexion contractures; paralysis; decreased respiratory exchange
Osteoporotic bones changes	Increased brittleness of bones; spontaneous fractures
Ossification of joint cartilage	Joint stiffness; ankylosis; impaired range of motion
Decreased muscle strength and endurance	Slowing and decreased endurance
Nutrition and Hydration	
Decreased metabolic rate: estimated at 1% per year after age 25	Changes in nutrition status, drug reaction, hypothermia; decreased caloric need in relation to physical activity
Water depletion	Increased risk of dehydration, constipation, urinary tract infection
Psychosocial Issues	
Increased inferiority and reflectiveness	Introspection, enjoyment of remembering past
Decreased self-image because of numerous losses and changes	Tendencies toward depression, paranoia, discouragement

5. Are normal lab tests and arterial blood gas (ABG) values the same for all adults?

They are basically the same. Slight increases may be seen in sedimentation rate, blood urea nitrogen (BUN), creatinine, thyroid-stimulating hormone, and alkaline phosphatase (ALP) because of age-related functional reduction in renal, pulmonary, and immune functions. In addition, slight decreases may be seen in hemoglobin, iron, and creatinine clearance. With ABG measurement, partial pressure of carbon dioxide (PCO_2) in arterial blood rises slightly and partial pressure of oxygen (PaO_2) in arterial blood falls slightly. Laboratory abnormalities should not be ascribed to normal aging until a thorough investigation into the patient's condition is made.

6. During the interview process, how can the nurse obtain the most accurate history?

To help communication, patients need to be comfortable and at ease. A warm, quiet environment with limited interruptions and traffic is imperative. Senior persons tend to be reluctant to share private information and need to feel trust to communicate openly. Avoid medical jargon, and speak slowly in low, clear tones. Directly face the patient to decrease the effects of hearing impairment. Seniors are sometimes mistakenly thought to be confused when they give inappropriate answers to questions they did not hear correctly. Closed-ended questions may focus the interview. Limitations of function or an inability to perform activities of daily living should be assessed. Particularly for cognitively impaired patients, family, medical records, primary physician, and pharmacy may be crucial to obtaining an adequate history.

7. Why must the index of suspicion for serious medical problems be higher in seniors?

Atypical presentations of disease are common in seniors. Experienced emergency nurses recognize that a myocardial infarction (MI) may be painless, sepsis may occur without fever, bacteriuria may be asymptomatic, pneumonia may present as confusion, and appendicitis may present with few localized symptoms. Anemia, tuberculosis, thyroid disease, and AIDS are commonly overlooked in seniors.

8. What are the most common diagnoses for seniors in the ED?

There is a tremendous difference between the diagnoses in general office practice and conditions seen on an emergency basis. The leading diagnoses in the ED are disorders in the respiratory system, including bronchitis, influenza, upper respiratory infection, aspiration, and pneumonia. Other frequent diagnoses include abdominal pain, MI, congestive heart failure (CHF), and electrolyte imbalance.

9. What may cause mental status changes in a senior person presenting to the ED?

Mental status changes are not a part of normal aging. Seniors may present with one of three mental status changes:
- **Dementia:** A chronic and progressive change in mental status.
- **Depression:** The most common psychiatric disorder in seniors, caused by the combination of decreased dopamine and serotonin along with the losses of aging. The suicide rate for men age 85 and older is 5.5 times the rate in the general population. Although not a typical "mental status change," acute depression can present with inability to concentrate or think and slowed speech.

- **Delirium or acute confusion:** A highly prevalent and life-threatening health problem for seniors. The emergency nurse should understand that delirium often has a treatable or reversible cause. The wide variety of causes of delirium are listed in the following box.

Causes of Delirium

Cardiac
Aneurysm
Arrhythmia
CHF
MI
Tamponade

Central Nervous System
CVA
Postictal status
TIA
Tumor

Drugs
Anticholinergics
Anticonvulsants
Antidepressants
Antihistamines
Antihypertensives
Antiparkinson's agents
Antipsychotics
Digitalis

Diuretics
Drug interactions
Drug withdrawal
NSAIDs
Opiates
Sedatives
Tranquilizers

Infectious
Bacteremia
Cellulitis
Meningitis
Pneumonia
Sinusitis
UTI

Metabolic
Acidosis
Alkalosis
Azotemia
Dehydration
Hepatic failure

Hypercalcemia
Hypercarbia
Hyperglycemia
Hypernatremia
Hyperthyroidism
Hypoglycemia
Hyponatremia
Hypothyroidism
Hypoxia
SIADH

Miscellaneous
Dehydration
Fecal impaction
Hypothermia
Nutritional
Restraint
Sensory deprivation
Urinary retention

SIADH, *syndrome of inappropriate secretion of antidiuretic hormone;* UTI, *urinary tract infection;* MI, *myocardial infarction;* CHF, *congestive heart failure;* CVA, *cerebrovascular accident;* TIA, *transient ischemic attack;* NSAIDs, *nonsteroidal antiinflammatory drugs.*

10. **What effect does polypharmacy have on the emergency treatment of seniors?**

Emergency nurses must be aware that medications taken by seniors may be the cause of the presenting problem. Use of multiple medications may increase administration errors, decrease compliance, and cause an increase in drug interactions and side effects. The four most problematic medications are aspirin, digoxin, warfarin, and diuretics. Some dangers of these drugs are outlined in the following table.

Common Problematic Medications

Medication	Dangers
Aspirin	GI irritation or bleeding; bruising and increased chance of hemorrhage; tinnitus; acidosis
Digoxin	Digoxin toxicity: nausea, vomiting, diarrhea, weakness, arrhythmia; psychosis
Warfarin	Hemorrhage with chest, abdomen, joint, or other pain; shock; allergic reactions; liver damage; gangrene of toes; inflammatory skin rash
Diuretics	Hypokalemia; anemias; constipation; dizziness; hypotension; muscle spasms; skin rash

In addition, many seniors use herbal medications. Nurses should be aware of the risk of undeclared pharmaceuticals in herbal products and should be cognizant of the potential for herb-drug interactions. An online reference for drug-nutrient interaction can be found at www.vitaminherbuniversity.com/drug_nutrient.asp?dnid=1. Many symptoms, such as weakness, anorexia, dizziness, syncope, or history of a fall, should prompt a thorough medication assessment. Forty percent of geriatric patients leave the ED with a new prescription. This increase in medication complexity should heighten the emphasis on medication teaching and counseling for senior persons discharged from the ED. Seniors need to understand how to incorporate their new medications into their present medication regimen.

11. How may an MI present differently in seniors?

A completely asymptomatic MI is rare but may occur in people older than age 85, especially women. Generally seniors present with a sudden onset of dyspnea. Other presenting complaints include syncope, "flu," nausea, vomiting, confusion, and weakness. Although many seniors may complain of classic chest pain, the nurse should be aware that atypical presentations occur in 25% of MIs. An error in triage or delay in recognition of cardiac problems leads to a large increase in the mortality rate of MI among seniors.

12. Are seniors more prone to infection than younger adults?

Yes. Although age-related decrease in immune response is a contributing factor, chronic illness and institutionalization are the most significant causes of the increased risk of infection. Several infections are more common in seniors, such as pneumonia and urinary tract infection (UTI). Infection and sepsis may be undetected because fever and elevated white blood cell (WBC) and band counts are not always evident in seniors.

13. What are the most frequent causes of acute abdominal pain in seniors?

Two of the most common causes of acute abdominal pain in seniors include diverticulitis and appendicitis. Inflammation of the diverticula is seen in 9% of all acute surgical admissions and rarely occurs before age 40. The abdominal pain with diverticulitis is generally on the left side and is characteristically mild to moderate, dull, aching, and persistent or crampy. Although appendicitis is most common in the second and third decades of life, the appendix has become an important and often overlooked site of disease in older people. Most seniors with appendicitis exhibit classic symptoms. However, pain may be less severe, guarding and rebound tenderness diminished, fever less pronounced, and WBC elevation less sensitive. Seniors may not have decreased bowel sounds, rectal tenderness, or positive psoas sign (in which the patient experiences abdominal pain when the thigh is flexed against resistance). The major difference in presentation between young and old patients is that appendicitis in older persons tends to progress more rapidly to perforation with less overt evidence of the advanced stage of disease. The incidence of perforation in seniors is approximately 65% and leads to higher rates of morbidity and mortality. Part of the reason for delayed diagnosis is that chronic conditions may confuse the diagnosis. Constipation, diverticulosis, liver disease, obesity, obstruction, and diabetes complicate the presentation. Forty percent of the causes of abdominal pain are surgical in seniors.

14. Is major trauma common in seniors?

Major trauma is relatively uncommon in seniors, constituting only 8% to 15% of all cases of major trauma per year. However, trauma in seniors causes higher mortality and poorer functional recovery compared with younger patients. Motor vehicle crashes may be caused by medical circumstances such as MI, arrhythmias, syncope, medication side effects, transient ischemic attacks (TIAs), stroke, or complications of diabetes. These medical problems require simultaneous diagnosis and treatment in the setting of a traumatic event.

The most common injuries among seniors are subdural hematomas after relatively minor trauma, cervical spine fractures because of decreasing bone density, pulmonary contusions caused by preexisting pulmonary pathology, and skeletal fractures and easily fractured ribs. Among seniors, hip fractures often result in death; about 30% of patients die from related complications within 6 months. If they do not die, they frequently lose their independence and have drastic lifestyle changes.

Falls remain the most common mechanism of injury for seniors. The fall needs to be investigated thoroughly for underlying causes. Unsafe home environments can be corrected, and physiological conditions such as orthostatic hypotension, arrhythmias, occult blood loss, and medication side effects can be identified and treated. Always consider physical abuse as a possible cause for a fall.

15. How should seniors with syncope be assessed? What are its causes?

Dizziness and syncope are frequent presenting complaints in seniors. Syncope in seniors is often multifactorial and calls for a multisystem assessment. A careful history can dictate in which direction and with what urgency an assessment should proceed. The nurse should determine the circumstances surrounding the event. Seniors may describe being "dizzy," "lightheaded," or "passed out." Weakness, if transient, may actually be an episode of syncope.

In seniors, the most common causes of syncope are arrhythmia, MI, hypovolemia secondary to gastrointestinal (GI) bleeding, vomiting, diarrhea, side effects of diuretic use, seizure, stroke, and vertebrobasilar insufficiency. In addition, the nurse should look for evidence of trauma that may have resulted from the syncopal episode.

Always consider medications as a cause of syncope. The most common offending medications are beta blockers, calcium channel blockers, phenothiazines, antihypertensives, and vasodilators.

16. How can the emergency nurse help the family of seniors in crisis?

When a crisis, either physical or social, occurs, family members of a senior person often come to the ED for help. The emergency nurse can be a beneficial member of the healthcare team by providing professional concern, advice, and hope. Grieving within the family may begin with an acute illness. Family members are directly involved in decision making about matters such as withholding of life support and do not attempt resuscitation (DNR) orders. Intrafamilial conflicts may be evident. Family members may second-guess themselves for not seeing the signs of the illness or decline in function sooner. Others may feel guilty for not visiting more often or being more attentive. There may be a great deal of fear that the senior will die or concern about care that the patient may need in the future. Family members may display anger at the staff when the illness cannot easily be diagnosed and treated.

The nurse should determine the family spokesperson and decision maker early in the interaction. Together, difficult decisions can be made about the future care of seniors. Gender and cultural heritage may affect decision making. For example, an African-American, Mexican, or Native-American man may not perceive himself as a provider of personal care to a parent. The nurse should keep in mind the balance between doing what is needed and doing more than what is actually required. "Taking over" infantilizes senior persons. In addition, the legal and civil rights of older persons are not always considered or respected. In crisis situations, medical social workers and case managers operate in consultant and collaborative roles to enhance the problem-solving capacities of families. The emergency nurse should use all available resources to assist both the family and patient during times of crisis.

17. What ethical issues surround the care of seniors in the ED?

The management of seniors in the ED is at times controversial and not well defined. Issues such as advance healthcare directives and healthcare rationing based on chronological age are controversial. The effectiveness of continued ED resuscitation of out-of-hospital arrests has been found to be of little benefit, but the practice continues. The economical burden to society and the individual resulting from high-technology emergency care for elderly people also has been a topic of debate. Restrictive admission criteria contribute to the conflict. These complex ethical issues require honest discussion between healthcare professionals and clients. As society ages, emergency nurses will be caring for more older adults who may be extremely frail and complex patients. Nurses must prepare themselves to answer the ethical questions posed by caring for senior patients.

Key Points

- Because older persons may have multiple underlying medical and social problems, the ED nurse should look at the total picture when evaluating the acute problem. Chronic problems complicate the evaluation and management of the acute problem.

- When assessing the older patient, the ED nurse must understand the difference between normal age-related physiological changes and pathology.

- Forty percent of older persons leave the ED with a new prescription. ED nurses must be sure that patients can integrate new medications into their already complex medication regimens.

- Mental status change is not a part of normal aging.

- Falls are the most common cause of trauma in an elderly person. Though more rare, major trauma in an older adult causes much higher mortality and disability than in younger adults.

- Atypical presentation of disease is common in older adults. Major health conditions such as MI, pneumonia, or acute abdomen may present with simple complaints such as fatigue.

Internet Resources

Emergency Nurses Association Position Statement, *Care of Older Adults in the Emergency Setting* (pdf document, Adobe Acrobat Reader software required):
www.ena.org/about/position/PDFs/Care-of-OlderAdults.pdf

The John A. Hartford Foundation Institute for Geriatric Nursing:
www.hartfordign.org

Society for Academic Emergency Medicine, *Emergency Care of the Elder Person: Instructor's Manual:*
www.saem.org/services/geriatoc.htm

Bibliography

Aminzadeh F, Dalziel W: Older adults in the emergency department: A systematic review of patterns of use, adverse outcomes, and effectiveness of interventions, *Ann Emerg Med* 39:3, 2002.

Birnbaumer D: The geriatric patient. In Marx J, Hockberger R, Walls R, editors: *Rosen's emergency medicine: Concepts and clinical practice,* ed 5, St Louis, 2002, Mosby.

Cassel C et al, editors: *Geriatric medicine: An evidence-based approach,* ed 4, New York, 2003, Springer-Verlag.

Eliopoulos C: *Gerontological nursing,* ed 6, Philadelphia, 2004, Lippincott.

Hayes KS: Research with elderly patients: Do we have any answers? *J Emerg Nurs* 26:3, 2000.

Richardson B: Overview of geriatric emergencies, *Mt Sinai J Med* 70:2, 2003.

Infants and Children

Donna Ojanen Thomas and Nancy L. Mecham

1. ### What is the definition of a pediatric patient?

   The definition of a pediatric patient varies widely in the literature. The American Heart Association (AHA), in the *Pediatric Advanced Life Support* manual, defines the pediatric patient by the following age groups:
   - **Newly born:** Infants in the first minutes to hours after birth
   - **Neonate:** Infants in the first 28 days (4 weeks) of life
   - **Infant:** The neonatal period up to 12 months or approximately 1 year
   - **Child:** Those between the ages of 1 and 8 years

   The term "child" can be further broken down into toddlers (1 to 3 years), preschoolers (3 to 5 years), and school age (5 to 11 years). Adolescents include those age 11 to 18 years.

   All of these different age groups have maturing physiological and psychosocial systems. Emergency nurses must be knowledgeable about these maturing systems and the common illnesses and injuries occurring in these age groups.

2. ### What are some important physiological differences to keep in mind when caring for pediatric patients?

   - Neonates have immature immune systems, although they gain some passive immunity from the mother in utero and in breast milk. Diminished concentrations of immunoglobulins and other immunological factors involved in the response to infection have been demonstrated in infants until 5 to 6 months of age.
   - Children have a higher baseline metabolic rate that translates into a higher oxygen and glucose demand.
   - Children have a tenuous fluid and electrolyte balance that puts them at higher risk for dehydration.

   The parents or caregivers of pediatric patients should also be regarded as patients. Caregivers vary in their level of knowledge about the child's condition and will respond differently depending on their coping mechanisms and prior experiences. One universal truth may be that caregivers always react out of concern for their child. Children, based on their ages, will respond differently to the emergency department (ED) staff and to the treatment they receive. The emotional needs of an individual child must be based on the child's particular stage of development.

3. What are the characteristics of the pediatric airway?

Because a child's airway is small in diameter, it is more easily occluded by blood, vomit, mucus, or any foreign materials. Infants have a large tongue, which can obstruct the airway as well. Therefore, assessing and clearing the airway should be foremost in the emergency nurse's mind when approaching the pediatric patient. Infants prefer nasal breathing up until the age of 6 months and any increase in nasal airflow resistance increases the work of breathing. When nasal mucus is increased, frequent suctioning may be necessary.

4. What are the characteristics of pediatric breathing?

The small diameter of the lower airways predisposes children to lower airway obstruction with mucus plugs and ventilation perfusion mismatch. Infants have fewer alveoli and thus a smaller area for gas exchange to occur. Infants and small children are diaphragmatic breathers with a very compliant chest wall and underdeveloped intercostal muscles. All of these differences can lead to early signs of respiratory distress in children.

Early respiratory distress is observed through tachypnea, retractions (substernal, suprasternal, intercostal, and supraclavicular), nasal flaring, grunting, stridor, and adventitious sounds (wheezing, rhonchi). Bradypnea can be a late sign of respiratory compromise or failure.

5. What are the characteristics of pediatric circulation?

A child's circulating blood volume is 80 ml/kg (90 ml/kg in infants). Because children have higher extracellular water content, a higher metabolic rate, immature renal function, and often are developmentally unable to meet their own intake needs, even a small amount of fluid or blood loss can lead to circulatory compromise. Capillary refill is an important indicator for circulatory status; a delay of longer than 2 seconds is cause for further evaluation. Cool skin temperature, mottling, decreased capillary refill, and changes in mental status are suspicious signs for circulatory compromise (shock). Children increase their heart rate to increase cardiac output when they need to compensate for circulatory compromise; thus tachycardia is an early sign of shock. Blood pressure initially remains normal or slightly elevated. If circulatory compromise is untreated or unrecognized, the heart rate decreases, cardiac output decreases, blood pressure decreases, and bradycardia with subsequent cardiac arrest is imminent.

6. Why is obtaining an accurate weight and temperature so important in the care of a pediatric patient?

Children have a high body surface area to weight ratio. The child's weight is needed for calculating medication doses and intravenous (IV) fluid amounts that are based on mg/kg dosage. Therefore, always obtain the child's weight in kilograms on arrival at the ED. To decrease the possibility of dosing errors, pediatric scales should be set to weigh only in kilograms. When weighing is not possible, always use a standardized measure such as a length-based resuscitation tape because estimations of weight are often inaccurate.

Obtaining a temperature in the pediatric patient is important and should be done at triage. This is because fever in an infant or neonate may have an impact on the triage decision. In infants 3 months of age or younger, a body temperature of 101.5° F (38.5° C) requires further evaluation and should be triaged at a higher level of acuity even if the infant looks well. Fever can be indicative of a serious bacterial infection in this age group. A temperature of 104° F (40° C) or higher in any age group should be considered a red flag and warrants a higher triage classification. A rectal temperature should be taken in children younger than 3 months of age except for children who are immunocompromised, have a rectal abnormality, or have had rectal surgery. Tympanic thermometers may not be as reliable in this age group if proper technique is not used, and an inaccurate measurement could result in failure to detect a serious infection.

7. **What are some tips to help with rapidly triaging a pediatric patient?**

The initial assessment occurs while assessing the child from "across the room." The Pediatric Assessment Triangle (PAT) is used during this assessment to rapidly determine how sick a child is and how quickly treatment is required. The PAT assesses the following parameters using the visual and auditory skills of the nurse:
- **General impression:** Does the child look ill or well? Is the child playful? What is the child's response to the environment and caregiver?
- **Work of breathing:** What is the position of comfort? Are there audible abnormal airway sounds such as wheezing or stridor? Is the child drooling?
- **Circulation to skin:** What is the child's skin color? Is there any obvious bleeding? Is the child diaphoretic?

The PAT allows for an overall general impression; that is, whether the child looks good or bad. Approach the child slowly and look at the child before doing anything that requires touching, such as assessing vital signs.

Always look at the child, no matter how busy at triage. Look under a blanket if necessary. When asking about the chief complaint, ask, "What worries you the most about your child?" While doing the assessment, ask, "How does your child usually look? How does he look to you now?" Do not say, "Is he always this blue (or pale)?" This will alarm the caregiver. Obtain a history, because the history may change your triage decision. Listen to the parents. Tell them what is being done and what the findings are. Let them know what will happen next. If concerned about the child and a room is not available, place the child in an area near the triage desk within sight. Provide pain relief, if possible, at triage. If a child is in severe pain, he or she should be triaged with a more urgent acuity. The chief complaints in a pediatric patient that require a more urgent triage rating are different than those of an adult. For example, chest pain in a child is not usually an emergent condition, but in an adult it usually is. Fever in an adult, on the other hand, is not by itself an emergent condition, but it is in an infant younger than 30 days old. Common causes of lawsuits result from missed diagnoses such as appendicitis and meningitis. Never discourage a visit in the ED even if it is suspected that the child's complaint is minimal. Frequently check on pediatric patients waiting in the waiting room, and keep the family updated about the waiting time. It is not wise to reassure a parent that his or her child will be fine. This may give a false sense of security and cause the patient to leave before seeing the doctor. Instead, apologize for the waiting time and encourage the family to stay.

Make sure the hospital has a separate section in the triage orientation devoted to the different assessment parameters in pediatrics and specific emergent and urgent complaints at triage. A pediatric hospital or ED in the area may be willing to help. Also consider the resources listed at the end of this chapter.

8. **How should the clinician assess a child from a developmental standpoint?**

Before performing an assessment, introduce yourself to the child and family. Call the child by name, an action that demonstrates respect for the child as an individual. Using the child's name also assists with the assessment of neurological functioning. Keep the child and family together as much as possible. Separation from familiar faces and voices is frightening to the child, who may have pain or discomfort. Older children or adolescents may want to be assessed without the parent in attendance; offer that option. Neonates, infants, and young children can be assessed on the parent's lap, whereas older children and adolescents may sit in a chair or on an exam table. Offer distractions, such as an age-appropriate toy, on which the child can focus attention. Finally, always tell the child what is being done to avoid surprises and promote trust. Offer choices, such as, "I have to count your heart beat and measure your blood pressure. Which one do you want me to do first?" Such choices allow the child to feel a sense of control in a strange environment.

Use nonthreatening language when talking with the child. Young children, especially those of preschool age, have a limited, literal understanding of words and their meanings. For example, "taking" a temperature may lead the child to believe that something will be taken from him or her. The statement, "I will measure your temperature," is less threatening to the child and is actually the correct interpretation of that nursing action. Never use terms such as, "This will just be a bee sting," because not many children think a bee sting is okay.

In general, children feel vulnerable in the supine position; when possible, perform assessments with the child in a sitting or standing position. Having the young child stand on the exam table and hug the parent during the measurement of rectal temperature gains the child's cooperation and simultaneously allows the parent to hold and comfort the child.

Adolescents should be allowed to choose whom they want to have with them during an examination. They may choose a parent or friend. Avoid asking probing questions about pregnancy, sexual activity, or drug or mental health issues in the presence of a parent or guardian; such questions are best asked in private. It is the adolescent's choice to share such information with the parent. Be familiar with the state laws concerning emancipated minors and informed consent.

9. **What common chief complaints bring pediatric patients to the ED?**

Children often present to the ED with a variety of vague, puzzling complaints, which may represent a major illness or a normal variant. The nurse needs to have good assessment skills, including listening to the parent and knowing which symptoms may represent a life-threatening emergency. Fever is one of the most common chief complaints seen in the ED and is discussed in question 10.

Abdominal pain is another common complaint and is discussed in question 13. Both fever and abdominal pain are "high risk" and "problem prone," which means that they are common but it is sometimes hard to diagnose a cause. Other common complaints include upper airway complaints, gastrointestinal (GI) complaints, rashes, and limping. Injury accounts for 43% of all ED visits made by children, and falls are the leading cause of unintentional injury.

10. What should an ED nurse know about pediatric fever?

Fever is an elevated body temperature that is necessary for the body to fight infection. The ED focus is on the underlying source of the fever rather than its treatment. The management of fever in young children is a controversial topic and much variation in management occurs even within the pediatric ED. Several practice guidelines exist describing ED management based on age. Some of these can be found in the National Guideline Clearinghouse (www.guidelines.gov). Guidelines published by Baraff et al (1993) continue to serve as a model for more recent guidelines.

The child's physical appearance, activity level, and other signs ("looks sick") should be taken into consideration when fever is present. A history of sickle cell disease or a child with fever and known neutropenia should be seen immediately. The following children are at risk for serious illness associated with fever and should be categorized as emergent:

- Toxic appearing children (lethargy, poor perfusion, respiratory distress)
- Children younger than 60 days who have a temperature above 38.0° C (100.4° F)
- Children younger than 4 years who have a temperature above 41.0° C (106° F)

Acetaminophen and ibuprofen can be administered for fever and may make the child feel better; however, the fever will persist until the underlying infection is resolved. When treating fever, nurses should discuss fever management as opposed to fever control. Parents often have misconceptions about fever, and the term "fever control" will lead them to believe the fever will actually go out of control. Teach parents that fever is treated to make a child more comfortable and not to keep it from going "out of control."

A sudden temperature elevation may result in a febrile seizure, which is frightening to parents. Parents need to be reassured that brain damage rarely occurs from prolonged, high temperatures or febrile seizures. Teaching parents about fever and its management are an important part of treating the child in the ED.

Finally, remember that sponging a child to reduce fever is an outdated practice. Sponging may cause the child to shiver and raise the temperature even more. Instead have the parent unbundle the child to reduce the temperature. The practice of sponging with alcohol should never be done because alcohol toxicity through skin absorption can occur.

11. What should an ED nurse know about dehydration in children?

Gastroenteritis is the most common underlying cause of dehydration in young children in the United States. Gastroenteritis can be caused by a bacterial, viral, or parasitic infection.

Weight loss is the most sensitive indicator for dehydration in young children, especially infants. Thus it is important to obtain the nude weight of an infant and the weight of all children with a history of vomiting or diarrhea.

A careful focused assessment of circulatory status is important to determine the severity of dehydration. Assessment of skin color, strength of peripheral pulses, capillary refill time, mental status assessment, and evaluation of heart rate and blood pressure all may help to determine the level of dehydration or hypovolemic shock.

In obtaining a history, ask the parent about the amount of urine output. Infants with fewer than six wet diapers per day or no urine for longer than 6 to 8 hours or older children with no urine for longer than 12 hours should raise a high level of suspicion for dehydration.

Other indicators of dehydration include the absence of tears, dry mucous membranes, dry cracked lips, sunken eyes, sunken anterior fontanel in infants, and tenting of the skin.

Oral rehydration solution can be given in the ED at 60 to 80 ml/kg over 4 hours with regular evaluations for improvement (heart rate, respiratory rate, blood pressure, level of consciousness, intake and output). This approach works best when the patient has only diarrhea and is not vomiting. However, vomiting alone is not a contraindication to attempting oral rehydration. Some general guidelines that can be used with children are to wait at least 2 hours after the last emesis (no waiting period if patient has diarrhea only) and offer small (10 to 15 ml) frequent (every 15 to 20 minutes) amounts of an oral rehydration solution (e.g., Pedialyte, Rehydrate). In the older child or adolescent, sports drinks can be used. This small amount can be given in 1-oz medicine cups or oral syringes so that the amounts can be easily documented. The triage nurse can even start an oral rehydration trial in the waiting area.

When signs of moderate to severe dehydration (hypovolemic shock) are identified, rapidly administering a fluid bolus and then reassessing the child is recommended. IV rehydration, starting at 20 ml/kg of normal saline or lactated Ringer's solution administered over 10 to 20 minutes, is the appropriate initial crystalloid infusion. Do not give large volumes of dextrose-containing solution during fluid resuscitation. This will result in a hyperglycemia that may induce an osmotic diuresis and produce or aggravate hypokalemia.

12. What should an ED nurse know about respiratory distress in children?

Children are prone to respiratory distress for anatomical and physiological reasons. Children who present to the ED with a respiratory complaint should have an assessment that focuses on the signs and symptoms of respiratory distress. Children in respiratory distress should be approached as gently as possible to avoid upsetting the child and further compromising their respiratory status. A focused exam should include assessment of airway patency, respiratory rate, work of breathing, auscultation of breath sounds, skin changes, or any changes in mental status.

Recognition of increased work of breathing includes:

- Increased respiratory rate
- Presence of stridor (inspiratory or expiratory)
- Absent or diminished breath sounds; inspiratory or expiratory wheezes

- Retractions
- Nasal flaring
- Grunting
- Fatigue

After respiratory distress is recognized in any child, the ED nurse must intervene quickly to prevent deterioration of the child's condition. Initial intervention for respiratory distress includes frequent focused respiratory assessments, including pulse oximetry monitoring, clearing of the airway with suction or repositioning, and placement of supplemental oxygen. If the respiratory distress progresses without intervention to respiratory failure or cardiopulmonary arrest, there is a high likelihood of a poor outcome. Keep in mind that acute heart failure can mimic respiratory distress. Consider that a child in respiratory distress who is not responding to usual interventions may be presenting with an underlying cardiac condition. Evaluate the heart rate and rhythm in all pediatric patients with respiratory distress.

Respiratory distress in the pediatric patient is most often categorized as being an upper airway illness such as croup or a lower airway illness such as bronchiolitis or asthma. Asthma is the most common chronic disease of childhood, affecting more than 5 million children younger than 21 years. Asthma accounts for 5% to 12% of annual ED visits. Some illnesses commonly seen in the adult population are not commonly seen in pediatrics because of the physiological differences between children and adults. An example of this is bronchitis.

13. What should an ED nurse know about abdominal pain in children?

Abdominal pain is a common complaint that brings children to the ED, especially the school-age child and adolescent. Certain causes of abdominal pain are more often associated with specific age groups. In the infant serious conditions such as volvulus and intussusception need to be considered. As the child gets older, conditions such as gastroenteritis, appendicitis, urinary tract infection (UTI), and constipation need to be considered. Adolescent abdominal pain brings new challenges. In the adolescent female ectopic pregnancy, pelvic inflammatory disease (PID), and inflammatory bowel disorders need to be considered. Respiratory illnesses such as pneumonia often have an abdominal pain component. This is because of muscle fatigue from the increased work of breathing and diaphragmatic irritation from coughing.

Constipation can be present when a child of any age has a problem with bowel movements because of a functional bowel problem or abnormal character of the stool. Frequency of stool should be determined for that particular patient, because stool frequency is very individualized. Bowel patterns reflect social, cultural, dietary, and familial patterns. Some caregivers might report that their infant "struggles, grunts, and turns red with bowel movements." Some infants will even cry with bowel movements. These parental concerns can all be normal and not diagnostic of constipation if the infant's stool is soft and the child has a normal exam.

Appendicitis is one of the most common pediatric surgical emergencies seen in the ED. It can occur in all age groups but is most difficult to diagnosis in the infant and toddler. Children with appendicitis classically have a progression of symptoms that initially may present with poorly localized complaints of mida-bdominal pain, anorexia, vomiting (in the younger child), low-grade fever, and pain radiating to the right lower quadrant. However, because of the varied location of the appendix in children, depending on age and size of the patient, location of pain and tenderness may also vary. Serial exams over time with consistent findings are often the key to a positive clinical exam. Laboratory testing of a complete blood count (CBC) is generally obtained as a minimum for screening. An elevated white blood cell (WBC) count and a positive clinical exam are suggestive of the need for a surgery consultation. The emergency nurse's ability to understand and explain to families the sometimes long process of examination and reexamination can be a vital part of this challenging diagnosis. Keeping the child NPO, controlling pain, and assisting in preparation of the family for the possibility of surgery are key nursing responsibilities.

14. **What are some ways to get children to cooperate with care and procedures in the ED?**

It is difficult for children of any age to remain still and cooperative for short or extended time periods. Ask the parents about the child's prior experiences with treatments and procedures. Also ask the parents for suggestions on gaining the child's trust and cooperation. For example, if the child likes to hold a particular toy or blanket, have it near the child. Keep in mind that many times children are very fearful of the unknown. Often the concerned and overstressed adults around a sick child will misinterpret this fear as uncooperativeness or pain.

Be honest with the child. If a procedure or treatment will cause discomfort, say so. Older children and adolescents can comprehend time, and explaining that a procedure will take 5 minutes is understandable to them. Young children, who do not have a concept of time, are best given a task to accomplish. For example, "The pinch [from an injection] will be over when we count to 10" or "This will take as long as it takes to make toast." Offer verbal praise and a tangible reward, such as a sticker or drink of juice, after the procedure is completed.

Be honest about the amount of time required for a procedure. Five minutes should not stretch into 20 minutes; at this point, the child and family become upset and frustrated, leading to anger and a struggle between the family and ED staff. Children should receive sedation and analgesia for procedures requiring extended time. Videotapes or DVDs, audiotapes, soap bubbles, and other distraction techniques can be helpful for procedures of short duration. Proper positioning and securing during procedures also help the child to remain still. No person is more valued than the "holder" during a procedure. Even the most experienced nurse has difficulty starting an IV line on a moving target.

For future reference, try these suggestions:

- Set limits with the child who is biting or kicking, but allow the child to scream if necessary.
- The nurse should not escalate the situation. Often, the more the child struggles and the louder the child gets, the louder the nurse speaks and the more upset the caregiver becomes. The situation can quickly escalate out of control.
- Focus on the task at hand rather than the child's behavior.

15. **What are some tips for caring for children with special healthcare needs?**

Up to about 25% of all visits to the pediatric ED are for complaints associated with chronic illnesses, and many children come to the ED with "hardware" such as shunts, tracheostomy tubes, venous access devices, and gastrostomy tubes. Some tips for dealing with these children are:
- Common illnesses affect these children just like other children. Do not ignore the device, but do not focus on it.
- The child with a device is predisposed to infection related to the device itself. Look for signs and symptoms of infection.
- Listen to the family, because they are familiar with the child's care, previous history, and subtle changes.
- Children with devices have a higher likelihood of being admitted to the hospital; care should be expedited.
- Latex allergies need to be considered.

16. **Should families be allowed to stay with their child at all times?**

Family presence during assessments, treatments, and procedures has been shown to be beneficial to the child, family, and ED staff. Research has shown that the majority of families would prefer to be present during the resuscitation of a loved one. There is much literature available on the pros and cons of family presence. In 1993, the Emergency Nurses Association (ENA) became the first professional organization to develop a position statement endorsing family presence during invasive procedures and resuscitations. Before offering this practice, all members of the emergency medical team must have input into a process for how and when this should occur. The process should include giving the parents a brief explanation of any procedure and asking their preference for staying or leaving. If the parents choose to leave, a consistent member of the staff should update them frequently with information about the child's condition and progress. If the parents choose to stay, a number of factors should be considered, including the invasiveness and urgency of the procedure, the staff's comfort level with performing certain procedures in the parents' presence, and the family's ability to comfort and support the child during the procedure. An ED staff member, such as a social worker, should focus exclusively on the family's needs when they are present in a treatment room. This support person can answer parents' questions, explain procedures and treatments, and assist them in supporting their child.

The ED should have a family presence protocol that guides staff and parents in making the decision. The policy should take into consideration the ethical, legal, and moral obligations of the hospital to serve as advocates for the child and family.

17. **What should be done for a family when their child dies in the ED?**

Dealing with the death of a child in the ED is never easy. The most important skill of the healthcare provider at the time of death is to communicate in a clear, honest, and empathetic manner. Although you are unable to make things better for the family, saying "I am sorry" may be comforting. Checklists have been developed to guide staff in what to say and do, but remember that there is no right way to grieve and everyone does it differently. Offer support by saying "I am sorry" and providing mementos such as a handprint or a lock of hair. Do not use platitudes such as "It is God's will," or "You can have another baby." Make sure the department provides education for staff on how to deal with death and that the support of a social worker or hospital chaplain is available. Offer organ donation according to the hospital's protocol. Give the family a chance to see their child and time to say goodbye, and let them know what will happen next. Finally, have a process for taking care of yourself. Sometimes debriefing with other staff members in an informal way is helpful. A formal debriefing process may be available and helpful to some.

18. What type of equipment should be available in the ED to care for the seriously ill or injured child?

The organization of a pediatric crash cart is individualized according to preference and availability of medications and equipment. A crash cart can be organized according to age and weight. For example, color-code a crash cart that matches colors with the Broselow tape. Some companies sell such products; check a medical supply catalog for details. Keep pediatric defibrillator paddles and external pacers marked separately and near the unit defibrillator. Quick reference guides should be accessible to help guide the choice of equipment. If you do not have a crash cart, keep medications and equipment in designated cabinets or drawers for quick access. Because such equipment and medications can be used infrequently, periodic checks should be initiated to eliminate outdated materials. Including a pediatric mock code scenario in annual training/skills days is another important way to prepare for the care of seriously ill or injured children.

19. What are the most common causes of cardiac arrest in children?

Pulseless cardiac arrest is rarely a sudden event in the pediatric population. Usually the cause results from prolonged unrecognized respiratory failure. This is why it is so imperative for emergency nurses to be proficient in recognizing respiratory distress, respiratory failure, and shock and to intervene quickly and appropriately.

Children who may present in cardiac arrest unrelated to respiratory failure are those with congenital heart disease and, after 1 year of age, trauma.

20. What are the most common types of arrhythmias in children?

Most pediatric patients that present in cardiac arrest will have asystole or bradycardia that is often wide complex. As mentioned in question 19, cardiopulmonary arrest has most often been preceded by a progression of respiratory failure and shock that has gone unrecognized and untreated.

In a previously healthy child with a sudden collapse, arrhythmic cardiac arrest may be the cause. Conditions that are high risk for arrhythmias are myocarditis or any other underlying acquired heart disease, congenital heart disease, history of arrhythmias, a sudden blow to the chest, prolonged QT syndrome, profound hypothermia, drug intoxication, or profound electrolyte imbalance.

Bradycardia in an infant or child is defined as a heart rate less than 60 beats per minute. Because this rhythm is most often caused by hypoxemia, immediate airway and ventilatory measures should be initiated. Chest compressions should be initiated in the setting of bradycardia associated with clinical signs of poor perfusion.

Supraventricular tachycardia (SVT) is the most common tachyarrhythmia that can cause a cardiovascular compromise in infants and children. It is most commonly caused by a reentry mechanism that involves the atrioventricular (AV) conduction system or an accessory pathway. It is a narrow complex tachycardia that can produce a heart rate as rapid as 300 beats/min. SVT can be fairly well tolerated for a period of time in most infants and children, but it will eventually lead to congestive heart failure (CHF) and clinical signs of shock if left untreated.

21. What are some ways to prevent errors in caring for the pediatric patient?

Always weigh the child in kilograms. Drug doses in the pediatric patient are based on mg/kg dosage; weighing in pounds can cause an overdose of drugs if the weight in pounds is mistaken for kilograms. Use a volumetric pump on all infusions to prevent fluid overload, and use a syringe pump for antibiotics. Double-check the drug, strength, and dosages of all medications with another staff member, and never second-guess spelling or dosages. Make sure a good history is obtained from the family concerning which drugs (prescription and over the counter) that the child has been taking. It is important to have pediatric supplies; never try to rig adult equipment for use on pediatric patients.

Like all ED patients, pediatric patients should have appropriate name bands on an extremity. It is not okay to put the identification band on the bed or on the parent. Make sure to check for allergies and document them on the chart, and provide an "allergy alert" name band. Finally, *listen* to the parent or caregiver. Caregivers know their children better than anyone else. Do not assume the family is "difficult" if they question you. If they feel uncomfortable about a medication or an order, double-check it.

22. How should discharge instructions be given?

Both verbal and written discharge instructions are often necessary. The Joint Commission on Accreditation of Healthcare Organizations (JCAHO) requires that all ED patients receive written instructions. Written instructions allow the parent and child a reference for future directions. Verbal instructions allow the parent to hear and repeat to the nurse the home care and required follow-up. The ED may use a computerized set of discharge instructions, which are disease or condition specific. They can be printed on discharge and given to the parents. These instructions allow continuity among patients with similar conditions; they also may be tailored to a child's specific condition. Both written and verbal instructions may require translation into another language or communication format, and the ED should have these capabilities. When discharging a pediatric patient, ask the family, "Do you have any further questions?" and "Do you feel comfortable caring for your child at home?" Make sure the family knows the number to call back (if the ED allows parents to call back within a certain amount of time after the ED visit) and always tell them that they can come back if they are concerned. Make sure they understand the follow-up care necessary.

Key Points

- Children increase their heart rate to increase cardiac output when they need to compensate for circulatory compromise; thus tachycardia is an early sign of shock.

- The child's weight is needed for calculating medication doses and IV fluid amounts and should always be measured in kilograms.

- In infants younger than 2 months of age, any fever should be triaged at a more urgent acuity level even if the infant looks well. Fever can be indicative of a serious bacterial infection in this age group.

- Always tell the child what you are going to do to avoid surprises and promote trust.

- When treating fever, nurses should discuss fever management as opposed to fever control.

- Loss of weight is the most sensitive indicator for dehydration in young children, especially infants; thus it is important to obtain the nude weight of an infant and weights of all children with a history of vomiting or diarrhea.

- Consider that a child in respiratory distress who is not responding to usual interventions may be presenting with an underlying cardiac condition. Evaluate the heart rate and rhythm in all pediatric patients with respiratory distress.

- Children with medical devices have a higher likelihood of being admitted to the hospital.

- Research has shown that families would prefer to be present during the resuscitation of a loved one.

- Pulseless cardiac arrest is rarely a sudden event in the pediatric population.

- When discharging a pediatric patient, ask the parents, "Do you feel comfortable caring for your child at home?"

Internet Resources

American Academy of Pediatrics:
www.aap.org

Emergency Medical Services for Children:
www.ems-c.org

National Association of Children's Hospitals and Related Institutions:
www.childrenshospitals.net

National Guideline Clearinghouse:
www.guidelines.gov

Pediatric Emergency Care Applied Research Network:
www.pecarn.org

Bibliography

Armon K et al: An evidence and consensus based guideline for acute diarrhea management, *Arch Dis Child* 85(2): 132-142, 2001.

Baraff LF et al: Practice guidelines for the management of infants and children 0-36 months of age with fever without source, *Pediatrics* 92(1): 1-12, 1993.

Bergeson PS, Shaw JC: Are infants really obligatory nasal breathers? *Clin Pediatr* 40(1): 567-568, 2001.

Cincinnati Children's Hospital Medical Center: *Evidenced-based clinical practice guidelines for fever of uncertain source in infants 60 days of age or less*, Cincinnati, 2003, Children's Hospital Medical Center.

Conway A: Developmental and psychosocial considerations. In Thomas D, Bernardo L, Herman B: *Core curriculum for pediatric emergency nursing*, Boston, 2003, Jones & Bartlett.

Crocetti M, Serwint J: Fever: Separating fact from fiction, *Contemp Pediatr* 22(1): 34-42, 2005.

Fein JA, Cronan K, Possner JC: Approach to the care of the technology dependent child. In Fleisher G, Ludwig S, editors: *Textbook of pediatric emergency care*, ed 4, Baltimore, 2000, Williams & Wilkins.

Hawkins S, editor: *Emergency nursing pediatric course*, ed 3, Des Plaines, Ill, 2004, Emergency Nurses Association.

Hazinski M, editor: *Textbook of pediatric advanced life support*, Chicago, 2002, American Academy of Pediatrics and American Heart Association.

Henderson D: Coping with asthma: The national institute of health asthma guidelines, *J Emerg Nurs* 26(1): 70-75, 2000.

Isaacman DJ et al: Comparative practice patterns of emergency medicine physicians and pediatric emergency medicine physicians managing fever in young children, *Pediatrics* 108(2): 354-358, 2001.

Jardine J: Respiratory emergencies. In Thomas D, Bernardo L,Herman B, editors: *Core curriculum for pediatric emergency nursing*, Boston, 2003, Jones & Bartlett.

Markowitz J, Ludwig S: Constipation. In Fleisher G, Ludwig S, editors: *Textbook of pediatric emergency medicine*, ed 4, Philadelphia, 2000, Lippincott Williams & Wilkins.

Mecham N: Acute viral myocarditis in the ED pediatric patient: Three case presentations, *J Emerg Nurs* 30(2): 179-182, 2004.

Moreland P: Family presence during invasive procedures and resuscitation in the emergency department: A review of the literature, *J Emerg Nurs* 31(1): 58-72, 2005.

Nelson DS: Emergency treatment of fever phobia, *J Emerg Nurs* 24(1): 83-84, 1998.

Schnaufer L, Mahboubi S: Abdominal emergencies. In Fleisher G, Ludwig S, editors: *Textbook of pediatric emergency medicine*, ed 4, Philadelphia, 2000, Lippincott Williams & Wilkins.

Soud T: Gastrointestinal emergencies. In Thomas D, Bernardo L, Herman B, editors: *Core curriculum for pediatric emergency nursing*, Boston, 2003, Jones & Bartlett.

Stephens L: Encounter at triage results in legal liability, *J Emerg Nurs* 29(1): 55-57, 2003.

Stoll B: Infections of the neonatal infant. In Behrman RE et al, editors: *Nelson textbook of pediatrics*, ed 17, Philadelphia, 2004, Elsevier.

Thomas D: Special considerations for pediatric triage in the emergency department, *Nurs Clin North Am* 37(1): 143-159, 2002.

Thomas D, Soud T, Karp T: Common chief complaints. In Thomas D, Bernardo L, Herman B, editors: *Core curriculum for pediatric emergency nursing*, Boston, 2003, Jones & Bartlett.

Underserved Patients

Ruth E. Malone and Angela Hackenschmidt

1. **The ED is not a soup kitchen or a shelter. What can emergency nurses do for homeless people who come to the emergency department (ED)?**

   Even in cities with shelters, some homeless people frequent EDs because the shelters are perceived as unsafe, shelter space is inadequate, or EDs are more accessible by public transportation. In addition to their roles in emergency medical treatment, EDs function as a safety net for people who have nowhere else to go. Myriad factors related to homelessness and poverty contribute to increased health risks, and an estimated third of homeless persons have chronic mental illness. Homeless patients may present with acute medical conditions in addition to requesting social services, and careful assessment is a must. When possible, allowing a patient to bathe or shower in the ED makes caregiving more pleasant for both patient and staff, and many EDs keep a stock of clean used clothing on hand. Nurses can engage administration in dialogue about ways to meet social needs that lie behind some repeated ED visits. For example, intensive case management can help patients locate resources and services and has been shown to be effective in reducing unnecessary ED visits. Nurses also may be powerful spokespersons in advocating for policy changes to address underlying issues related to poverty.

2. **Should intoxicated people be taken to detoxification units or sobering centers instead of to the ED?**

   Problems such as occult head trauma, diabetes, and seizure disorders can cause symptoms that may be confused with alcohol intoxication. Acute alcohol intoxication also puts patients at risk for aspiration, falls, and other injuries. Even when the diagnosis is clear, a detoxification unit or sobering center may not be appropriate for particular patients. For example, some patients may require pharmacological management as they withdraw from alcohol, to avert seizures and other potentially dangerous sequelae. This may or may not be available in detoxification units. If such centers are available, strict referral criteria should be observed and patient outcomes measured.

3. **Some welfare mothers bring the whole family in for a checkup when one child has an upper respiratory infection. How can this behavior be stopped?**

   Such behavior is understandable if the mother has limited or no access to primary medical care because she can find no one to accept Medicaid coverage or she is uninsured. She also may be unable to take the child to a clinic during regular hours because of work or because she has no funds to pay for babysitters for other children. Learning about the context of the patients' lives may help the nurse be more innovative in assisting them and provides more career satisfaction in the long term than attempts to keep people from coming to the ED. A hospital social worker or a community health nurse may share information about what programs are available to help such families.

4. Many ED patients have drinking problems, smoke, do not wear seat belts, use drugs, etc. Is it a waste of energy and resources to treat patients who may continue unhealthy behaviors?

It is frustrating to feel that efforts to educate and support do not make a real difference, but there may be incremental changes that cannot be seen. Self-destructive behavior is often a reflection of and a way to cope with devaluation, which could be related to poverty or other life stressors. The ability to sustain a positive self-image and overcome addictions and other obstacles is hampered when one is blinded by depression or despair. There is no "quick fix" for socially embedded problems, but nurses can help by treating patients with kindness and respect, even when they are dirty, abusive, and difficult. Patients who have recovered from drug or alcohol addiction often recall one person who believed in them, even when they could not believe in themselves. Education may be helpful, if it is targeted to a particular moment of patient readiness, but learning what one *should* do is different from mobilizing the inner strength to do it. It can be helpful for nurses to view themselves as supporters in a *process* that could lead to patients harnessing the resources necessary for positive lifestyle changes.

5. Some Medicaid patients are demanding and unappreciative. Why should the nurse be nice to them when it feels like they are taking advantage of the system and tax dollars help pay for their care?

Think about a time when you may have been demanding. It was probably a time when you felt that your concerns were not being heard or that you had been treated unjustly. Patients with Medicaid often find that no doctor in the community will accept them. By the time they arrive at the ED after repeated and futile calls to doctors' offices (often using pay phones, because they may not be able to afford a home telephone), they may feel that they have been "through the mill" and are angry and defensive in general. It may have nothing to do with you. However, if negative feelings interfere with providing good care in a particular case, the most professional option may be to ask a colleague to care for the patient.

The larger question is whether feelings about an entire group of patients (in this case, people with Medicaid) represent a bias that interferes with the ability to give good care. Nursing has an ethical mandate to care for patients without regard to their financial circumstances. Taxes help support services that are important to the community; healthcare for everyone contributes to a healthy community.

6. **Is it acceptable not to get a translator if the nurse thinks he or she understands the problem of a patient who speaks little or no English?**

No, unless the nurse is fluent in the patient's language. Misunderstandings can be life threatening. For example, an Asian-American immigrant presented with weakness, shortness of breath, and dizziness. When asked about her medication, she was understood to say "Humulin." Clinicians treated her with fluids, thinking that she was a diabetic taking Humulin insulin and possibly in ketoacidosis. Her condition worsened significantly, and she spoke those dreaded words: "I feel like I'm going to die." Only then did the ED staff learn that she was taking *Coumadin* for a stenotic cardiac condition. The fluid had worsened her heart failure. Fortunately, the mistake was corrected in time and the woman recovered. Timely use of translator services could have averted this life-threatening mistake. Caution should be exercised with using a patient's family member to translate, because patients may not give complete or accurate information because of privacy concerns. Patients are more at ease when they are addressed in their own language. If any of us were sick or injured in a foreign country where the health services were unfamiliar, we would certainly be greatly relieved to find someone fluent in English.

7. **What should be done about illegal immigrants coming to the ED?**

Welfare reform in 1996 placed limitations on the ability of undocumented immigrants to access health services. However, everyone presenting to an ED is entitled to emergency medical screening and treatment, regardless of financial or immigration circumstances. Undocumented persons may delay seeking care out of fear of being reported or because of financial concerns. This group is sometimes blamed as the "cause" of complex problems, such as ED overcrowding and the economical crises of the U.S. healthcare system. However, research suggests that such problems are multifactorial. Some states have dedicated funding to pay for some basic and preventive care for undocumented persons to try to avoid reliance on more costly ED visits. Immigrants, both documented and undocumented, live and work in society, and their health affects the health of the community.

8. **The same people keep coming back to the ED repeatedly. What should be done to prevent this?**

A small percentage of ED users account for a disproportionately large percentage of total ED visits. Research has shown that such patients have elevated morbidity and mortality rates compared with non-ED users or infrequent users and also are more likely to be poor, unemployed, or homeless and to have one or more chronic conditions in addition to any acute condition with which they may present. Familiarity with such patients may lead nurses to assume that they know what is going on or to minimize the seriousness of these patients' complaints. To guard against this danger, emergency nurses should regard frequent users as a high-risk category of patients and consider strategies such as intensive case management to address their often complex and multifaceted clinical and social problems.

9. **What do nurses need to know about caring for lesbian, gay, bisexual, and transgendered (LGBT) patients?**

    It can be easy to assume that all ED patients are heterosexual or to make assumptions about health risk factors or behaviors of LGBT patients. It is important to approach each patient with respect and openness. LGBT persons may be hesitant to disclose pertinent health information because of having experienced discrimination or heterosexist views, and they may be at higher risk for health problems because of avoidance of routine preventive care. Transgendered persons are particularly at risk for and may experience high levels of discrimination, violence, and social isolation. Recommendations for caring for LGBT patients include recognizing that there is great diversity among sexual minority persons; using inclusive language when interviewing patients; recognizing and involving significant others and family in patient care and teaching; and promoting a supportive, nonjudgmental environment to encourage disclosure of health history and concerns.

10. **Are there racial and ethnic disparities in emergency care and health outcomes? What are the implications for ED clinicians?**

    Yes. Statistically, nonwhite persons have significantly higher morbidity rates for multiple chronic diseases and are more likely to experience delays in treatment. The causes for this are complex and not entirely understood. One recent study found that most of the differences in time to treatment were related to differences between hospitals, rather than differential racial treatment within a hospital. However, qualitative research has also shown how individuals' marginalization experiences shape responses to symptoms, care-seeking behavior, and interpretation of care activities. This highlights the importance of sensitivity to the experiences of marginalized groups and advocating for high-quality ED and hospital care throughout communities, because hospitals serving disproportionate numbers of racial and ethnic minorities tend to be in poorer areas with fewer resources.

11. **There are more uninsured patients then ever who have no primary care provider. What is the nurse's role, and how can using clinics rather than the ED be encouraged?**

    About 45 million people in the United States, most of whom are working and poor, are uninsured, have little access to care, and suffer worse health outcomes compared with those who have insurance. In some cases EDs can screen and refer stable patients to an urgent care clinic or provide information about available free or sliding-scale community clinics. State budget crises result in ongoing cuts to local services, including closure of outpatient health programs and public health services. ED nurses can engage local and state officials to advocate maintaining outpatient resources in communities and can participate in healthcare reform efforts. The United States remains the only major developed country without universal health insurance.

12. How can an emergency nurse keep from getting burned out when the numbers of poor patients are increasing, their problems seem worse, and resources are increasingly limited?

Long-term, expert, caring nurses learn to reinvent their practice periodically; that is, to make an effort to see some new aspect of the job or something they do in a different light. This process is a kind of refocusing. For example, the technical and bureaucratic aspects of emergency nursing are only one part of the work. Helping people feel truly acknowledged and cared for in rapidly changing and difficult situations is an art. No one wants to be "treated like a case"; everyone wants to be recognized as a human being, no matter what the circumstances. A useful exercise is to focus on the difference between *care* and *control*. When trying to control the uncontrollable, obstacles arise and the nurse may become frustrated and angry with patients, co-workers, or families. A focus on care means that even when things are going awry, the nurse tries to sustain engagement with patients (and co-workers) as individuals and accept them as they are. Emergency nurses are constantly reminded that life is short and that nothing can be taken for granted. This in itself can be a kind of gift.

 Key Points

- "Underserved" patients are often poor; uninsured or underinsured; may be from racial, ethnic, or sexual minority groups; and experience multiple challenges to accessing health services.

- There are no quick fixes for complex societal problems (e.g., poverty, racism, homophobia) that affect patients presenting to EDs, but emergency nurses have a unique perspective that can be used to advocate for patients and confront problems on a policy and system level.

- Engaging patients and "meeting them where they are" can be an effective way to offer positive support and hope to patients who struggle with addiction and social problems. This approach is more likely to produce professional satisfaction than trying to control others' behavior or decisions.

- Patients who are considered "underserved" may also be at higher risk for illness and poor health outcomes. Careful history taking and assessment by the ED nurse contribute to quality care for these individuals.

Internet Resources

Academic Emergency Medicine, Special Issue: Disparities in Emergency Health Care:
www.aemj.org/content/vol10/issue11

Centers for Disease Control and Prevention, Office of Minority Health: Eliminating Racial & Ethnic Health Disparities:
www.cdc.gov/omh/AboutUs/disparities.htm

Gay and Lesbian Medical Association (Choose "Advocacy" tab, then Healthy People 2010 Companion Document for LGBT Health):
www.glma.org

The Henry J. Kaiser Family Foundation, Health Coverage & the Uninsured:
www.kff.org/uninsured

National Coalition for the Homeless:
www.nationalhomeless.org

Bibliography

Banks A, Malone RE: Accustomed to enduring: Experiences of African American women seeking care for cardiac symptoms, *Heart Lung* 34:13-21, 2005.

Bonvicini KA, Perlin MJ: The same but different: Clinician-patient communication with gay and lesbian patients, *Patient Educ Couns* 51:115-122, 2003.

Bradley EH et al: Racial and ethnic differences in time to acute reperfusion therapy for patients hospitalized with myocardial infarction, *JAMA* 292:1563-1572, 2004.

Kushel MB et al: Emergency department use among the homeless and marginally housed: Results from a community-based study, *Am J Public Health* 92:778-784, 2002.

Malone RE: Dimensions of vulnerability in emergency nurses' narratives, *Adv Nurs Sci* 23:1-11, 2000.

Malone RE: Underserved patients. In Oman KS, Koziol-McLain J, Scheetz LJ, editors: *Emergency nursing secrets*, Philadelphia, 2000, Hanley & Belfus.

Malone RE: Whither the almshouse? Overutilization and the role of the emergency department, *J Health Polit Policy Law* 23:795-832, 1998.

Ruger JP et al: Analysis of costs, length of stay, and utilization of emergency department services by frequent users: Implications for health policy, *Acad Emerg Med* 11:1311-1317, 2004.

Abused and Neglected Patients

Karen Hayes, Jane Koziol-McLain, and Marilyn K. Johnson

ELDER ABUSE

1. Is elder abuse a significant problem?

Unfortunately, older adults are not immune from the violence in society. Abuse, neglect, and mistreatment are significant and growing problems for older adults. Lack of reporting makes the incidence of abuse difficult to measure accurately; however, it is estimated that as many as 2 million elders each year suffer some form of abuse. In 80% of abuse cases, violence recurs. The abuser is a family member in 86% of cases. Elder abuse victims have numerous interactions with emergency departments (EDs), and these visits frequently result in hospital admission.

2. What is considered elder abuse?

The definition of elder abuse is broad. It includes a variety of violent and nonviolent acts such as brutal beatings, burns, fractures, and neglect.

Types of Elder Abuse

Type	Description
Physical	Physical contact that causes trauma, pain, or mental distress
Psychological	Systematic efforts to provoke fear of abuse, fear of removal from home, isolation, or loss of self-esteem
Sexual	Sexual contact by coercion, threat, or force
Neglect	Failure of able caretakers to meet elder's physical or mental needs
Abandonment	Purposefully deserting the elder or withdrawing care, such as "dropping off" in the ED
Financial	Taking advantage of an elder for monetary or material gain or profit

3. Which elders are at risk?

    Studies have identified a pattern in the risk of elder abuse. Risk factors include advanced age (older than age 75); females; lower socioeconomic status; dementia, or multiple medical problems requiring many medications; and elders who need others to provide for activities of daily living. The risk applies particularly to elders with incontinence, which may be viewed by a caretaker as purposeful behavior. In addition, elders who experienced abusive or violent lifestyles are at risk. Abused elders may have been abusers of their children.

4. What parts of the history and review of systems may show warning signs of abuse?

    Emergency nurses must develop a "sixth sense" in assessing elder abuse. Always maintain a high level of suspicion. Be alert when the caregiver or elder is reticent to discuss the problem. A common red flag is a long delay between the illness or injury and presentation to the ED. A cognitively intact abused elder may behave in a passive, elusive way or show signs of depression.

    The assessment begins with a history that includes a review of risk factors. Look particularly for dependence on a caregiver, social isolation, and recent household conflicts. The review of systems may uncover symptoms such as dehydration, wasting subcutaneous tissue, contractures, or untreated injuries.

5. What changes should the nurse look for in the physical assessment?

    Note carefully the general appearance, including condition of clothing, hair, skin, and nails. Look for unusual areas of hair loss, bruising, broken teeth, skin tears, scars, burns, skin breakdown, or lesions with unusual markings, such as teeth marks. The emergency nurse must be knowledgeable about normal age-related changes (see Chapter 35) to diagnose neglect or abuse.

6. How should findings be documented?

    Various standardized assessment tools are available for documenting abuse findings. Whether or not these tools are used, details must be noted carefully. Verbatim reports from both the victim and suspected perpetrator should be recorded. Physical exam findings should be documented in objective descriptive terms; pictures may be helpful.

7. Do diagnostic tests help to identify abuse or neglect?

    Radiographs may reveal occult fractures, multiple old fractures in various stages of healing, or transverse or oblique fractures of long bones. Metabolic screenings may show malnutrition or electrolyte imbalance. Drug levels should be obtained for overmedication or undermedication. If sexual assault is suspected, testing for assault or sexually transmitted diseases (STDs) is indicated.

8. What is the emergency nurse's role in the management of elder abuse?

    The most important role for the emergency nurse is to detect abuse and to treat the immediate problem. Elders may need treatment for bleeding, head injury, hypothermia, dehydration, fractures, or burns. Generally, these patients are admitted to the hospital. Patient safety is the goal. Elder abuse is a volatile situation that requires a multidisciplinary approach. If the patient will be returned to a potentially abusive environment, referral to social service, case management, or primary care provider (PCP) is important. In many states, reporting of elder abuse or neglect is mandatory. In fact, many abused elders refuse help. They may fear retaliation or feel that their current situation is better than removal from the home. It is the patient's right to choose to remain in the abusive situation. However, it is the emergency nurse's role to make an appropriate referral so that an elder will be aware of available resources and can make an informed choice.

DOMESTIC VIOLENCE

9. Few women come to ED for domestic violence. Why is domestic violence such an important issue?

Domestic violence (partner violence, wife abuse, or battering) in society is well hidden. But studies show that up to 55% of women seen in EDs report that they have been a victim of partner violence at some time in their life. Asked about violence in the past year, 15% to 30% of women seen in EDs respond affirmatively. Over their adulthoods, domestic violence affects over 50% of women seen in the ED. Violence also occurs against men and women in gay and lesbian relationships.

Not only are the numbers substantial, but negative health outcomes are numerous. Substantial morbidity and mortality are associated with partner violence. Abused women are more likely to have chronic headaches, gynecological problems, depression, substance abuse problems, suicide attempts, and posttraumatic stress disorder (PTSD). All too often, women are killed; 40% to 50% of all women who are murdered in the United States are murdered by a current or ex-partner. Children in the home are also at risk; children who witness violence demonstrate internalizing and externalizing behaviors, including PTSD. The large numbers and the negative health consequences of partner abuse mean that it is a major concern.

10. Should screening for partner violence only happen when a woman comes to the ED for injuries?

No. Physical violence is only one way of exerting power and control over an intimate partner. In one instance, a woman told of never having been physically hurt, yet she recounted how one day her partner shot a gun past her head into the wall, exclaiming, "Next time I won't miss." Emotional abuse (e.g., threats, put-downs, name calling), forced sex (e.g., unwanted roughness, demeaning sex acts), financial abuse, using the children (e.g., "I'll report you to children's services, and you'll never see your kids again"), harassment, and stalking are examples of ways to unnerve an intimate partner's sense of self and ability to consider options.

Screening, then, is not just for the injured. Research indicates that women with non–injury-related ED visits are just as likely to screen positive for partner violence as women with injury-related visits. Therefore, all patients should be screened. Women who screen positive for violence in the past year are at high risk for repeated violence, especially if they are trying to separate from an abusive partner.

Screening is also appropriate for both men and women. Although the overwhelming majority of injuries related to partner violence involve women abused by a male partner, women may abuse male partners, and males in homosexual relationships may abuse their partners. One colleague shared that one of the first "positive" screens following implementation of routine screening was a man in his 40s whose wife was beating him. Some women will respond to a routine screen saying, "I'm the one who is abusive." Although the majority of the literature and advocacy work has focused on heterosexual male violence against women, it is important to be open and nonjudgmental to the abuse that can occur to anyone, regardless of gender, gender identity, age, race, education, or socioeconomic status.

11. What should the patient be asked?

Before considering what to ask, stop and reflect. Is it possible to be nonjudgmental and culturally sensitive when you bring up the subject of abuse? Consider your own experience with abuse; if you know someone who has been abused by a partner, listen to that person's story. Learn about partner abuse. It is not simple to leave an abusing partner; learn about the process that one struggles through to make the necessary life changes to be free from violence. Consider the nurse's role as a healthcare provider. By not asking, the nurse conspires to keep problems hidden. Documenting "hit in head with pipe" is insufficient; if appropriate, document "hit in head with pipe by John Doe, her ex-boyfriend." Consider learning about partner abuse from a perspective other than that of the ED. Spend some time with a women's advocate, at a shelter for battered women, in women's support groups, or perhaps at the courthouse where orders of protection (restraining orders, no contact orders) are judged.

Emergency nurses are in a strategic position to provide compassionate, supportive, culturally sensitive care to battered persons who are otherwise isolated. Be aware, however, that a traditional approach to emergency care focused on "immediate" cures does not work in the case of partner violence. Consider approaching the issue from an empowerment model, focusing on coping strategies and strengths. Base nursing care on principles such as sharing information, giving choices, and brainstorming solutions.

After a decision is made to act, the following checklist will help patients (and the nurse) talk about abuse:

- Be aware of department policy for identifying and treating domestic violence (this is a requirement of the Joint Commission on Accreditation of Healthcare Organizations [JCAHO]).
- Put up posters to let people know it is okay to talk about abuse.
- Have brochures and referrals available; put brochures in the waiting room and bathrooms.
- Take safety measures; make it routine to have a few private moments with each patient.

Once prepared, use an "ice breaker" to bring up the topic, such as, "We have found that many of the people we see are experiencing abuse in their homes, so we now ask everyone some screening questions." The ice breaker is then followed with direct screening questions such as those listed in the following box. Ask in private, because how the questions are asked often affects whether a person chooses to disclose violence. Studies and experience show that women do not mind being asked about abuse; they prefer straightforward questions.

Examples of Screening Questions for Partner Abuse

1. In the past year, have you been hit, slapped, kicked, raped, or otherwise physically hurt by someone you know or knew intimately?
2. Have you been emotionally or physically abused by your partner or someone important to you?
3. Is there a current or past partner making you feel unsafe?
4. Has someone close to you forced you to have sex when you did not want to?
5. Many women seen in the ED have been abused by a partner. Is that the case for you?
6. Is there a partner physically hurting or threatening you?
7. When women say they are under a lot of stress, it is sometimes because they are being hurt or threatened by their partner. Is that the case with you?

---

12. **What are the nurse's responsibilities if the patient indicates that he or she is a victim of abuse?**

At a minimum, nurses should be prepared to do the following:
Assess risk:
- Immediate safety: Determine whether the perpetrator is in the ED; ask whether children are at risk.
- Injuries and other health effects: Document all injuries using a body map; photograph injuries.
- Lethality: Have the person complete a Danger Assessment form to increase his or her awareness of risk.
- Support system: Determine whether the person has someone close to him or her with whom he or she has talked about the abuse.

Offer support:
- Actively listen. Focus on the person's strengths. Let him or her know it is not acceptable to be hit, that he or she is not to blame, that he or she is not alone ("Many people experience this; you are not alone"), and that he or she does not have to end the relationship unless it is his or her choice.

Plan for safety:
- Help the patient decide where to go in an emergency.
- Tell the patient to let a neighbor know when to call the police.
- Instruct the patient to pack a bag that includes important papers (e.g., birth certificates, car title, social security card, children's immunization records),

keys, medications, and things for the children (such as a special toy, blanket, or pillow).
- Suggest that the patient put some money aside (hidden).
- Tell the patient to remove firearms and ammunition from the home.

Offer options:
- Identify resources and make referrals as needed, such as legal, safe housing (shelter), and counseling.

13. Many states have a mandatory reporting law for domestic violence. What should be done if the person insists on not reporting but it is mandatory in the state?

This is not an easy question to answer. Many issues are involved in mandatory reporting. Laws differ across states, as does their implementation. Resources available for abused women (and men) and mandatory arrest policies vary locally. The goal of advocacy is based on empowering the person to make informed choices. Yet partner violence should not be tolerated; it is a crime and there should be consequences for the batterer. It is a difficult dilemma. Consider the individual circumstances. Know about the law, how it is applied in the community, and what resources are available. Then, consider what the person has told you. A report should not be made without first having a discussion with the person.

SEXUAL ASSAULT

14. When should a patient be asked about sexual assault?

Routinely ask about "forced sex." Forced sex occurs when someone (female or male) is physically forced or coerced to participate in a sexual act when it is unwanted. About 40% of battered women also experience forced sex. Many women participate in sex with a violent partner to avoid possibly worse outcomes (such as threats against the children). In some cases, women are forced by their intimate partners to engage in sex with others. A partner may refuse to engage in safe sex, putting the woman at risk for sexually transmitted infections (STIs), including HIV.

15. In some EDs no protocol exists for sexual assault victims. Women often have to wait a long time in the crowded waiting room, and exams are not standardized. What can be done about this?

Take action. Begin by gathering an interdisciplinary team to address substandard care delivery for women who have been sexually assaulted. Contact advocates in the community to support and provide resources as a plan is developed and put into action. Investigate the Sexual Assault Nurse Examiner (SANE) program. SANE members are trained to provide forensic examination of the sexual assault victim; training programs are in place in many communities. SANE nurses complete advanced specialized training to qualify to examine prepubertal children.

CHILD ABUSE AND NEGLECT

16. **When was the public's attention drawn to the plight of abused children?**

The famous case of "Mary Ellen," a battered child who could be protected only if the Society for the Prevention of Cruelty to Animals was invoked, sparked interest in the topic of child abuse in the United States in the 1870s. People realized that abused children had fewer protections than animals. In the 1940s and 1950s Caffey and Silverman, two radiologists, recognized that subdural hematomas and fractures had a relationship to the intentional injury of children. In 1962, C. Henry Kempe described the "battered child syndrome." Thereafter, states began enacting mandatory reporting laws.

Currently, all 50 states have mandatory reporting laws for suspicions of child abuse. The laws' intent is to protect children from harm and to mandate that allegations be investigated by specific agencies, using appropriate methods. Some states also place misdemeanor sanctions for failure to report suspicion of abuse. The JCAHO requires that all EDs have policies for reporting child abuse and neglect.

Despite mandatory reporting laws and hospital policies, experts believe that the detected cases of abuse represent only the tip of the iceberg. Undoubtedly, many children who suffer the consequences of abuse go unrecognized. In the ED, a full-body inspection is important to discover easily missed trauma, which usually is covered by clothing.

17. **What are the types and methods of abuse against children?**

The four recognized types of child abuse are physical abuse, sexual abuse, emotional abuse, and neglect. Often, children have overlays of more than one type of abuse. Examples are sexual abuse and neglect or emotional abuse with physical abuse.

Implements that are used in physical abuse include belts, straps, cords, and hands. Burns may be inflicted to "teach" a child about fire or hot objects. Cigarettes, incense sticks, or heated implements can leave burn marks that may be found in areas not easily recognized (e.g., between fingers or toes). Other methods could include hot liquid splash scalds, hot water immersion burns, chemical burns, and bites.

Many injuries occur because of poor parenting techniques. Challenges such as parental sleep deficits, plus an environment of high stress, accompanied by a trigger such as a child crying or misbehaving, may lead to loss of control resulting in harm to the child. Emotional abuse results in damaging a child's psyche, which can lead to deeper problems as the child grows.

Sexual abuse is often perpetrated by someone the child knows. Children are many times told that the activity is a secret between the perpetrator and the child or are threatened if they tell.

18. **Do all marks seen on children indicate abuse?**

No. Accidental injuries, religious or cultural practices, and disease processes can produce marks that can be misinterpreted as abuse. In evaluating a religious or cultural practice, the general rule of thumb is that intention to cause harm is abuse. A practice consistent with the caretaker's spiritual belief system and not intended to harm is usually not considered abuse. However, some practices, such as female genital mutilation (including female circumcision and suturing of the labia), are considered abusive by international standards. Examples of processes that "imitate" abuse are listed in the following table.

Possible Imitators of Child Abuse

Category	Name	Description
Folk remedies	Cao Gio	A treelike pattern on the back and/or chest as a result of fluid that is applied and vigorously rubbed with a coin or shell
	Moxibustion/Maquas	Burns inflicted as therapy
	Cupping/spooning	Cultural practice causing bruising
Vasculitis	Henoch-Schölein purpura	No patterned bruises
Bleeding disorders	von Willebrand's disease	No patterned bruises
	Hemophilia	
	Leukemia	
	Idiothrombocytopenic purpura	
Birthmarks, other marks, or rashes	Mongolian spots	Usually in sacral area but also can be widely disseminated on back, legs, and arms; generally disappear by 10 years of age; if pressing on the spot produces pain, a bruise might be underneath; spots do not fade when pressure is applied
	Phytophotodermatitis	When the juice from limes, lemons, figs, or celery is left on the skin and exposed to sunlight, a discoloration or burn results
	Erythema multiforme	Ecchymotic lesions

19. Can bruises be accurately dated (number of days) by noting the coloration?

No. People have different bruising and healing capacities. A bruise results when capillaries fracture and blood escapes into the interstitial tissue. The skin is the window to see the bruise. The depth, location, and skin complexion affect the time of appearance and the color of the bruise. Deep abdominal trauma may not show a bruise until much later or not at all because of the depth of the injury. Developmental capabilities of the child and history given for a bruise may not match, leading one to consider abuse. Falls usually result in bruises to one plane of the body. Multiple bruises of varying ages, in areas such as the face, trunk of the body, or arms should raise concerns. Some bruises may also match an object or implement that was used in an abusive act.

20. **If child abuse is suspected, should a skeletal survey be ordered?**

When child abuse is suspected, children younger than 2 years of age should have a skeletal survey. A skeletal survey involves taking two views of each body area; each area is x-rayed separately. If a survey is done, a follow-up x-ray is recommended in 2 weeks to look for ossification of subtle fractures, which may not have been visible on the original survey.

"Babygrams" are never appropriate. A babygram involves placing an infant or small child on a single large x-ray plate, which results in a full-body antero-posterior (AP) film. Babygrams expose the child to unnecessary radiation and are not helpful in discovering the subtle fractures of child abuse.

With a verbal child, the child's symptoms and capability to tell what is hurting are better indications that an injury requires an x-ray. Only the areas of concern may need to be x-rayed. Pediatric radiologists have a better chance of diagnosing subtle findings that some adult specialists may miss. Today, most x-rays are digital, allowing an off-site radiologist to read them.

21. **Many children present to the ED with fractures. When should abuse be suspected?**

It is estimated that 11% to 55% of all childhood fractures are a result of abuse. With certain fractures, the proportion attributed to abuse is much greater. For example, 60% of long-bone fractures in a nonambulatory child (younger than 1 year of age) are caused by abuse. Fractures that should be evaluated by medical providers with expertise in pediatric radiology and child abuse include:
- Metaphyseal corner fractures on the distal portion of the long bones
- "Bucket handle" fractures from shaking or twisting
- Rib fractures in infants (anterior, posterior, first and second ribs, some lateral fractures)
- Multiple fractures of different ages
- Periosteal elevation from shaking or twisting
- Long-bone fractures (in nonambulatory child) without a history of an accidental cause, osteogenesis imperfecta, metabolic cause, infection, or neoplasms

22. **Given an injury, on what basis should the nurse be concerned about abuse?**

Look at the plausibility of accidental injury. Evaluate the child's development and capacity for self-injury. Is the child able to "cruise" (move about independently)? Many abuse-related fractures may not be discovered because the medical staff believes the caretaker's story or the fracture is misdiagnosed.

When gathering information about the mechanism, ask caretakers only open-ended questions, such as, "How did it happen?" Asking leading questions can assist a caretaker (and child) in fabricating a possible explanation. Leading questions would contain part of an answer and may contaminate or create problems for later disclosures to an investigator. Discrepancies or changes in explanations are important data in investigations. Triage and primary nurses should document statements made by the child or caretaker about the injury. Always document, in quotations, both the questions that were posed and the responses. Limit questions to those that are necessary to direct nursing and medical care. Finally, even if there is a high index of suspicion, remain objective and nonjudgmental in interactions with caretakers.

23. **How can a nurse "remain objective and nonjudgmental" when someone has caused a child to suffer?**

It is natural to feel anger when caring for a traumatized child. But it is not acceptable to direct anger at the caregiver who brought the child to the ED. The emergency nurse should consider several issues. First, in most cases, determining who inflicted harm is not immediately apparent. For example, the person in the ED who acts "unusual" may be covering for someone else.

Second, when a caregiver abuses a child, it is usually in response to a set of circumstances that began long before the event. Perhaps they were abused as a child or utilize negative or abusive parenting styles. Abusive acts are typically responses to a trigger in the setting of various socioeconomic, parenting, and child-produced stressors. Triggers may be related to unrealistic expectations of the child, such as bed wetting or crying.

Third, the courts strive to keep children with their primary caregiver. By providing respect and perhaps even compassion, the nurse keeps the door open for future therapeutic change. Many believe that people who admit they are wrong have a good chance of avoiding future bad incidents. Even in the worst cases when a child is removed from the care of parents, it is realistic to assume that they will have other children. Hopefully other children within that family unit will be free from abuse.

Caring for a child who is severely harmed is one of the most stressful experiences that an emergency nurse faces. For healthcare providers, talking in a confidential setting with other members of the health team may be helpful for emotional and spiritual healing. Consider what actions are needed to foster change in communities and what role nurses have. For example, some nurses are involved in teaching parenting classes and role-modeling nonviolence.

24. **A child who had a life-threatening abdominal hollow organ injury was seen in the ED. He did not cry. Why?**

Some children have been abused frequently and are told that they will be hurt worse if they cry. Such children may dissociate when exposed to abuse. Dissociation is a normal protective mechanism in the face of an abnormal situation (abuse). The demeanor that is seen may not be the way that the child truly feels. Abused children learn not to trust adults and may not interact with clinicians as one would expect.

A false, misleading history given by a caretaker, delay in seeking medical care, and a child's stoicism contribute to missed or delayed diagnosis and treatment of abdominal injury. Abdominal injury is the second most common cause of fatality from abuse. Central nervous system injuries are the leading cause of death from abuse. CNS injuries are misdiagnosed in 30% of cases. Hollow and solid organ injuries are best diagnosed by computed tomography (CT) with contrast studies, which are better for detecting a duodenal hematoma (commonly caused by blunt abdominal trauma). Surgical intervention is often needed. Studies ordered may include alanine aminotransferase (ALT), aspartate aminotransferase (AST), amylase, and urinalysis.

25. What is shaken baby syndrome (SBS), now referred to as abusive head trauma (AHT)?

SBS or AHT is a pattern of injuries that results from violent manual shaking. Signs and symptoms are classically seen without evidence of external trauma. AHT is characterized by intracranial injury (usually subdural hematoma) and retinal hemorrhages (60% to 80% of cases). Bony fractures are also possible. The most characteristic newborn fractures are corner fractures of the long bones and posterior rib fractures. The injuries are believed to result from forceful acceleration, deceleration, and rotation of the head (because of a child's weak neck muscles). Sometimes the addition of an impact enhances the force with sudden deceleration.

To explain the cause of a child's neurological impairment or death, caretakers may give the history that the child fell from a couch or bed or developed sudden apnea and that the caretaker shook the child to revive him or her. These stories prove to be fabricated because it takes a forceful shake to produce the damage seen with AHT.

When AHT is suspected, a dilated eye exam with an indirect ophthalmoscope to look for retinal hemorrhage should be performed by an experienced pediatric ophthalmologist. A CT scan is used for acute diagnosis, but magnetic resonance imaging (MRI) is more sensitive and assists with dating the bleeds. Other studies should include a skeletal survey and bleeding studies.

26. Is there always physical evidence of child sexual abuse?

No. Often, the crime involves activities that do not result in tissue damage. Although a child may say something has gone "inside," intralabial contact may or may not leave any evidence. Even with significant trauma, healing can occur in a short time. There have been cases seen in child sex abuse clinics when a teen has given birth and still had her hymen intact. The genitals are highly vascular and heal very rapidly. The old adage about a hymen, "once broken, it never heals," is a myth.

Over 90% of child sexual abuse victims have no physical evidence. Remember that physical evidence is only a part of the picture. Investigative experts should conduct careful interviews, and behavioral issues must be considered. Child sexual abuse is often perpetrated by an adult, most often known to the child, who gradually builds a relationship of trust, facilitating abuse of the child, and may describe their special relationship as "our secret."

27. When should a child come to the ED for forensic collection of evidence after sexual assault?

The guidelines in the following box were developed by a team of medical experts in Utah who are members of the American Professional Society on the Abuse of

Children (APSAC). Children are not small adults, and national experts recommend that children need to be evaluated by a midlevel provider or physician with pediatric experience.

When Children Need Medical Exams for Suspected Sex Abuse

Whenever there is a concern about sexual abuse of a child, a medical examination is needed. The child's PCP can perform an initial screening examination. Referral to those with specialized expertise in performing sexual abuse examination may be necessary. Except in cases of a true medical emergency, the ED is often not the optimal location to assess sexual abuse, because it is crowded and there is less time for an evaluation. The following guidelines help to determine the urgency of the medical examination.

1. **Immediate medical examination:** If the following are present, the child should be seen as soon as possible that day:
   - History of inappropriate sexual contact within 72 hours (rape, fondling, sodomy, fellatio, cunnilingus, and incidents in which children are found in unusual circumstances with adults or older children, such as naked or undressed, with clothing ripped or missing; possibility of pregnancy; abdominal pain or bleeding in a known pregnancy).
   - Need for forensic evidence collection for rape kit (contact within 72 hours).
   - Acute vaginal or rectal bleeding, vaginal or rectal pain, and/or genital or anal trauma, unexplained or thought to be related to sexual abuse (includes blood found on diaper or underwear).
   - If a drug-facilitated rape is suspected within 96 hours of drugging, the collection of blood and urine specimens should be considered.
2. **Urgent medical examination:** If the following are present, the child should be examined as soon as possible. Referral to a specialist in child sexual abuse may be appropriate:
   - Delayed disclosure of inappropriate sexual contact more than 72 hours ago and within the past 2 weeks.
   - Vaginal or penile discharge and possibility of STI or history suggestive for STIs. Vaginal or penile discharge may not cause symptoms but may be noticed by caretakers on diaper or underwear. Other concerns for STI include history of genital ulcers or blisters or any unusual rash in the genital area.
   - The sexual contact occurred more than 72 hours ago, and the possibility of pregnancy exists.
3. **Nonurgent medical examination:** Children who do not meet the above criteria and do not require an immediate or urgent examination should have an examination as soon as possible. Exams conducted in a non-ED setting can reduce the anxiety surrounding sexual abuse investigations. Referral to a specialist in child sexual abuse may be appropriate. Following are examples of children for whom a nonurgent medical examination is appropriate:
   - Delayed disclosure of sexual abuse, which occurred more than 2 weeks ago.
   - Behavioral changes suspicious for abuse.
   - Siblings of known abuse victims and children exposed to domestic violence, if, after evaluation, sexual abuse is a concern.

28. When a report of suspected child abuse is made, should the parents be told?

When there is concern and immediate risk, it is best to allow one person to inform the caretakers. Timing is important. Often in EDs there are multiple ways to stall or place the child in a safe place for "just one more test" while waiting for child protective services or law enforcement. The investigating agent needs to use forensic interviewing techniques. In most states, it is only the investigators who can question children or parents about a concern for child abuse. Many states have Children's Justice Centers where children can be interviewed in a child-friendly environment. Limit questions to what is necessary for nursing and medical care. The nurse's role is to care for the child and offer support to the caretakers, without discussing abuse. If comments are made by the child or caregiver that seem relevant to the case, document them and share them with the investigators.

29. What does "medical neglect" mean?

Medical neglect applies to a child who is harmed or at risk of serious harm because of lack of healthcare or a child who does not receive healthcare that would offer a significant benefit. The child's basic needs are adequate food, clothing, healthcare, supervision, protection, education, and nurturance. Many physical effects of neglect can result in injuries, ingestions, illnesses, dental problems, malnutrition, neurological challenges, and fatalities.

30. Some children who come to the ED have been exposed to methamphetamine labs. Is care for them different than normal ED care? Most of these children don't seem to have any medical problems.

Care relates to:
- ABCs (airway, breathing, circulation)
- Possibility of chemical burns to the skin
- Ingestion
- Toxicity

Meth labs are becoming increasingly more common across the country. Methods of "cooking" meth include mixing red phosphorous (from matchbox strips), pseudoephedrine from cold tablets, iodine, and other chemicals such as ether; the Nazi method uses anhydrous ammonia (which farmers use for fertilizer). Both methods are extremely dangerous with possibilities of explosions and burns or children drinking the chemicals stored in their juice containers or baby bottles by the caregivers trying to hide what they are doing.

It is uncertain what the long-term effects of meth lab exposure are on children. There is a great deal of concern for neurotoxicity, respiratory effects, lead poisoning, psychological trauma, and learning challenges. The National Alliance for Drug Endangered Children (NADEC) lists emergency actions and suggestions for lab exposures and has organized specialists to address actions and responsibilities needed for care of the children. The majority of exposed children do not have medical symptoms but do need a comprehensive evaluation done by a healthcare provider who understands the issues around drug-exposed children. Referrals to specialties relating to medical, psychological, and neglectful needs are imperative.

There is also concern for children who reside in environments where there is drug use, commonly along with drug paraphernalia, guns, pornography, and other dangers. A study done by the National Jewish Medical and Research Center in Denver, Colorado, quantified the dangers in these clandestine settings, demonstrating significant environmental toxicity in environments where children reside with their drug-abusing parents (findings summarized at the Colorado Alliance for Drug Endangered Children website). Internet sites for more information about drug-endangered children include:

- National Alliance for Drug Endangered Children (NADEC): www.nationaldec.org
- Colorado Alliance for Drug Endangered Children: www.colodec.org
- Office of National Drug Control Policy, Drug Endangered Children: www.whitehousedrugpolicy.gov/enforce/dr_endangered_child.html
- Methamphetamine Fact Sheet: www.whitehousedrugpolicy.gov/publications/factsht/methamph/index.html
- National Institute on Drug Abuse (NIDA): www.nida.nih.gov (see also NIDA Notes: www.drugabuse.gov/NIDA_Notes/NNInfo2.html)

31. What are some long-term effects of child abuse?

Numerous studies have documented effects of child abuse on later adult health. These include social, emotional, and cognitive impairment; adoption of health-risk behaviors; disease; disability; and death. There is an increased incidence of depression, alcoholism, drug abuse, and severe obesity. The economical effects, both short- and long-term, are massive. In 2001 Suzette Fromm conservatively estimated the costs of child abuse at $94 billion per year in the United States. The costs she included were hospitalization, chronic healthcare, mental healthcare, child welfare system, law enforcement, and the judicial system.

The Adverse Childhood Experiences (ACE) Study is one of the largest studies examining the link between child maltreatment and later health and well-being. The study confirms that childhood experiences of abuse, neglect, and family dysfunction are "major risk factors for the leading causes of illness and death as well as poor quality of life in the United States." (For more information about the ACE Study, go to www.cdc.gov/nccdphp/ace/about.htm.)

32. Child abuse resulting in a fatality affects everyone in the ED emotionally. How frequently does this happen?

Dealing with the emotional impact of the loss of a child is not to be taken lightly. Many hospitals have peer support teams that help all people involved in the care of the child to debrief and find support. Debriefing may be helpful for nurses, physicians, and others who work directly with these patients.

According to the National Child Abuse and Neglect Data System (NCANDS), 1500 children were estimated to have died because of child abuse or neglect in 2003. It is believed that many more child abuse fatalities occur but go unreported. Among reported child abuse fatalities, most are related to neglect (36%), multiple maltreatment types (29%), or physical abuse only (28%).

33. Do children suffer ill effects from living in homes with domestic violence?

Yes. Even if children only hear the violence (but do not see it), they worry about their parents being hurt or dying. Children living in homes with domestic violence are commonly victims of physical abuse (80%) and sexual abuse (40%) themselves. Whenever partner abuse is disclosed, there should be an inquiry about whether children are living in the home. Minimally, these children should be provided services for "witnessing" abuse. A referral should include investigation for protecting children from harm, providing education to caregivers about domestic violence effects on children, and counseling for the children themselves.

34. **What can be done to stop the cycle of violence?**

Children learn how to deal with life by the nurturing they receive and the environment they live in. Promoting healthy, caring environments for all children should be a priority. Positive parenting needs to be part of every parent's skills checklist. And if abuse occurs, investigation and therapeutic intervention for child victims are necessities.

 ## Key Points

- Elder abuse extends beyond physical abuse to neglect, exploitation, and abandonment.
- Signs of abuse in an elderly ED patient include obvious physical signs of trauma, poor hygiene, decubiti, strained or tense relationships with caregivers, or withdrawn behavior.
- The only way to know if someone is being abused by a partner is to ask. When screened for partner violence in the past year, up to 30% of women in EDs respond affirmatively. Reliable rates for men have yet to be reported.
- Women who screen positive for violence in the past year are at high risk for repeated violence, especially if they are trying to separate from an abusive partner.
- Emergency nursing care for abuse is based on empowerment; that is, focusing on coping strategies and strengths. Assess risk, provide support, plan for safety, and offer options.
- When gathering information about mechanism of injury for children, ask only open-ended questions. Avoid leading questions.
- Do not make assumptions in assigning responsibility for child maltreatment to a specific individual.
- Have a high index of suspicion for reporting child maltreatment; reporting triggers a thorough investigation, risk assessment, and intervention toward promoting child safety.
- Child maltreatment, in all its forms, has profound negative long-term effects on children's health and well-being.
- Family support and therapeutic intervention for child maltreatment victims may interrupt the cycle of violence.

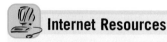
Internet Resources

Centers for Disease Control and Prevention, Adverse Childhood Experiences Study:
www.cdc.gov/nccdphp/ace

Centers for Disease Control and Prevention, Injury and Violence:
www.cdc.gov/node.do/id/0900f3ec8000e539

Centers for Disease Control and Prevention, National Center for Injury Prevention and Control, Child Maltreatment links:
www.cdc.gov/ncipc/factsheets/cmlinks.htm

eMedicine, Elder Abuse:
www.emedicine.com/emerg/topic160.htm

Emergency Department Nurse, Intimate Partner Violence Screening:
www.ednurse.org

Emergency Nurses Association Position Statement, *Care of Sexual Assault Victims* (pdf document, Adobe Acrobat Reader software required):
www.ena.org/about/position/PDFs/Care-Sexual-Assault-Victims.PDF

Emergency Nurses Association Position Statement, *Domestic Violence, Maltreatment, and Neglect* (pdf document, Adobe Acrobat Reader software required):
www.ena.org/about/position/PDFs/DomesticViolence.PDF

Family Violence Prevention Fund, Health Care:
www.endabuse.org/programs/healthcare

National Center on Elder Abuse:
www.elderabusecenter.org/default.cfm

U.S. Department of Health & Human Services, Administration for Children & Families, National Clearinghouse on Child Abuse and Neglect Information:
www.nccanch.acf.hhs.gov

U.S. Department of Justice, Office on Violence Against Women:
www.usdoj.gov/ovw

World Health Organization, *Female Genital Mutilation* (pdf document, Adobe Acrobat Reader software required):
www.who.int/gender/other_health/en/teachersguide.pdf

Bibliography

Cabinum-Foller E, Frasier L: Bruising in children, *Lancet* 365(9468):1369-1370, 2005.

Campbell JC, Humphreys J, editors: *Family violence and nursing practice*, Philadelphia, 2003, Lippincott Williams & Wilkins.

DeVoe ER, Faller KC: Questioning strategies in interviews with children who may have been sexually abused, *Child Welfare* 81(1):5-31, 2002.

Felitti VJ: The relationship of adverse childhood experiences and adult health: Turning gold into lead, *Permanente J* 6:44-47, 2002. Available at xnet.kp.org/permanentejournal/winter02/goldtolead.html.

Forbes BJ: Inflicted childhood neurotrauma (shaken baby syndrome): Ophthalmic findings, *J Pediatr Ophthalmol Strabismus* 41(2):80-88, 2004.

Fromm S: *Total estimated cost of child abuse and neglect in the United States,* Chicago, 2001, Prevent Child Abuse America. Available at www.preventchildabuse.org/learn_more/research_docs/cost_analysis.pdf.

Graham-Bermann S, Seng J: Violence and traumatic stress symptoms as additional predictors of health problems in high-risk children, *J Pediatr* 146:349-354, 2005.

Gushurst CA: Child abuse: Behavioral aspects and other associated problems, *Pediatr Clin North Am* 50:4, 2003.

Hansen KK: Folk remedies and child abuse: A review with emphasis on caida de mollera and its relationship to shaken baby syndrome, *Child Abuse Negl* 22:117-127, 1998.

Heymann WR: Cutaneous signs of child abuse, *J Am Acad Dermatol* 53:1, 2005.

Jenny C et al: Analysis of missed cases of abusive head trauma, *JAMA* 281:621-626, 1999.

Kleinman PL, Kleinman PK, Savageau JA: Suspected infant abuse: Radiographic skeletal survey practices in pediatric health care facilities, *Radiology* 233(2):477-485, 2004.

Levine LM: Pediatric ocular trauma and shaken infant syndrome, *Pediatr Clin North Am* 50(1):137-148, 2003.

Maguire S et al: Are there patterns of bruising in childhood which are diagnostic or suggestive of abuse? *Arch Dis Child* 90:182-186, 2005.

Maguire S et al: Can you age bruises accurately in children? *Arch Dis Child* 90:187-189, 2005.

Monk M: Interviewing suspected victims of child maltreatment in the emergency department, *J Emerg Nurs* 24:31-34, 1998.

Straus MA, Kantor GK: Definition and measurement of neglectful behavior: Some principles and guidelines, *Child Abuse Negl* 29:19-29, 2005.

Sugar NF, Taylor JA, Feldman KW: Bruises in infants and toddlers: Those who don't cruise rarely bruise, *Arch Pediatr Adolesc Med* 153:339-403, 1999.

Taliaferro EH: Abuse in the elderly and impaired. In Tintinalli JE, Kelen GD, Stapczynski JS, editors: *Emergency medicine: A comprehensive study guide,* New York, 2004, McGraw-Hill.

US Department of Health and Human Services, Administration on Children, Youth and Families: *Child Maltreatment 2003,* Washington, DC, 2005, US Government Printing Office. Available at www.acf.hhs.gov/programs/cb/pubs/cm03/index.htm

Wang GJ et al: Partial recovery of brain metabolism in methamphetamine abusers after protracted abstinence, *Am J Psychiatry* 161(2):242-248, 2004.

Drug- and Alcohol-Impaired Patients

Anne M. Felton and Bari K. Platter

1. **What are the most common emergencies related to drug and alcohol impairment?**

   Common emergency presentations related to drug and alcohol impairment can be divided into several categories. There are complications of the substance itself, such as acute intoxication, overdose, or withdrawal. There are presentations exacerbated by substances, such as mental illness and medical conditions such as diabetes. Finally, there are cases with inferred causal relationships between the presenting complaint and the presence of a substance (e.g., motor vehicle crashes, assaults, other injuries).

2. **How prevalent are alcohol- or drug-impaired patients in the emergency department (ED)?**

   The Drug Abuse Warning Network (DAWN) provides estimates of drug-related ED visits. Based on data compiled from participating hospitals across the nation in the third and fourth quarter of 2003, DAWN estimated the following for drug-related ED visits:
   - Out of 52 million ED visits, 630,000 (or 1.2%) were drug or alcohol related. Because DAWN does not track ED visits for adults over the age of 21 who abuse alcohol only, this number may be much higher.
   - One in five (20%) cases of drug-related ED visits involved cocaine. Marijuana-related ED visits may be as common as cocaine.
   - Heroin visits accounted for 8% of drug-related ED visits.
   - Seven percent of drug-related ED visits involved stimulants such as amphetamines and methamphetamines.
   - Other illicit drugs, such as lysergic acid diethylamide (LSD), phencyclidine (PCP), and inhalants, appeared at much lower frequencies.
   - Current data from major U.S. trauma centers reflects as much as 50% to 60% of all trauma cases involve one or more drugs (including alcohol).
   - Six percent of these drug- or alcohol-related visits involved a suicide attempt.

3. **What should be known about suicide and substance abuse?**

   Current data show a relationship between substance abuse (especially alcohol) and suicide. This is not a new phenomenon. There have been many studies, both old and new, attempting to demonstrate a causal relationship between substance use and suicide. Causal relationships are difficult to establish because there are multiple and complex variables involved in both substance abuse and suicide attempts.

It is important for the emergency nurse to be aware of the high rate of patients who attempt suicide while impaired. Both the substance abuse history and the mental health history of the patient should be considered when developing the plan of care.

4. What drugs of abuse are seen in the ED?

- **Alcohol:** Alcohol is absorbed quickly into the bloodstream, with effects on mental status evident in as little as 10 minutes and peak effects typically seen 1 hour after consumption. Alcohol is also a central nervous system depressant.
- **Opiods:** Opioids are naturally occurring and synthetic drugs that act at specific opioid receptors in the brain and in the body. Opioids induce feelings of both relaxation and euphoria. Examples of opioids include opium, morphine, heroin, and hydromorphone.
- **Stimulants:** Stimulant drugs increase the action of dopamine and norepinephrine, causing the user to feel a rush of energy, vigor, and feelings of well-being. The most common types of stimulants are cocaine, amphetamines, and methamphetamines. Cocaine can be used pharmaceutically as a local anesthetic but is usually obtained illicitly in a powder or crystallized ("crack") form. Amphetamines are available as an oral prescription and illicitly in powdered or crystallized forms.
- **Hallucinogens and inhalants:** Hallucinogens are those drugs that are used to alter one's perception of reality. The desired effects of hallucinogens include euphoria and the enhancement of sensory perceptions, including induction of hallucinations and illusions. This group of drugs includes both natural and synthetic substances, such as LSD, PCP, and marijuana. Inhalants include psychoactive nonpharmaceutical substances that are inhaled, sniffed, or snorted. Inhalants fall into three categories, which the following table describes.

Inhalants

Category	Examples
Volatile solvents	Adhesives (airplane glue, rubber cement, household glue)
	Aerosols (spray paint, hairspray, air freshener, deodorant)
	Solvents and gases (nail polish remover, paint thinner, toxic markers, gasoline, propane, helium)
	Cleaning agents (dry-cleaning fluid)
	Food products (vegetable oil cooking spray, dessert topping spray)
Nitrites	Amyl nitrites ("poppers," "snappers")
	Butyl nitrites ("rush," "locker room," "bolt")
Chlorofluorohydrocarbons (freons)	Anesthetic gases (nitrous oxide, ether, chloroform)

- **Sedative-hypnotics:** These drugs are used to sedate or tranquilize, to induce sleep, as anticonvulsants, and as muscle relaxants. Classes include benzodiazepines, barbiturates, and barbiturate-like drugs such as methaqualone (Quaalude) and ethchlorvynol (Placidyl).

5. How can alcohol abuse be recognized in a patient?

Many patients present to the ED with alcohol-related problems. Patients may present because of injury or accidents related to alcohol consumption or with a medical condition such as hypertension directly related to their abuse. There are also many conditions, such as pregnancy, for which teaching regarding the risks associated with alcohol consumption is crucial.

The CAGE questionnaire is a simple tool to use to identify patients that would benefit from additional screening and education. CAGE refers to:
- Have you ever felt you should **cut** down on your drinking?
- Have people **annoyed** you by criticizing your drinking?
- Have you ever felt bad or **guilty** about your drinking?
- Have you **ever** had a drink first thing in the morning to steady nerves or to rid a hangover?

A "yes" response indicates possible alcohol problems. The patient should be screened during the ED visit for possible withdrawal and provided appropriate education and referral upon discharge.

6. What are the signs and symptoms of alcohol intoxication?

The signs and symptoms of intoxication differ based on the patient and the level of alcohol in the blood. The following effects are common as blood alcohol concentration increases:
- Initial stimulant effects with decreased inhibition and facilitation of social interactions
- Ataxia and slurred speech
- A sense of euphoria and mood lability
- Poor judgment
- Decreased concentration, poor memory, and confusion
- Stupor and coma; respiratory paralysis and death are associated with blood alcohol levels (BALs) above 0.5 mg/dl
    Other physical findings associated with alcohol intoxication include:
- Enlarged pupils
- Nystagmus
- Facial flushing

Alcohol-intoxicated patients should be monitored for adequate ventilation and perfusion, as well as altered mental status. Intoxication may also mask underlying signs and symptoms of closed head injury. Occasionally, alcohol-intoxicated patients require aggressive airway management, including intubation and mechanical ventilation.

7. **How is alcohol withdrawal recognized in a patient?**

The severity of withdrawal symptoms is relative to the length of time a patient has had alcohol dependence. A patient with a high tolerance (high BAL required before experiencing signs of intoxication) and long history of dependence may begin to experience withdrawal symptoms simply by decreasing the amount consumed. Typically, withdrawal symptoms begin 4 to 24 hours after the last drink and will peak between 36 and 48 hours. The following box describes symptoms of alcohol withdrawal by severity.

Alcohol Withdrawal

Mild
Irritability
Insomnia
Upset stomach
Anxiety

Moderate
Nausea, vomiting, diarrhea
Diaphoresis
Tremor
Tachycardia and hypertension

Severe
Fever
Confusion and agitation
Hallucinations and delusions
Grand mal seizures

---

8. **What are delirium tremens (DTs)?**

DTs are a severe syndrome experienced by a small percentage of patients in alcohol withdrawal. DTs are also referred to as alcohol withdrawal delirium. Symptoms usually begin within 24 to 72 hours of alcohol abstinence. Patients with DTs experience fever generally followed by extreme agitation and psychosis lasting as long as several days. DTs are a medical emergency with a mortality rate of 5% to 15%. With early detection and initiation of appropriate treatments, this rate may be reduced to 1%.

9. **What is important to know about alcohol withdrawal seizures?**

Alcohol withdrawal seizures occur in approximately 10% of patients in active withdrawal. Seizures are typically grand mal and begin within the first 48 hours of withdrawal, lasting 6 to 12 hours. The risk for withdrawal seizures increases dramatically if the patient has a past history of seizures during withdrawal.

10. How are alcohol withdrawal and DTs managed in the ED?

Many patients with alcohol dependence are also dehydrated and malnourished, complicating withdrawal symptoms in the ED. There are also many medical complications of chronic alcohol abuse that may have to be addressed during a patient presentation to the ED for withdrawal. Many alcoholics come to the ED for a different complaint, and then during their evaluation in the ED begin to experience withdrawal symptoms. It is important for the ED nurse to recognize early signs of alcohol withdrawal and begin treatment when necessary. Regardless of whether the patient in alcohol withdrawal is seeking detoxification, the ED nurse must treat the withdrawal symptoms to prevent further medical complications.

Benzodiazepines have been found to be the most beneficial drugs for management of many symptoms associated with alcohol withdrawal. Benzodiazepines are sedatives that target the symptoms of agitation, insomnia, hypertension, and tachycardia (symptoms characterized as hyperexcitability). Benzodiazepines are also used to prevent seizures. There are many benzodiazepines available (e.g., clorazepate, lorazepam, oxazepam, diazepam, chlordiazepoxide) that can be used to target different symptoms; they are practical because of ease of administration. Long-acting benzodiazepines (clorazepate, chlordiazepoxide) are recommended when a patient can be monitored in early withdrawal. Short-acting benzodiazepines (e.g., lorazepam, oxazepam) are generally considered to be of greater therapeutic benefit to patients who are already experiencing significant withdrawal symptoms. Patients requiring benzodiazepines for withdrawal management should have their liver function evaluated. Those patients with severely compromised liver function should be treated with lorazepam, which is not metabolized in the liver.

History of alcohol consumption should be obtained from all patients presenting to the ED. With this history, the nurse can then develop a plan of care that includes interventions to manage alcohol withdrawal. If it is determined that the patient is experiencing withdrawal, the Canadian Addiction Research Foundation (ARF) Clinical Institute Withdrawal Assessment for Alcohol, revised (CIWA-Ar) is a valid and easily administered tool for the nurse to assess risk and determine an appropriate course of treatment.

Addiction Research Foundation Clinical Institute Withdrawal Assessment-Alcohol (CIWA-Ar)
This scale is not copyrighted and may be used freely.

Patient: _____ Date: /___/___/___ Time: ___:_____ (24-hour clock; midnight=00:00)

NAUSEA AND VOMITING
Ask: "Do you feel sick to your stomach? Have you vomited?"

Observation:
0   No nausea and no vomiting
1   Mild nausea with no vomiting
2
3
4   Intermittent nausea with dry heaves
5
6
7   Constant nausea; frequent dry heaves and vomiting

TACTILE DISTURBANCES
Ask: "Have you any itching, pins and needles sensations, burning, or numbness? Do you feel bugs crawling on or under your skin?"

Observation:
0   None
1   Mild itching, pins and needles, burning or numbness
2   Mild itching, pins and needles, burning or numbness
3   Moderate itching, pins and needles, burning or numbness
4   Moderately severe hallucinations
5   Severe hallucinations
6   Extremely severe hallucinations
7   Continuous hallucinations

TREMOR
Arms extended and fingers spread apart

Observation:
0   No tremor
1   Not visible; can be felt fingertip to fingertip
2
3
4   Moderate with patient's arms extended
5
6
7   Severe even with arms not extended

AUDITORY DISTURBANCES
Ask: "Are you more aware of sounds around you? Are they harsh? Do they frighten you? Are you hearing anything that is disturbing to you? Are you hearing things you know are not there?"

Observation:
0   Not present
1   Very mild harshness or ability to frighten
2   Mild harshness or ability to frighten
3   Moderate harshness or ability to frighten
4   Moderately severe hallucinations
5   Severe hallucinations
6   Extremely severe hallucinations
7   Continuous hallucinations

PAROSYSMAL SWEATS

Observation:
0   No sweat visible
1   Barely perceptible sweating, palms moist
2
3
4   Beads of sweat obvious on forehead
5
6
7   Drenching sweats

VISUAL DISTURBANCES
Ask: "Does the light appear to be too bright? Is its color different? Does it hurt your eyes? Are you seeing anything that is disturbing to you? Are you seeing things you know are not there?"

Observation:
0   Not present
1   Very mild sensitivity
2   Mild sensitivity
3   Moderate sensitivity
4   Moderately severe hallucinations
5   Severe hallucinations
6   Extremely severe hallucinations
7   Continuous hallucinations

Clinical Institute Withdrawal Assessment for Alcohol, revised (CIWA-Ar). *Adapted from the Canadian Addiction Research Foundation Clinical Institute Withdrawal Assessment for Alcohol, revised (CIWA-Ar).*

Continued

ANXIETY
Ask: "Do you feel nervous?"
 	
Observation:
0 No anxiety, at ease
1
2
3
4 Moderately anxious, or
   guarded, so anxiety is inferred
5
6
7 Equivalent to acute panic
   states as seen in severe
   delirium or acute schizo-
   phrenic reactions
	HEADACHE, FULLNESS IN HEAD
	Ask: "Does your head feel different? Does it feel like there is
	a band around your head?"
	   Do not rate for dizziness or lightheadedness. Otherwise,
	rate severity.
	
	Observation:
	0 Not present
	1 Very mild
	2 Mild
	3 Moderate
	4 Moderately severe
	5 Severe
	6 Very severe
	7 Extremely severe

AGITATION
 	
Observation:
0 Normal activity
1 Somewhat more than normal
   activity
2
3
4 Moderately fidgety and
   restless
5
6
7 Paces back and forth during
   most of the interview or
   constantly thrashes about
	ORIENTATION AND CLOUDING OF SENSORIUM
	Ask: "What day is this? Where are you? Who am I?"
	
	Observation:
	0 Oriented and can do serial additions
	1 Cannot do serial additions or is uncertain about date
	2 Disoriented for date by no more than 2 calendar days
	3 Disoriented for date by more than 2 calendar days
	4 Disoriented for place and/or person

Total CIWA-A score _____
Rater's initials _____
Maximum possible score 67

11. How are DTs managed in the ED?

Prevention is the best treatment for DTs. Management of alcohol withdrawal should include intravenous (IV) fluids and correction of any electrolyte imbalance. Vitamin therapy should be administered to account for likely nutritional deficiencies. Benzodiazepines remain the drug of choice for managing the symptoms of psychotic agitation associated with DTs. Many EDs and critical care units traditionally administer large doses of haloperidol and benzodiazepines to patients who are experiencing DTs. Haloperidol is contraindicated for psychotic agitation resulting from DTs because it lowers the seizure threshold and has been linked with further electrolyte disturbances.

12. What are the effects of alcohol abuse on different body systems?

The complications from alcohol abuse are multisystemic. Symptoms vary from mild to chronic and severe based on consumption. Many symptoms are reversible with abstinence from alcohol; others, such as cirrhosis, are not.

The following common medical presentations are often seen in patients with alcohol abuse:

- **Gastrointestinal:** GI bleeds associated with gastric ulcers, esophagitis, and esophageal varices; pancreatitis; and cirrhosis
- **Cardiovascular:** Hypertension and alcoholic cardiomyopathy
- **Hematopoietic:** Anemia, thrombocytopenia, elevated mean corpuscular volume (MCV), and decreased ability of the platelets to clump together; as a result, minor injuries may cause increased bleeding
- **Endocrine:** Decreased testosterone levels in men and increased estrogen levels in both men and women, resulting in impotence and menstrual irregularities

13. What are Wernicke-Korsakoff syndrome and hepatic encephalopathy?

Wernicke-Korsakoff syndrome is an encephalopathic disease process character-ized by a progression of symptoms ranging from short-term memory loss, drowsiness, and confusion, leading to stupor, ataxia, and psychosis. Dementia-like symptoms can develop if the patient is not treated rapidly. This syndrome is caused in large part by chronic thiamine deficiency. Treatment is immediate intramuscular (IM) administration of 100 mg thiamine. IM administration is preferred to oral administration for better absorption and tolerance. Thiamine should be administered before glucose, because glucose depletes B vitamins.

Hepatic encephalopathy is a potentially fatal disorder. It is caused by a buildup of neurotoxins, such as ammonia and manganese, that are normally cleared from the blood by a healthy liver. Ammonia and manganese are able to cross the blood-brain barrier, with signs and symptoms of hepatic encephalopa-thy developing as toxic levels rise in the blood. Signs and symptoms include personality changes and mood swings, changes in sleep patterns, cognitive dysfunction, and incoordination. A classic symptom of hepatic encephalopathy is asterixis, which is a flapping tremor of the hands. Final symptoms (hepatic coma) may be fatal, with patients no longer able to respond to stimuli. Treatment for hepatic encephalopathy is centered around attempts to lower blood ammonia levels or to counter their effects in the brain. Liver transplantation is also consid-ered an option for patients with end-stage liver disease. Because most of these treatment options are not available to the emergency nurse, the management of symptoms becomes the focus for care.

14. How does the emergency nurse differentiate between opioid intoxication and opioid overdose?

The following box contrasts the differences between opioid intoxication and opioid overdose.

Opiod Intoxication vs. Overdose

Intoxication
Shallow respirations
Constricted pupils
Depression
Drowsiness to somnolence
Euphoria
Nausea
Slurred speech

Overdose
Respiratory depression or apnea
Clammy skin
Convulsions and seizures
Hypotension
Cyanosis
Pulmonary edema
Coma
Pinpoint pupils

15. How does the ED nurse manage opioid overdose?

Because the most common cause of death from opioid overdose is respiratory depression, aggressive airway and ventilatory management are essential until the narcotic's respiratory depressant effects can be reversed. Naloxone (Narcan) is used to reverse the effects of opioid overdose. Initial dosing is 2 mg, given via IV, IM injection, or subcutaneously. Subsequent doses are titrated at 2 mg, up to a total dose of 10 mg, until the patient's respiratory status is stabilized and the patient is alert.

16. What are the signs and symptoms of opioid withdrawal?

The following symptoms are seen at all stages of withdrawal:
- Dilated pupils
- Anxiety and panic
- Irritability
- Paranoia

Early   Late

Rhinitis   Diaphoresis   Fever   Hypertension   Hyperventilation

Lacrimation   Myalgia   Chills   Vomiting   Tachycardia

The progression of opioid withdrawal symptoms.

17. How is opioid withdrawal managed in the ED?

Opioid withdrawal is not a life-threatening event, although it may feel that way to those addicted to opioids. Treatment of opioid withdrawal does not generally begin in the ED. The role of the nurse in the ED is to provide comfort measures to assist the patient in easing the symptoms of withdrawal until the patient can be transferred to a treatment facility to begin a detoxification treatment program.

The most effective way to alleviate opioid withdrawal is by using another opioid drug. Methadone is the most common drug used to withdraw patients from opioids. Other medications, such as clonidine and buprenorphine, are less commonly used.

18. **What are the signs and symptoms of stimulant intoxication?**

Common signs and symptoms of stimulant intoxication (e.g., cocaine, amphetamines, methamphetamines) include tachycardia, hypertension, and hyperreflexia. Patients report feelings of euphoria, with increased energy and decreased appetite and need for sleep. Patients are hypertalkative, over-alert, and grandiose. Physical symptoms include GI distress, such as nausea, vomiting, stomach cramps, and diarrhea. With higher doses or prolonged use, patients begin to experience symptoms of psychosis and may begin to pick at their skin because they feel as if insects are crawling on them. This psychosis is often linked with extreme paranoia and more common with methamphetamine abuse. Methamphetamines have become increasingly problematic because of their toxic effects on the brain.

19. **How is sedative-hypnotic abuse recognized?**

Benzodiazepines, a common group of sedative-hypnotic drugs, are frequently prescribed to manage anxiety and sleep disorders. Although sedative-hypnotics are prescription drugs, they are also favored by illicit drug users for use in combination or alone. Many illicit drug users "self-medicate" with sedative-hypnotics to control the adverse effects from their drugs of choice. For example, an amphetamine (speed) user commonly uses benzodiazepines to induce sleep and avoid agitation after bingeing on amphetamines.

The effects of sedative-hypnotics are similar to that of alcohol. A noticeable difference with sedative-hypnotic users is that the patient may have marked sedation.

20. **What is the treatment for sedative-hypnotic overdose?**

Both benzodiazepines and barbiturates cause respiratory depression. In overdose, benzodiazepines alone are not likely to cause severe medical complications. When combined with central nervous system depressants, such as alcohol, benzodiazepines are more likely to lead to significant respiratory depression and hypotension. Barbiturates, on the other hand, are often lethal in overdose. This group of medication causes severe respiratory depression that is less responsive to medical intervention. The ED nurse must focus on airway and ventilatory management as the first priority. Fluid replacement should be considered to address symptoms of hypotension. Activated charcoal may be indicated but airway protection is of major importance. Aspiration of charcoal can result in serious complications. Flumazenil is a benzodiazepine antagonist that may be used to counteract a benzodiazepine overdose.

21. **How are patients experiencing withdrawal from sedative-hypnotics managed?**

Symptoms of sedative-hypnotic withdrawal range from tachycardia and restlessness to extreme agitation. Patients can also experience influenza-like symptoms, such as diaphoresis, nausea, and vomiting. Seizure is also possible during withdrawal from sedative-hypnotics, especially high-dose, long-acting medications. As with alcohol withdrawal, patients should be closely monitored for electrolyte imbalance, cardiac abnormalities, and seizure activity and treated appropriately as symptoms arise.

22. What are the signs and symptoms of inhalant intoxication?

Patients who use inhalants experience a rapid onset and short-lived euphoria. In addition to experiencing the desired effect of disinhibition and lightheadedness, patients may also experience nausea, vomiting, headache, and blurred vision. Patients may present to the ED with a rash around the nose and mouth; the patient may smell of solvents. The majority of inhalant-intoxicated patients presenting to the ED are also under the influence of other substances, most commonly stimulants. The presentation, therefore, may be clouded by the presence of other mind-altering substances.

23. How does the emergency nurse manage patients under the influence of hallucinogens?

Patients under the influence of hallucinogens (LSD, PCP, marijuana) most commonly present to the ED with injuries sustained secondary to impaired judgment. Patients may believe that they have supernatural powers and can exhibit self-injurious behaviors such as jumping off of buildings and running through traffic.

Patients can also present to the ED with a "bad trip" (anxiety, agitation, and paranoia). Nursing interventions include:
- Placing the patient in a quiet room away from busy areas of the ED
- Decreasing stimulation; closing doors, lowering the lights
- Providing reassurance and reorientation
- Medicating patients with extreme agitation and panic with benzodiazepines

Hallucinogens can produce a prolonged psychotic state that can last for several days. Treatment includes use of antipsychotic medications. Carbamazepine has also been successfully used to decrease psychosis related to hallucinogen use.

24. What are "designer drugs," and how are patients under the influence of these drugs managed?

"Designer drugs" or "club drugs" are those drugs that are used recreationally, typically by youth in nightclub settings. Examples of these drugs include 3,4-methylenedioxymethamphetamine (MDMA; also know as Ecstasy), gamma hydroxybutyrate (GHB), flunitrazepam (Rohypnol), and ketamine. Patients under the influence of "designer" or "club" drugs initially experience euphoria and disinhibition. Complications can range from severe psychotic reaction to fatal overdose. Ecstasy commonly causes hypertension, hyperthermia, and tachycardia. GHB overdose affects temperature regulation, glucose metabolism, and blood flow, and GHB crosses the blood-brain barrier. There is no reversal agent for GHB overdose. The ED nurse should focus care on ventilatory support and management of bradycardia. Patients who have taken Rohypnol or ketamine may be at risk of respiratory depression and aspiration of gastric contents. Overdose of these drugs may require aggressive airway and ventilatory management.

Nursing management in the ED is similar to management of patients under the influence of hallucinogens. Place the patient in a quiet room away from busy areas of the ED, and provide reassurance and reorientation. Benzodiazepines and low-potency neuroleptic medications are helpful in decreasing anxiety and psychosis. Baseline laboratory tests to measure electrolyte balance are helpful because many patients under the influence of "designer" or "club" drugs experience electrolyte imbalance.

25. What are the treatment options for drug- and alcohol-impaired patients?

Treatment options vary, depending on the patient's internal motivation for treatment, the patient's financial resources, the type of drug(s) of abuse, and available community treatment programs. Many patients will need to complete a detoxification program before entering treatment.

Examples of treatment options include:

- **Inpatient treatment:** This model of treatment is the most intensive and the least common.
- **Residential treatment:** Traditional models are 30-day programs. Many patients benefit from a dual diagnosis program that addresses both substance use and mental illness. Some communities have residential programs for specialized populations such as those for women, youth, the homeless, HIV-positive patients, and Native Americans.
- **Partial programs:** This type of program provides structure during the day and/or evening for patients who require increased monitoring but are either unable to attend a residential program or are waiting to enter a residential program.
- **Outpatient programs:** There are a wide variety of outpatient programs, from those specializing in individual and group therapy to those that dispense methadone. Outpatient programs can include individual, couples, and group therapy. Many programs may include only medication management.
- **Self-help programs:** The most widely recognized self-help programs are Alcoholics Anonymous (AA) and Narcotics Anonymous (NA). These programs are widely available. AA and NA meetings can be specialized for certain populations, such as gender, sexual orientation, trauma, language, smoking or nonsmoking, and cultural background.

Key Points

- Drug- and alcohol-impaired patients often have complex presentations complicated by mental illness, accident and other traumas, and various medical conditions.
- Suicidal ideation is a common co-morbid condition and should be assessed when taking a history from a drug- and alcohol-impaired patient.
- Consider drug and alcohol history with all patients admitted to the ED.
- Dehydration and nutritional and electrolyte imbalances are common conditions of alcoholism. Any patient with significant alcohol consumption history should be monitored carefully for withdrawal symptoms and treated appropriately.
- Stimulant withdrawal syndrome is often accompanied by severe dysphoria and suicidal ideation.
- Respiratory depression is the most common and life-threatening complication related to sedative-hypnotic overdose.
- Hallucinogen-impaired patients most commonly present to the ED with personal injuries secondary to impaired judgment.

Internet Resources

American Academy of Child & Adolescent Psychiatry, *Teens: Alcohol and Other Drugs:*
www.aacap.org/publications/factsfam/teendrug.htm

Drug Abuse Warning Network:
www.DAWNinfo.samhsa.gov

Emergency Nurses Association, Position Statement, *Alcohol Screening and Brief Intervention* (pdf document, Adobe Acrobat Reader software required):
www.ena.org/about/position/PDFs/AlcoholScreening.PDF

National Association on Alcohol, Drugs and Disability:
www.naadd.org

National Institute on Drug Abuse:
www.drugabuse.gov

National Institute on Drug Abuse, ClubDrugs.org:
www.clubdrugs.org

U.S. Department of Health & Human Services and SAMHSA's National Clearinghouse for Alcohol & Drug Information Straight Facts About Drugs and Alcohol:
www.health.org/govpubs/rpo884

Bibliography

Asplund CA, Aaronson JW, Aaronson HE: Three regimens for alcohol withdrawal and detoxification, *J Fam Pract* 53:545, 2004.

Butterworth RF: Hepatic encephalopathy: A serious complication of alcoholic liver disease, *Alcohol Res Health* 27:143, 2003.

Cohen ST, Jacobson AM: Dual diagnosis: Substance abuse and psychiatric illness. In Jacobson JL, Jacobson AM, editors: *Psychiatric secrets*, ed 2, Philadelphia, 2000, Hanley & Belfus.

Desai RA et al: Suicidal ideation and suicide attempts in a sample of homeless people with mental illness, *J Nerv Ment Dis* 191:363, 2003.

Harris JT, Thornton R, Thornton J: A role for valproate in the treatment of sedative-hypnotic withdrawal and for relapse prevention, *Alcohol Alcohol* 35:319, 2000.

Kennedy JA: Alcohol use disorders. In Jacobson JL, Jacobson AM, editors: *Psychiatric secrets*, ed 2, Philadelphia, 2000, Hanley & Belfus.

Kennedy JA: Cocaine and amphetamine use disorders. In Jacobson JL, Jacobson AM, editors: *Psychiatric secrets*, ed 2, Philadelphia, 2000, Hanley & Belfus.

Kennedy JA: Marijuana, hallucinogens, phencyclidine, and inhalants. In Jacobson JL, Jacobson AM, editors: *Psychiatric secrets*, ed 2, Philadelphia, 2000, Hanley & Belfus.

Kennedy JA: Opioid use disorders. In Jacobson JL, Jacobson AM, editors: *Psychiatric secrets*, ed 2, Philadelphia, 2000, Hanley & Belfus.

Kennedy JA: Sedative-hypnotic use disorders. In Jacobson JL, Jacobson AM, editors: *Psychiatric secrets*, ed 2, Philadelphia, 2000, Hanley & Belfus.

Kosten TR, O'Connor PG: Management of drug and alcohol withdrawal, *N Engl J Med* 348:1786, 2003.

Lisanti P: Adult health: Acute care. In Naegle MA, D'Avanzo CE, editors: *Addictions and substance abuse: Strategies for advanced practice nursing*, New York, 2001, Prentice Hall.

Lombardo DM: Substance abuse. In Newberry L, Sheehy SB, editors: *Sheehy's emergency nursing principles and practice*, ed 5, St Louis, 2003, Mosby.

Mayo-Smith MF et al: Management of alcohol withdrawal delirium: An evidence-based practice guideline, *Arch Intern Med* 164:1405, 2004.

National Institute on Drug Abuse: *Cocaine*. Available at www.nida.nih.gov/DrugPages/Cocaine.html.

National Institute on Drug Abuse: *Heroin*. Available at www.nida.nih.gov/DrugPages/Heroin.html.

National Institute on Drug Abuse: *Marijuana*. Available at www.nida.nih.gov/DrugPages/Marijuana.html.

National Institute on Drug Abuse: *NIDA InfoFacts: Hospital Visits*. Available at www.nida.nih.gov/infofacts/HospitalVisits.html.

Rossow I, Groholt B, Wichstrom L: Intoxicants and suicidal behavior among adolescents: Changes in levels and associations from 1992 to 2002, *Addiction* 100:79, 2005.

Saitz R: Unhealthy alcohol use, *N Engl J Med* 352:596, 2005.

Smith-Alnimer M, Watford MF: Alcohol withdrawal and delirium tremens: Fast recognition may save a patient from the worst of withdrawal, *Am J Nurs* 104:72A, 2004.

Sporer KA: Acute heroin overdose, *Ann Intern Med* 130:584, 1999.

Index

Page numbers in **boldface type** indicate complete chapters; b indicates box; f indicates figure; t indicates table.

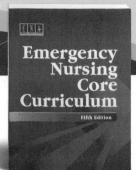

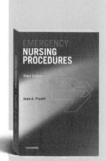
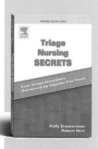